Learning Disabilities Sourcebook, 3rd Edition

Leukemia Sourcebook

Liver Disorders Sourcebook

Lung Disorders Sourcebook

Medical Tests Sourcebook, 3rd Edition

Men's Health Concerns Sourcebook, 2nd Edition

Mental Health Disorders Sourcebook, 4th Edition

Mental Retardation Sourcebook

Movement Disorders Sourcebook, 2nd Edition

Multiple Sclerosis Sourcebook

Muscular Dystrophy Sourcebook

Obesity Sourcebook

Osteoporosis Sourcebook

Pain Sourcebook, 3rd Edition

Pediatric Cancer Sourcebook

Physical & Mental Issues in Aging Sourcebook

Podiatry Sourcebook, 2nd Edition

Pregnancy & Birth Sourcebook, 2nd Edition

Prostate & Urological Disorders Sourcebook

Prostate Cancer Sourcebook

Reconstructive & Cosmetic Surgery Sourcebook

Rehabilitation Sourcebook

Respiratory Disorders Sourcebook, 2nd Edition

Sexually Transmitted Diseases Sourcebook, 3rd Edition

Sleep Disorders Sourcebook, 3rd Edition

Smoking Concerns Sourcebook

Sports Injuries Sourcebook, 3rd Edition

Stress-Related Disorders Sourcebook, 2nd Edition

Stroke Sourcebook, 2nd Edition

Surgery Sourcebook, 2nd Edition

Thyroid Disorders Sourcebook

Transplantation Sourcebook

Traveler's Health Sourcebook

Urinary Tract & Kidney Diseases & Disorders Sourcebook, 2nd Edition

Vegetarian Sourcebook

Women's Health Concerns Sourcebook, 3rd Edition

Workplace Health & Safety Sourcebook

Worldwide Health Sourcebook

Teen Health Series

Abuse & Violence Information for Teens

Accident & Safety Information for Teens

Alcohol Information for Teens, 2nd Edition

Allergy Information for Teens

Asthma Information for Teens, 2nd Edition

Body Information for Teens

Cancer Information for Teens

Complementary & Alternative Medicine Information for Teens

Diabetes Information for Teens

Diet Information for Teens, 2nd Edition

Drug Information for Teens, 3rd Edition

Eating Disorders Information for Teens, 2nd Edition

Fitness Information for Teens, 2nd Edition

Learning Disabilities Information for Teens

Mental Health Information for Teens, 3rd Edition

Pregnancy Information for Teens

Sexual Health Information for Teens, 2nd Edition

Skin Health Information for Teens, 2nd Edition

Sleep Information for Teens

Sports Injuries Information for Teens, 2nd Edition

Stress Information for Teens

Suicide Information for Teens, 2nd Edition

Tobacco Information for Teens, 2nd Edition

Sleep Disorders SOURCEBOOK

Third Edition

Health Reference Series

Third Edition

Sleep Disorders SOURCEBOOK

Basic Consumer Health Information about Sleep Disorders, Including Insomnia, Sleep Apnea and Snoring, Jet Lag and Other Circadian Rhythm Disorders, Narcolepsy, and Parasomnias, Such as Sleepwalking and Sleep Paralysis, and Featuring Facts about Other Health Problems that Affect Sleep, Why Sleep Is Necessary, How Much Sleep Is Needed, the Physical and Mental Effects of Sleep Deprivation, and Pediatric Sleep Issues

Along with Tips for Diagnosing and Treating Sleep Disorders, a Glossary of Related Terms, and a List of Resources for Additional Help and Information

Edited by
Sandra J. Judd

Omnigraphics

P.O. Box 31-1640, Detroit, MI 48231

Bibliographic Note

Because this page cannot legibly accommodate all the copyright notices, the Bibliographic Note portion of the Preface constitutes an extension of the copyright notice.

Edited by Sandra J. Judd

Health Reference Series

Karen Bellenir, *Managing Editor*
David A. Cooke, MD, FACP, *Medical Consultant*
Elizabeth Collins, *Research and Permissions Coordinator*
Cherry Edwards, *Permissions Assistant*
EdIndex, Services for Publishers, *Indexers*

* * *

Omnigraphics, Inc.

Matthew P. Barbour, *Senior Vice President*
Kevin M. Hayes, *Operations Manager*

* * *

Peter E. Ruffner, *Publisher*

Copyright © 2010 Omnigraphics, Inc.

ISBN 978-0-7808-1084-6

Library of Congress Cataloging-in-Publication Data

Sleep Disorders sourcebook : basic consumer health information about sleep disorders, including insomnia, sleep apnea and snoring, jet lag and other circadian rhythm disorders, narcolepsy, and parasomnias, such as sleepwalking and sleep paralysis, and featuring facts about other health problems that affect sleep, why sleep is necessary, how much sleep is needed, the physical and mental effects of sleep deprivation, and pediatric sleep issues, along with tips for diagnosing and treating sleep disorders / edited by Sandra J. Judd. -- 3rd ed.
    p. cm. -- (Health reference series)
    Includes bibliographical references and index.
    ISBN 978-0-7808-1084-6 (hardcover : alk. paper) 1. Sleep disorders. 2. Consumer education. I. Judd, Sandra J.
    RC547.S536 2011
    616.8'498--dc22

                                                2010040484

Table of Contents

Visit www.healthreferenceseries.com to view *A Contents Guide to the Health Reference Series*, a listing of more than 15,000 topics and the volumes in which they are covered.

Part II: The Causes and Consequences of Sleep Deprivation

Part V: Preventing, Diagnosing, and Treating Sleep Disorders

Part VI: A Special Look at Pediatric Sleep Issues

Part VII: Additional Help and Information

Preface

About This Book

According to the National Sleep Foundation, nearly fifty million Americans chronically suffer from sleep problems that can affect their careers, their personal relationships, and their safety. The effects of sleep loss are broad-ranging: 29 percent of polled adults had fallen asleep or become very sleepy at work; 36 percent had nodded off or fallen asleep while driving; and 14 percent had missed family events, work functions, or leisure activities due to sleepiness. Furthermore, studies have shown that a lack of sleep impacts the immune system, mood, memory, the ability to learn and process new information, and even weight.

Sleep Disorders Sourcebook, Third Edition, offers basic consumer health information about common sleep disorders, including insomnia, sleep apnea, narcolepsy, circadian rhythm disorders, and parasomnias, and other health problems that affect sleep, such as cancer, gastroesophageal reflux disorder, pain, and respiratory disorders. It explains how much sleep is needed, the causes and consequences of sleep deprivation, and the methods used to prevent, diagnose, and treat sleep disorders. A section about pediatric sleep issues discusses concerns that impact children from infancy through the teen years. A glossary of terms related to sleep disorders and a list of resources for further help and information are also included.

How to Use This Book

This book is divided into parts and chapters. Parts focus on broad areas of interest. Chapters are devoted to single topics within a part.

Part I: Sleep Basics presents facts about why and how people sleep, including an explanation of circadian rhythms, the stages and physical characteristics of sleep, the benefits of napping, and what is known about dreaming. It describes gender differences in sleep, and it explains how aging affects sleep patterns.

Part II: The Causes and Consequences of Sleep Deprivation defines sleep deprivation, explains how it occurs, and discusses its physical effects, including how loss of sleep can contribute to the of development coronary artery disease, diabetes, obesity, and other physical disorders. It also describes the effects sleepiness has on memory, problem solving, learning, working, and driving.

Part III: Sleep Disorders describes disorders that directly affect the ability to get a good night's sleep. These include breathing disorders, such as sleep apnea and snoring, insomnia, circadian rhythm disorders, and parasomnias—disorders that disrupt sleep as a result of abnormal arousals or movements. Narcolepsy and disorders associated with excessive sleeping are also discussed.

Part IV: Other Health Problems that Often Affect Sleep provides information about disorders that often impact sleep quality, including cancer, fibromyalgia, gastroesophageal reflux disease, headaches, respiratory disorders, and mental health concerns. The symptoms that disrupt sleep are described, and suggestions for lessening their impact are provided.

Part V: Preventing, Diagnosing, and Treating Sleep Disorders identifies common sleep disruptors and explains the importance of a proper sleep environment. It describes how sleep studies work and details treatment options, including medications, dietary supplements, cognitive behavioral therapy, bright light therapy, continuous positive airway pressure and other devices, and surgery.

Part VI: A Special Look at Pediatric Sleep Issues describes sleep disturbances in infancy, childhood, and adolescence. It discusses safe sleeping environments for infants and explains sudden infant death syndrome. It provides suggestions for getting children into bed and offers facts about bedwetting, sleepwalking, and teeth grinding. It also discusses problems associated with sleep deprivation in teenagers, especially school difficulties, drowsy driving, and mental health concerns.

Part VII: Additional Help and Information includes a glossary of terms related to sleep and sleep disorders and a directory of resources for additional help and support.

Bibliographic Note

This volume contains documents and excerpts from publications issued by the following U.S. government agencies: Centers for Disease Control and Prevention; National Cancer Institute; National Center for Complementary and Alternative Medicine; National Center for Post-traumatic Stress Disorder; National Heart, Lung, and Blood Institute; National Highway Traffic Safety Administration; National Institute of Diabetes and Digestive and Kidney Diseases; National Institute of Mental Health; National Institute of Neurological Disorders and Stroke; National Institute on Aging; National Institute on Alcohol Abuse and Alcoholism; National Institutes of Health; National Library of Medicine; Office of Dietary Supplements; Substance Abuse and Mental Health Services Administration; U.S. Department of Justice; and the U.S. Food and Drug Administration.

In addition, this volume contains copyrighted documents from the following organizations and publications: AAA Foundation for Traffic Safety; A.D.A.M., Inc.; Allied Media; Alzheimer's Association; American Academy of Dental Sleep Medicine; American College of Chest Physicians; American Parkinson Disease Association; American Psychological Association; American Sleep Apnea Association; Anxiety Disorders Association of America; Australian Broadcasting Corporation; Better Sleep Council; Biological Sciences Curriculum Study; *Chest*; Cincinnati Children's Hospital Medical Center; Cleveland Clinic; Columbia University Medical Center; Department of Health, Government of Western Australia; Dove Medical Press; Duke University Medical Centers News Office; Endocrine Society; Helpguide (c/o Center for Healthy Aging); Illinois Neurological Institute; InterMDnet Corporation; International Association for the Study of Dreams; Johns Hopkins Bayview Medical Center; Lippincott Williams and Wilkins; Lung Association of Saskatchewan; MediZine LLC; National Association for Continence; National Multiple Sclerosis Society; Natural Standard; Nemours Foundation; North Carolina Healthy Start Foundation; Northwestern University News Center; PsychCentral; Quadrant HealthCom, *Neuropsychiatry Reviews*; Rush University Medical Center; Scottsdale Sleep Center;

Talk About Sleep; Somerset Medical Center—Sleep for Life Program; University of California San Diego News Center; University of Chicago Medical Center; University of Chicago News Office; University of Cincinnati News; University of Minnesota Academic Health Center; University of Pennsylvania Health System; Wake Forest University Baptist Medical Center; Washington University in St. Louis School of Medicine, Office of Medical Public Affairs; Washington University Sleep Medicine Center; and Weight Watchers.

Full citation information is provided on the first page of each chapter or section. Every effort has been made to secure all necessary rights to reprint the copyrighted material. If any omissions have been made, please contact Omnigraphics to make corrections for future editions.

Acknowledgements

Thanks go to the many organizations, agencies, and individuals who have contributed materials for this *Sourcebook* and to medical consultant Dr. David Cooke and document engineer Bruce Bellenir. Special thanks go to managing editor Karen Bellenir and permissions coordinator Liz Collins for their help and support.

About the Health Reference Series

The *Health Reference Series* is designed to provide basic medical information for patients, families, caregivers, and the general public. Each volume takes a particular topic and provides comprehensive coverage. This is especially important for people who may be dealing with a newly diagnosed disease or a chronic disorder in themselves or in a family member. People looking for preventive guidance, information about disease warning signs, medical statistics, and risk factors for health problems will also find answers to their questions in the *Health Reference Series*. The *Series*, however, is not intended to serve as a tool for diagnosing illness, in prescribing treatments, or as a substitute for the physician/patient relationship. All people concerned about medical symptoms or the possibility of disease are encouraged to seek professional care from an appropriate healthcare provider.

A Note about Spelling and Style

Health Reference Series editors use *Stedman's Medical Dictionary* as an authority for questions related to the spelling of medical terms and the *Chicago Manual of Style* for questions related to grammatical structures, punctuation, and other editorial concerns. Consistent adherence is not always possible, however, because the individual volumes within the *Series* include many documents from a wide variety of different producers and copyright holders, and the editor's primary goal is to present material from each source as accurately as is possible following the terms specified by each document's producer. This sometimes means that information in different chapters or sections may follow other guidelines and alternate spelling authorities. For example, occasionally a copyright holder may require that eponymous terms be shown in possessive forms (Crohn's disease *vs.* Crohn disease) or that British spelling norms be retained (leukaemia *vs.* leukemia).

Locating Information within the Health Reference Series

The *Health Reference Series* contains a wealth of information about a wide variety of medical topics. Ensuring easy access to all the fact sheets, research reports, in-depth discussions, and other material contained within the individual books of the series remains one of our highest priorities. As the *Series* continues to grow in size and scope, however, locating the precise information needed by a reader may become more challenging.

A Contents Guide to the Health Reference Series was developed to direct readers to the specific volumes that address their concerns. It presents an extensive list of diseases, treatments, and other topics of general interest compiled from the Tables of Contents and major index headings. To access *A Contents Guide to the Health Reference Series*, visit www.healthreferenceseries.com.

Medical Consultant

Medical consultation services are provided to the *Health Reference Series* editors by David A. Cooke, MD, FACP. Dr. Cooke is a graduate of Brandeis University, and he received his M.D. degree from the University of Michigan. He completed residency training at the University of Wisconsin Hospital and Clinics. He is board-certified in Internal Medicine. Dr. Cooke currently works as part of the University of Michigan Health System and practices in Ann Arbor, MI. In his free time, he enjoys writing, science fiction, and spending time with his family.

Our Advisory Board

We would like to thank the following board members for providing guidance to the development of this series:

Dr. Lynda Baker, Associate Professor of Library and Information Science, Wayne State University, Detroit, MI

Nancy Bulgarelli, William Beaumont Hospital Library, Royal Oak, MI

Karen Imarisio, Bloomfield Township Public Library, Bloomfield Township, MI

Karen Morgan, Mardigian Library, University of Michigan-Dearborn, Dearborn, MI

Rosemary Orlando, St. Clair Shores Public Library, St. Clair Shores, MI

Health Reference Series *Update Policy*

The inaugural book in the *Health Reference Series* was the first edition of *Cancer Sourcebook* published in 1989. Since then, the *Series* has been enthusiastically received by librarians and in the medical community. In order to maintain the standard of providing high-quality health information for the layperson the editorial staff at Omnigraphics felt it was necessary to implement a policy of updating volumes when warranted.

Medical researchers have been making tremendous strides, and it is the purpose of the *Health Reference Series* to stay current with the most recent advances. Each decision to update a volume is made on an individual basis. Some of the considerations include how much new information is available and the feedback we receive from people who use the books. If there is a topic you would like to see added to the update list, or an area of medical concern you feel has not been adequately addressed, please write to:

Editor
Health Reference Series
Omnigraphics, Inc.
P.O. Box 31-1640
Detroit, MI 48231
E-mail: editorial@omnigraphics.com

Part One

Sleep Basics

Chapter 1

Understanding Sleep

Chapter Contents

Section 1.1

Why Do We Sleep?

Sleep is a behavioral state that is a natural part of every individual's life. We spend about one-third of our lives asleep. Nonetheless, people generally know little about the importance of this essential activity. Sleep is not just something to fill time when a person is inactive. Sleep is a required activity, not an option. Even though the precise functions of sleep remain a mystery, sleep is important for normal motor and cognitive function. We all recognize and feel the need to sleep. After sleeping, we recognize changes that have occurred, as we feel rested and more alert. Sleep actually appears to be required for survival. Rats deprived of sleep will die within two to three weeks, a time frame similar to death due to starvation.[1]

Very few textbooks provide any scientific information about changes that occur in the body during sleep and how those changes affect our ability to move and think. Of course, we've heard that a good night's sleep will help us perform better on a test the next day, but is this based on scientific fact, or is it just a continuing myth? The lack of information in textbooks may be due to the fact that sleep research is only recently gaining recognition. A great deal remains to be learned through scientific studies, including an answer to the key question, "What is the function of sleep?" Although its function remains unclear, research is providing a great deal of information about what happens in the brain and body during sleep and how the body regulates sleep.

Functions of Sleep

Animal studies have demonstrated that sleep is essential for survival. Consider studies that have been performed with laboratory rats. While these animals will normally live for two to three years, rats deprived of rapid eye movement (REM) sleep survive an average of only five months. Rats deprived of all sleep survive only about three weeks.[1] In humans, extreme sleep deprivation can cause an apparent state of paranoia and hallucinations in otherwise healthy individuals. However, despite identifying several physiological changes that occur in the brain and body during sleep, scientists still do not fully understand the functions of sleep. Many hypotheses have been advanced to explain the role of this necessary and natural behavior.[1] The following examples highlight several of these theories.

Hypothesis: Restoration and Recovery of Body Systems. This theory recognizes the need of an organism to replenish its energy stores and generally repair itself after a period of energy consumption and breakdown (wakefulness). The brain remains active during sleep, and the low metabolic rate characteristic of sleep is thought to be conducive to biosynthetic reactions. There is little, if any, evidence that more repair occurs during sleep than during rest or relaxed wakefulness. In fact, whole-body protein synthesis decreases during sleep, which is consistent with sleep being a period of overnight fasting.

Hypothesis: Energy Conservation. This theory states that we sleep to conserve energy and is based on the fact that the metabolic rate is lower during sleep. The theory predicts that total sleep time and non–rapid eye movement (NREM) sleep time will be proportional to the amount of energy expended during wakefulness. Support for this theory is derived from several lines of evidence. For example, NREM and REM sleep states are found only in endothermic animals (that is, those that expend energy to maintain body temperature). Species with greater total sleep times generally have higher core body temperatures and higher metabolic rates. Consider also that NREM sleep time and total sleep time decrease in humans with age, as do body and brain metabolism. In addition, infectious diseases tend to make us feel sleepy. This may be because molecules called cytokines, which regulate the function of the immune system, are powerful sleep inducers. It may be that sleep allows the body to conserve energy and other resources, which the immune system may then use to fight the infection.

Hypothesis: Memory Consolidation. The idea here is that sleeping reinforces learning and memory, while at the same time helping us to forget or to clear stores of unneeded memories. During the course of a day we are inundated with experiences, some of which should be remembered while others need not be. Perhaps sleep aids in rearranging all of the experiences and thoughts from the day so that those that are important are stored and those that are not are discarded. A recent study of songbirds suggests that sleep may play an important role in learning.[2]

Young birds listened to the songs of adult birds and began to practice and refine their own songs. The scientists were able to monitor the firing of individual brain cells involved with singing. They found that if sleeping birds listened to a recording of their own song, their neurons would later fire in a pattern nearly identical to that of song production though no sound was produced. The researchers speculate that the birds dream of singing; they relay and rehearse their songs and strengthen the nerve patterns required for song production. Sleep appears to be important for human learning as well. People who get plenty of deep NREM sleep in the first half of the night and REM sleep in the second half improve their ability to perform spatial tasks. This suggests that the full night's sleep plays a role in learning—not just one kind of sleep or the other.

Hypothesis: Protection from Predation. Inactivity during sleep may minimize exposure to predators. At the same time, however, sleep decreases sensitivity to external stimuli and may, as a consequence, increase vulnerability to predation.

Hypothesis: Brain Development. This proposed function of sleep is related to REM sleep, which occurs for prolonged periods during fetal and infant development. This sleep state may be involved in the formation of brain synapses.

Hypothesis: Discharge of Emotions. Perhaps dreaming during REM sleep provides a safe discharge of emotions. As protection to ourselves and to a bed partner, the muscular paralysis that occurs during REM sleep does not allow us to act out what we are dreaming. Additionally, activity in brain regions that control emotions, decision making, and social interactions is reduced during sleep. Perhaps this provides relief from the stresses that occur during wakefulness and helps maintain optimal performance when awake.

Unfortunately, each of these hypotheses suffers from flaws. Most fail because they cannot offer a mechanism for why sleep is more valuable than simply resting while remaining awake. In others, the shortcomings are more subtle.

References

1. Rechtschaffen, A. 1998. Current perspectives on the function of sleep. *Perspectives in Biological Medicine, 41*: 359–90.

2. Dave, A.S., and Margoliash, D. 2000. Song replay during sleep and computational rules for sensoring vocal learning. *Science, 290*: 812–16.

Section 1.2

Circadian Rhythms

Excerpted from "Brain Basics: Understanding Sleep," National Institute of Neurological Disorders and Stroke, National Institutes of Health, NIH Publication No. 06-3440-c, May 21, 2007.

Circadian rhythms are regular changes in mental and physical characteristics that occur in the course of a day (circadian is Latin for "around a day"). Most circadian rhythms are controlled by the body's biological "clock." This clock, called the suprachiasmatic nucleus or SCN, is actually a pair of pinhead-sized brain structures that together contain about twenty thousand neurons. The SCN rests in a part of the brain called the hypothalamus, just above the point where the optic nerves cross. Light that reaches photoreceptors in the retina (a tissue at the back of the eye) creates signals that travel along the optic nerve to the SCN.

Signals from the SCN travel to several brain regions, including the pineal gland, which responds to light-induced signals by switching off production of the hormone melatonin. The body's level of melatonin normally increases after darkness falls, making people feel drowsy. The SCN also governs functions that are synchronized with the sleep/wake cycle, including body temperature, hormone secretion, urine production, and changes in blood pressure.

By depriving people of light and other external time cues, scientists have learned that most people's biological clocks work on a twenty-five-hour cycle rather than a twenty-four-hour one. But because sunlight or other bright lights can reset the SCN, our biological cycles normally follow the twenty-four-hour cycle of the sun, rather than our innate cycle. Circadian rhythms can be affected to some degree by almost any kind of external time cue, such as the beeping of your alarm clock, the clatter of a garbage truck, or the timing of your meals. Scientists call external time cues zeitgebers (German for "time givers").

When travelers pass from one time zone to another, they suffer from disrupted circadian rhythms, an uncomfortable feeling known as jet lag. For instance, if you travel from California to New York, you "lose" three hours according to your body's clock. You will feel tired when the alarm rings at 8 a.m. the next morning because, according to your body's clock, it is still 5 a.m. It usually takes several days for your body's cycles to adjust to the new time.

To reduce the effects of jet lag, some doctors try to manipulate the biological clock with a technique called light therapy. They expose people to special lights, many times brighter than ordinary household light, for several hours near the time the subjects want to wake up. This helps them reset their biological clocks and adjust to a new time zone.

Symptoms much like jet lag are common in people who work nights or who perform shift work. Because these people's work schedules are at odds with powerful sleep-regulating cues like sunlight, they often become uncontrollably drowsy during work, and they may suffer insomnia or other problems when they try to sleep. Shift workers have an increased risk of heart problems, digestive disturbances, and emotional and mental problems, all of which may be related to their sleeping problems. The number and severity of workplace accidents also tend to increase during the night shift. Major industrial accidents attributed partly to errors made by fatigued night-shift workers include the Exxon *Valdez* oil spill and the Three Mile Island and Chernobyl nuclear power plant accidents. One study also found that medical interns working on the night shift are twice as likely as others to misinterpret hospital test records, which could endanger their patients. It may be possible to reduce shift-related fatigue by using bright lights in the workplace, minimizing shift changes, and taking scheduled naps.

Many people with total blindness experience lifelong sleeping problems because their retinas are unable to detect light. These people have a kind of permanent jet lag and periodic insomnia because their circadian rhythms follow their innate cycle rather than a twenty-four-hour one. Daily supplements of melatonin may improve nighttime sleep for such patients. However, since the high doses of melatonin found in most supplements can build up in the body, long-term use of this substance may create new problems. Because the potential side effects of melatonin supplements are still largely unknown, most experts discourage melatonin use by the general public.

Section 1.3

Physical Characteristics of Sleep

Sleep is a cyclical process. During sleep, people experience repeated cycles of non–rapid eye movement (NREM) and rapid eye movement (REM) sleep, beginning with an NREM phase. This cycle lasts approximately 90 to 110 minutes and is repeated four to six times per night. As the night progresses, however, the amount of deep NREM sleep decreases and the amount of REM sleep increases. The term ultradian rhythm (that is, rhythm occurring within a period of less than twenty-four hours) is used to describe this cycling through sleep stages.

Physiological Changes during Sleep

Table 1.1 summarizes some basic physiological changes that occur in NREM and REM sleep.

The functions of many organ systems are also linked to the sleep cycle, as follows:

- **Endocrine system:** Most hormone secretion is controlled by the circadian clock or in response to physical events. Sleep is one of the events that modify the timing of secretion for certain hormones. Many hormones are secreted into the blood during sleep. For example, scientists believe that the release of growth hormone is related in part to repair processes that occur during sleep. Follicle stimulating hormone and luteinizing hormone, which are involved in maturational and reproductive processes, are among the hormones released during sleep. In fact, the sleep-dependent release of luteinizing hormone is thought to be the event that initiates puberty. Other hormones, such as thyroid-stimulating hormone, are released prior to sleep.

- **Renal system:** Kidney filtration, plasma flow, and the excretion of sodium, chloride, potassium, and calcium all are reduced during both NREM and REM sleep. These changes cause urine to be more concentrated during sleep.

- **Alimentary activity:** In a person with normal digestive function, gastric acid secretion is reduced during sleep. In those with an active ulcer, gastric acid secretion is actually increased and swallowing occurs less frequently.

Table 1.1. Comparison of Physiological Changes During NREM and REM Sleep

Physiological Process	During NREM	During REM
Brain activity	Decreases from wakefulness	Increases in motor and sensory areas, while other areas are similar to NREM
Heart rate	Slows from wakefulness	Increases and varies compared with NREM
Blood pressure	Decreases from wakefulness	Increases (up to 30 percent) and varies from NREM
Blood flow to brain	Does not change from wakefulness in most regions	Increases by 50 to 200 percent from NREM, depending on brain region
Respiration	Decreases from wakefulness	Increases and varies from NREM, but may show brief stoppages (apnea); coughing suppressed
Airway resistance	Increases from wakefulness	Increases and varies from wakefulness
Body temperature	Is regulated at lower set point than wakefulness; shivering initiated at lower temperature than during wakefulness	Is not regulated; no shivering or sweating; temperature drifts toward that of the local environment
Sexual arousal	Occurs infrequently	Increases from NREM (in both males and females)

Section 1.4

Stages of Sleep

Excerpted from "Your Guide to Healthy Sleep," National Heart, Lung, and Blood Institute, National Institutes of Health, NIH Publication No. 06-5271, November 2005. Reviewed by David A. Cooke, M.D., F.A.C.P., March 23, 2010.

What Is Sleep?

Sleep was long considered just a uniform block of time when you are not awake. Thanks to sleep studies done over the past several decades, it is now known that sleep has distinct stages that cycle throughout the night in predictable patterns. How well rested you are and how well you function depend not just on your total sleep time but on how much of the various stages of sleep you get each night.

Your brain stays active throughout sleep, and each stage of sleep is linked to a distinctive pattern of electrical activity known as brain waves.

Sleep is divided into two basic types: rapid eye movement (REM) sleep and non REM sleep (with four different stages). Typically, sleep begins with non-REM sleep. In stage 1 non-REM sleep, you sleep lightly and can be awakened easily by noises or other disturbances. During this first stage of sleep, your eyes move slowly, and your muscle activity slows. You then enter stage 2 non-REM sleep, when your eye movements stop. Your brain shows a distinctive pattern of slower brain waves with occasional bursts of rapid waves.

When you progress into stage 3 non-REM sleep, your brain waves become even slower, although they are still punctuated by smaller, faster waves. By stage 4 non-REM sleep, the brain produces extremely slow waves almost exclusively. Stages 3 and 4 are considered deep sleep, during which it is very difficult to be awakened. Children who wet the bed or sleep walk tend to do so during stages 3 or 4 of non-REM sleep. Deep sleep is considered the "restorative" part of sleep that is necessary for feeling well rested and energetic during the day.

During REM sleep, your eyes move rapidly in various directions, even though your eyelids remain closed. Your breathing also becomes more rapid, irregular, and shallow, and your heart rate and blood pressure increase. Dreaming typically occurs during REM sleep. During this type of sleep, your arm and leg muscles are temporarily paralyzed so that you cannot "act out" any dreams that you may be having.

The first period of REM sleep you experience usually occurs about an hour to an hour and a half after falling asleep. After that, the sleep stages repeat themselves continuously while you sleep. As the night progresses, REM sleep time becomes longer, while time spent in non-REM sleep stages 3 and 4 becomes shorter. By morning, nearly all your sleep time is spent in stages 1 and 2 of non-REM sleep and in REM sleep. If REM sleep is disrupted during one night, REM sleep time is typically longer than normal in subsequent nights until you catch up. Overall, almost one-half your total sleep time is spent in stages 1 and 2 non-REM sleep and about one-fifth each in deep sleep (stages 3 and 4 of non-REM sleep) and REM sleep. In contrast, infants spend half or more of their total sleep time in REM sleep. Gradually, as they mature, the percentage of total sleep time they spend in REM progressively decreases to reach the one-fifth level typical of later childhood and adulthood.

Why people dream and why REM sleep is so important are not well understood. It is known that REM sleep stimulates the brain regions used in learning and the laying down of memories. Animal studies suggest that dreams may reflect the brain's sorting and selectively storing important new information acquired during wake time. While this information is processed, the brain might revisit scenes from the day while pulling up older memories. This process may explain why childhood memories can be interspersed with more recent events during dreams. Studies show, however, that other stages of sleep besides REM are also needed to form the pathways in the brain that enable us to learn and remember.

Table 1.2. Types of Sleep

Non-REM Sleep	REM Sleep
Stage 1: Light sleep; easily awakened; muscle activity; eye movements slow down.	Usually first occurs about 90 minutes after you fall asleep; cycles along with the non-REM stages throughout the night. Eyes move rapidly, with eyelids closed. Breathing is more rapid, irregular, and shallow. Heart rate and blood pressure increase. Dreaming occurs. Arm and leg muscles are temporarily paralyzed.
Stage 2: Eye movements stop; slower brain waves, with occasional bursts of rapid brain waves.	
Stage 3: Considered deep sleep; difficult to awaken; brain waves slow down more, but still have occasional rapid waves.	
Stage 4: Considered deep sleep; difficult to awaken; extremely slow brain waves.	

Chapter 2

Napping: Benefits for All Ages

Chapter Contents

Section 2.1

Young Children Need Naps

"Naps," November 2009, reprinted with permission from www.kidshealth.org. Copyright © 2009 The Nemours Foundation. This information was provided by KidsHealth, one of the largest resources online for medically reviewed health information written for parents, kids, and teens. For more articles like this one, visit www.KidsHealth.org, or www.TeensHealth.org.

The Importance of Naps

Nap. It's a small word, but for most parents a hugely important one. Why? Sleep is a major requirement for good health, and for young kids to get enough of it, some daytime sleep is usually needed. Crucial physical and mental development occurs in early childhood, and naps provide much-needed downtime for growth and rejuvenation.

Naps also help keep kids from becoming overtired, which not only takes a toll on their moods but may also make it harder for them to fall asleep at night. And naptime gives parents a brief oasis during the day and time to tackle household chores or just unwind.

Sleep Needs by Age

There's no one-size-fits-all answer regarding how much daytime sleep kids need. It all depends on the age, the child, and the sleep total during a twenty-four-hour period. For example, one toddler may sleep thirteen hours at night with only some daytime catnapping, while another gets nine hours at night but takes a solid two-hour nap each afternoon.

Though sleep needs are highly individual, these age-by-age guidelines give an idea of average daily sleep requirements.

Birth to six months. Infants require about sixteen to twenty total hours of sleep per day. Younger infants tend to sleep on and off around the clock, waking every two or three hours to eat. As they approach four months of age, sleep rhythms become more established. Most babies sleep ten to twelve hours at night, usually with an interruption for feeding, and average three to five hours of sleep during the day (usually grouped into two or three naps).

Six to twelve months. Babies this age usually sleep about eleven hours at night, plus two daytime naps totaling three to four hours. At this age, most infants do not need to wake at night to feed, but may begin to experience separation anxiety, which can contribute to sleep disturbances.

Toddlers (one to three years). Toddlers generally require ten to thirteen hours of sleep, including an afternoon nap of one to three hours. Young toddlers might still be taking two naps, but naps should not occur too close to bedtime, as they may make it harder for toddlers to fall asleep at night.

Preschoolers (three to five years). Preschoolers average about ten to twelve hours at night, plus an afternoon nap. Most give up this nap by five years of age.

School-age (five to twelve years). School-age kids need about ten to twelve hours at night. Some five-year-olds might still need a nap, and if a regular nap isn't possible, they might need an earlier bedtime.

Signs of Insufficient Sleep

Most parents underestimate the amount of sleep kids need, so be sure to watch your child's behavior for signs of sleep deprivation, which can range from the obvious—like fatigue—to more subtle problems with behavior and schoolwork.

Ask yourself:

- Does my child act sleepy during the day?

- Does my child get cranky and irritable in the late afternoon?

- Is it a battle to get my child out of bed in the morning?

- Is my child inattentive, impatient, hyperactive, or aggressive?

- Does my child have trouble focusing on schoolwork and other tasks?

If you answered yes to any of these questions, consider adjusting your child's sleep or nap schedule. It may take several weeks to find a routine that works. Talk to your doctor if you have concerns about your child's sleep.

Naptime Routines and Other Concerns

The key to good napping can be as simple as setting up a good nap routine early on and sticking to it. With infants, watch for cues like fussing and rubbing eyes, then put your baby to bed while sleepy but not yet asleep. This teaches kids how to fall asleep themselves—a skill that only becomes more important as they get older. Soft music, dim lights, or a quiet story or rhyme at bedtime can help ease the transition to sleep and become a source of comfort for your child.

For toddlers and preschoolers, sticking to a naptime schedule can be more challenging. Though many do still love their nap, others don't want to miss out on a minute of the action and will fight sleep even as their eyes are closing. In this case, don't let naptime become a battle—you can't force your child to sleep, but you can insist on some quiet time. Let your child read books or play quietly in his or her room. Parents are often surprised by how quickly quiet time can lead to sleep time—but even if it doesn't, at least your child is getting some much-needed rest. If your child has given up daytime naps, consider adjusting to an earlier bedtime.

Many parents worry that naptime will interfere with kids' bedtime (and if a child takes a late-afternoon nap, this could be the case). But before you end naps entirely in an effort to wear out your child by bedtime, consider this: Well-rested kids are quicker to settle down at night than overtired ones. Overtired kids are often "wired" and restless, unable to self-soothe at bedtime, and more likely to wake through the night.

If you feel your child's late naptime is the cause of bedtime problems, try making the nap a little bit earlier, which may mean waking your child a little earlier in the morning so the nap can begin sooner.

You might also try waking your child from a nap earlier than usual so he or she has a longer active period before bedtime. In other words, try to make some adjustments before abandoning the nap—both you and your child will feel much better if there is one.

Section 2.2

Power Napping for Increased Productivity

Reprinted from "'Power Nap' Prevents Burnout; Morning Sleep Perfects a Skill," National Institute of Mental Health, July 2, 2002. Reviewed by David A. Cooke, M.D., F.A.C.P., March 23, 2010.

Evidence is mounting that sleep—even a nap—appears to enhance information processing and learning. New experiments by National Institute of Mental Health (NIMH) grantee Alan Hobson, M.D., Robert Stickgold, Ph.D., and colleagues at Harvard University show that a midday snooze reverses information overload and that a 20 percent overnight improvement in learning a motor skill is largely traceable to a late stage of sleep that some early risers might be missing. Overall, their studies suggest that the brain uses a night's sleep to consolidate the memories of habits, actions, and skills learned during the day.

The bottom line: we should stop feeling guilty about taking that "power nap" at work or catching those extra winks the night before our piano recital.

Reporting in the July 2002 *Nature Neuroscience*, Sara Mednick, Ph.D., Stickgold, and colleagues demonstrate that "burnout"—irritation, frustration, and poorer performance on a mental task—sets in as a day of training wears on. Subjects performed a visual task, reporting the horizontal or vertical orientation of three diagonal bars against a background of horizontal bars in the lower left corner of a computer screen. Their scores on the task worsened over the course of four daily practice sessions. Allowing subjects a thirty-minute nap after the second session prevented any further deterioration, while a one-hour nap actually boosted performance in the third and fourth sessions back to morning levels.

Rather than generalized fatigue, the researchers suspected that the burnout was limited to just the brain visual system circuits involved in the task. To find out, they engaged a fresh set of neural circuitry by switching the location of the task to the lower right corner of the computer screen for just the fourth practice session. As predicted, subjects experienced no burnout and performed about as well as they did in the first session—or after a short nap.

17

This led the researchers to propose that neural networks in the visual cortex "gradually become saturated with information through repeated testing, preventing further perceptual processing." They think burnout may be the brain's "mechanism for preserving information that has been processed but has not yet been consolidated into memory by sleep."

So how might a nap help? Recordings of brain and ocular electrical activity monitored while napping revealed that the longer one-hour naps contained more than four times as much deep, or slow wave, sleep and rapid eye movement (REM) sleep than the half-hour naps. Subjects who took the longer naps also spent significantly more time in a slow wave sleep state on the test day than on a "baseline" day, when they were not practicing. Previous studies by the Harvard group have traced overnight memory consolidation and improvement on the same perceptual task to amounts of slow wave sleep in the first quarter of the night and to REM sleep in the last quarter. Since a nap hardly allows enough time for the latter early morning REM sleep effect to develop, a slow wave sleep effect appears to be the antidote to burnout.

Neural networks involved in the task are refreshed by "mechanisms of cortical plasticity" operating during slow wave sleep, suggest the researchers. "Slow wave sleep serves as the initial processing stage of experience-dependent, long-term learning and as the critical stage for restoring perceptual performance."

The Harvard team has now extended to a motor-skill task their earlier discovery of sleep's role in enhancing learning of the perceptual task. Matthew Walker, Ph.D., Hobson, Stickgold, and colleagues report in the July 3, 2002, *Neuron* that a 20 percent overnight boost in speed on a finger tapping task is accounted for mostly by stage 2 non-rapid eye movement (NREM) sleep in the two hours just before waking.

Prior to the study, it was known that people learning motor skills continue to improve for at least a day following a training session. For example, musicians, dancers, and athletes often report that their performance has improved even though they haven't practiced for a day or two. But until now it was unclear whether this could be ascribed to specific sleep states instead of simply to the passage of time.

In the study, sixty-two right-handers were asked to type a sequence of numbers (4-1-3-2-4) with their left hand as rapidly and accurately as possible for thirty seconds. Each finger tap registered as a white dot on a computer screen rather than the number typed, so subjects didn't know how accurately they were performing. Twelve such trials separated by thirty-second rest periods constituted a training session, which was scored for speed and accuracy.

Regardless of whether they trained in the morning or the evening, subjects improved by an average of nearly 60 percent by simply repeating the task, with most of the boost coming within the first few trials. A group tested after training in the morning and staying awake for twelve hours showed no significant improvement. But when tested following a night's sleep, their performance increased by nearly 19 percent. Another group that trained in the evening scored 20.5 percent faster after a night's sleep, but gained only a negligible 2 percent after another twelve hours of waking. To rule out the possibility that motor skill activity during waking hours might interfere with consolidation of the task in memory, another group even wore mittens for a day to prevent skilled finger movements. Their improvement was negligible—until after a full night's sleep, when their scores soared by nearly 20 percent.

Sleep lab monitoring of twelve subjects who trained at 10 p.m. revealed that their improved performance was directly proportional to the amount of stage 2 NREM sleep they got in the fourth quarter of the night. Although this stage represents about half of a night's sleep overall, Walker said he and his colleagues were surprised at the pivotal role stage 2 NREM plays in enhancing learning of the motor task, given that REM and slow wave sleep had accounted for the similar overnight learning improvement in the perceptual task.

They speculate that sleep may enhance motor skill learning via powerful bursts of synchronous neuronal firing, called "spindles," characteristic of stage 2 NREM sleep during the early morning hours. These spindles predominate around the center of the brain, conspicuously near motor regions, and are thought to promote new neural connections by triggering an influx of calcium into cells of the cortex. Studies have observed an increase in spindles following training on a motor task.

The new findings have implications for learning sports, a musical instrument, or developing artistic movement control. "All such learning of new actions may require sleep before the maximum benefit of practice is expressed," note the researchers. Since a full night's sleep is a prerequisite to experiencing the critical final two hours of stage 2 NREM sleep, "life's modern erosion of sleep time could shortchange your brain of some learning potential," added Walker.

The findings also underscore why sleep may be important to the learning involved in recovering function following insults to the brain's motor system, as in stroke. They also may help to explain why infants sleep so much. "Their intensity of learning may drive the brain's hunger for large amounts of sleep," suggested Walker.

Chapter 3

Dreaming

Chapter Contents

Section 3.1

Dreaming and Rapid Eye Movement (REM) Sleep: The Science behind Dreams

Excerpted from "Brain Basics: Understanding Sleep," National Institute of Neurological Disorders and Stroke, National Institutes of Health, NIH Publication No. 06-3440-c, May 21, 2007.

We typically spend more than two hours each night dreaming. Scientists do not know much about how or why we dream. Sigmund Freud, who greatly influenced the field of psychology, believed dreaming was a "safety valve" for unconscious desires. Only after 1953, when researchers first described rapid eye movement (REM) in sleeping infants, did scientists begin to carefully study sleep and dreaming. They soon realized that the strange, illogical experiences we call dreams almost always occur during REM sleep. While most mammals and birds show signs of REM sleep, reptiles and other cold-blooded animals do not.

REM sleep begins with signals from an area at the base of the brain called the pons. These signals travel to a brain region called the thalamus, which relays them to the cerebral cortex—the outer layer of the brain that is responsible for learning, thinking, and organizing information. The pons also sends signals that shut off neurons in the spinal cord, causing temporary paralysis of the limb muscles. If something interferes with this paralysis, people will begin to physically "act out" their dreams—a rare, dangerous problem called REM sleep behavior disorder. A person dreaming about a ball game, for example, may run headlong into furniture or blindly strike someone sleeping nearby while trying to catch a ball in the dream.

REM sleep stimulates the brain regions used in learning. This may be important for normal brain development during infancy, which would explain why infants spend much more time in REM sleep than adults. Like deep sleep, REM sleep is associated with increased production of proteins. One study found that REM sleep affects learning of certain mental skills. People taught a skill and then deprived of non-REM sleep could recall what they had learned after sleeping, while people deprived of REM sleep could not.

Some scientists believe dreams are the cortex's attempt to find meaning in the random signals that it receives during REM sleep. The cortex is the part of the brain that interprets and organizes information from the environment during consciousness. It may be that, given random signals from the pons during REM sleep, the cortex tries to interpret these signals as well, creating a "story" out of fragmented brain activity.

Section 3.2

Common Questions about Dreams

Does everyone dream?

Yes. Laboratory studies have shown that we experience our most vivid dreams during a type of sleep called rapid eye movement (REM) sleep. During REM sleep the brain is very active, the eyes move back and forth rapidly under the lids, and the large muscles of the body are relaxed. REM sleep occurs every ninety to one hundred minutes, three to four times a night, and lasts longer as the night progresses. The final REM period may last as long as forty-five minutes. Less vivid dreams occur at other times during the night.

Why do people have trouble remembering their dreams?

Some people have no difficulty in remembering several dreams nightly, whereas others recall dreams only occasionally or not at all. Nearly everything that happens during sleep—including dreams, the thoughts which occur throughout the night, and memories of brief awakenings—is forgotten by morning. There is something about the phenomenon of sleep itself which makes it difficult to remember what has occurred and most dreams are forgotten unless they are written down. Sometimes a dream is suddenly remembered later in the day or on another day, suggesting that the memory is not totally lost but for some reason is very hard to retrieve. Sleep and dreams also are affected by a great variety of drugs and medications, including alcohol. Further, stopping certain medications suddenly may cause nightmares. It is advisable to discuss with your physician the effect of any drugs or medications you are taking.

How can I improve my dream memory?

Before you fall asleep, remind yourself that you want to remember your dreams. Keep a paper and pen or tape recorder by your bedside. As you awaken, try to move as little as possible and try not to think right away about your upcoming day. Write down all of your dreams and images, as they can fade quickly if not recorded. Any distractions will cause the memory of your dream to fade. If you can't remember a full dream, record the last thing that was on your mind before awakening, even if you have only a vague memory of it.

Are dreams in color?

Most dreams are in color, although people may not be aware of it, either because they have difficulty remembering their dreams or because color is such a natural part of visual experience. People who are very aware of color while awake probably notice color more often in their dreams.

Do dreams have meaning?

Although scientists continue to debate this issue, most people who work with their dreams, either by themselves or with others, find that their dreams are very meaningful for them. Dreams are useful in learning more about the dreamer's feelings, thoughts, behavior, motives, and values. Many find that dreams can help them solve problems. Further, artists, writers, and scientists often get creative ideas from dreams.

How can I learn to interpret my dreams?

The most important thing to keep in mind is that your dreams reflect your own underlying thoughts and feelings, and that the people, actions, settings, and emotions in your dreams are personal to you. Some dream experts theorize that there are typical or archetypal dreams and dream elements that persist across different persons, cultures, and times. Usually, however, the same image or symbol will have different meanings for different people. For example, an elephant in a dream can mean one thing to a zookeeper and something quite different to a child whose favorite toy is a stuffed elephant. Therefore, books which give a specific meaning for a specific dream image or symbol (or "dream dictionaries") are not usually helpful. By thinking about what each dream element means to you or reminds you of, by looking for parallels between these associations and what is happening in your waking life, and by being patient and persistent, you can learn to understand your dreams. It can be helpful to keep a dream diary and reflect on many dreams over a long period of time to get the truest picture of your unique dream life. Many good books exist that can help you get started interpreting your dreams.

What does it mean when I have the same dream over and over?

Recurrent dreams, which can continue for years, may be treated as any other dream. That is, one may look for parallels between the dream and the thoughts, feelings, behavior, and motives of the dreamer. Understanding the meaning of the recurrent dream sometimes can help the dreamer resolve an issue that he or she has been struggling with for years.

Is it normal to have nightmares?

Nightmares are very common among children and fairly common among adults. Often nightmares are caused by stress, traumatic experiences, emotional difficulties, drugs or medication, or illness. However, some people have frequent nightmares that seem unrelated to their waking lives. Recent studies suggest that these people tend to be more open, sensitive, trusting, and emotional than average.

Is it true that if you dream that you die or that you hit bottom in a falling dream, you will in fact die in your sleep?

No, these beliefs are not true. Many people have dreamed that they died or hit bottom in a fall and they have lived to tell the tale! You can explore the meaning of these kinds of images just as you would explore any others that might occur in your dreams. However, if any aspect of your dreams worries or distresses you, talk to a professional mental health practitioner about your concerns.

Can dreams predict the future?

There are many examples of dreams that seemed to predict future events. Some may have been due to coincidence, faulty memory, or an unconscious tying together of known information. A few laboratory studies have been conducted of predictive dreams, as well as clairvoyant and telepathic dreams, but the results were varied, as these kinds of dreams are difficult to study in a laboratory setting.

Is it possible to control dreams?

You often can influence your dreams by giving yourself pre-sleep suggestions. Another method of influencing dreams is called lucid dreaming, in which you are aware you are dreaming while still asleep and in the dream. Sometimes people experience this type of dreaming spontaneously. It is often possible to learn how to increase lucid dreaming, and thereby increase your capacity to affect the course of the dream events as they unfold. Some things are easier than others to control, and indeed complete control is probably never possible. Some professional dream workers question the advisability of trying to control the dream, and encourage learning to enjoy and understand it instead.

Section 3.3

Nightmares

A nightmare is a dream that occurs during sleep that brings out strong feelings of fear, terror, distress, or anxiety. Nightmares usually happen in the second part of the night and wake up the sleeper, who is able to remember the content of the dream.

Considerations

Nightmares tend to be more common among children and become less frequent toward adulthood. About 50 percent of adults have occasional nightmares, women more often than men.

Causes

Anxiety and stress are the most common causes of nightmares. A major life event occurs before the nightmare in some cases.

Other causes of nightmares include:

- abrupt alcohol withdrawal;

- breathing disorder in sleep (sleep apnea);

- death of a loved one (bereavement);

- excessive alcohol consumption;

- illness with a fever;

- recent withdrawal from a drug, such as sleeping pills;

- side effect of a drug;

- sleep disorder (for example, narcolepsy or sleep terror disorder);

- eating just before going to bed, which raises the body's metabolism and brain activity.

Home Care

If you are under stress, ask for support from friends and relatives. Talking about what is on your mind can help.

Follow a regular fitness routine, with aerobic exercise if possible. You will find that you will be able to fall asleep faster, sleep more deeply, and wake up feeling more refreshed.

Learn techniques to reduce muscle tension (relaxation therapy), which will help reduce your anxiety.

Practice good sleep hygiene. Go to bed at the same time each night, and wake up at the same time each morning. Avoid long-term use of tranquilizers, as well as caffeine and other stimulants.

If your nightmares started shortly after you began taking a new medication, contact your healthcare provider. He or she will let you know whether to stop taking that medication, and may recommend an alternative.

For nightmares caused by the effects of "street drugs" or regular alcohol use, ask for advice from your doctor on the safest and most successful ways to quit.

When to Contact a Medical Professional

Contact your health care provider if:

- you have nightmares more than once a week;
- nightmares stop you from getting a good night's rest, or from keeping up with your daily activities for a long period of time.

What to Expect at Your Office Visit

Your doctor will examine you, ask you questions, and possibly recommend tests. You may be asked any of the following questions:

- Time pattern:
  - How often do you have nightmares?
  - Do they occur in the second half of the night?
- Quality:
  - Do you wake up suddenly from sleep?
- Other issues:
  - Do the nightmares cause you intense fear and anxiety?
  - Can you remember a particular nightmare (one with vivid images and a story-like plot)?

- Aggravating factors:
  - Have you had a recent illness?
  - Did you have a fever?
  - Were you in a stressful situation recently?
- Other:
  - Do you use alcohol? How much?
  - What medications do you take?
  - Do you take "street drugs?" If so, which ones?
  - Do you take natural supplements or alternative remedies?
  - What other symptoms do you have?

Tests that may be done include:

- blood cell measurements;
- liver function tests;
- thyroid function tests;
- electroencephalogram (EEG), which painlessly measures brain waves with electrodes placed on the head.

If reducing stress, medication side effects, and substance use do not improve the nightmares, your healthcare provider may want to send you to a sleep medicine specialist for a sleep study (polysomnography). In some cases, certain medications may help reduce nightmares.

Alternative Names

Dreams—bad; bad dreams

References

Moore DP, Jefferson JW. Nightmare disorder. In: Moore DP, Jefferson JW, eds. *Handbook of Medical Psychiatry. 2nd ed.* Philadelphia, Pa: Mosby Elsevier; 2004:chap 123.

Moser SE, Bober JF. Behavioral problems in children and adolescents. In: Rakel RE, ed. *Textbook of Family Medicine. 7th ed.* Philadelphia, Pa: Saunders Elsevier; 2007:chap 33.

Section 3.4

Night Terrors

Night terrors are a sleep disorder in which a person quickly awakens from sleep in a terrified state.

Causes

Night terrors (sleep terrors) occur during deep sleep, usually during the first third of the night. The cause is unknown but night terrors may be triggered by fever, lack of sleep, or periods of emotional tension, stress, or conflict.

In contrast, nightmares are more common in the early morning. They may occur after someone watches frightening movies/TV shows or has an emotional experience. A person may remember the details of a dream upon awakening, and will not be disoriented after the episode.

Night terrors are most common in boys ages five to seven, although they also can occur in girls. They are fairly common in children ages three to seven, and much less common after that. Night terrors may run in families. They can occur in adults, especially with emotional tension and/or the use of alcohol.

Symptoms

Night terrors are most common during the first third of the night, often between midnight and 2 a.m.:

- Children often scream and are very frightened and confused. They thrash around violently and are often not aware of their surroundings.
- You may be unable to talk to, comfort, or fully awaken a child who is having a night terror.
- The child may be sweating, breathing very fast (hyperventilating), have a fast heart rate, and dilated pupils.
- The spell may last ten to twenty minutes, then normal sleep returns.

Most children are unable to explain what happened the next morning. There is often no memory of the event when they awaken the next day. Children with night terrors may also sleep walk.

Exams and Tests

In many cases, no further examination or testing is needed. If the night terror is severe or prolonged, the child may need a psychological evaluation.

Treatment

In many cases, a child who has a night terror only needs comfort and reassurance. Psychotherapy or counseling may be appropriate in some cases. Benzodiazepine medications (such as diazepam) used at bedtime will often reduce night terrors; however, medication is rarely recommended to treat this disorder.

Outlook (Prognosis)

Most children outgrow night terrors in a short period of time. They don't usually remember the event. Stress reduction and/or psychotherapy may be helpful for night terror in adults.

Possible Complications

- Insomnia (unusual)

When to Contact a Medical Professional

Call for an appointment with your health care provider if:

- the night terrors are persistent or frequent;
- they occur often enough to regularly disrupt sleep;
- other symptoms occur with the night terror;
- the night terror causes, or almost causes, injuries.

Prevention

Minimizing stress or using coping mechanisms may reduce night terrors. The number of episodes usually decreases after age ten.

Alternative Names

Pavor nocturnus; Sleep terror disorder

References

Owens JA. Sleep medicine: In: Kliegman RM, Behrman RE, Jenson HB, Stanton BF, eds. *Nelson Textbook of Pediatrics. 18th ed.* Philadelphia, Pa: Saunders Elsevier; 2007: chap 18.

Chapter 4

Gender Differences in Quality of Sleep

Even with growing progress toward gender equality in the workplace, women continue to carry the most responsibility for family care, a load that according to a new study could indicate why women report more sleep disruption than men.

The research led by David Maume, a University of Cincinnati professor of sociology and director of the UC Kunz Center for Research in Work, Family and Gender, UC graduate student Rachel A. Sebastian, and Miami University (Ohio) graduate student Anthony R. Bardo was presented August 10, 2009, at the 104th annual meeting of the American Sociological Association (ASA) in San Francisco.

Health researchers have traditionally dominated the field of sleep research, examining biological differences and their effects on sleep patterns. The University of Cincinnati study delved into the social issues of how work and family obligations could trigger tossing and turning when it came to a good night's sleep. "Drawing on scholarship on gender inequality on time use, we contend that sleep is an activity that is affected by gender inequality in waking role obligations," write the authors.

The UC researchers conducted a phone survey of 583 union workers represented by a Midwestern chapter of the United Food and Commercial Workers (UFCW). The phone survey took place between January and April of 2007. Sixty-two percent of the respondents were women.

33

Participants were asked about the number of hours they slept, as well as about sleep-related questions that healthcare workers would review in examining the health effects of sleep loss, such as, "In the past three months, did you never, rarely, sometimes or often":

- Have trouble falling asleep?
- Wake up before you wanted to?
- Wake up feeling refreshed?
- Get the right amount of sleep?
- Have sleep interrupted by another family member?
- Feel tired even on days when you weren't working?
- Sleep longer on days when you weren't working?
- Have trouble with memory?
- Feel sluggish or rundown at work?
- Fall asleep at work?

The researchers also factored in demographics such as age, race, and education, as well as health predictors such as pain frequency that would affect sleep, and body mass index (BMI).

To examine how family obligations would affect sleep, the researchers also differentiated between respondents married to nonworking spouses, part-time working spouses, and full-time working spouses as well as nonmarried respondents. Stress was also measured by asking participants about the stability of their relationships and having children.

In examining work demands on sleep, the researchers reviewed overnight shifts and rotating schedules as well as job satisfaction, number of years on the job, and job autonomy.

The researchers found that gender differences in health status accounted for a substantial portion (27 percent) of the gender gap in sleep disruption, with women more likely to report health effects on sleep disruption. Women were also more likely to report conflicts in balancing the demands of their work schedules with finding the time, energy, and enthusiasm to meet family responsibilities, accounting for 17 percent of the gender gap in sleep disruption, with parental status accounting for an additional 5 percent of the gender gap in sleep disruption.

The authors say that women were more likely than men to report more sleep disruption when they were concerned about their marriages, when they worked nonstandard schedules, when job demands spilled over into family lives, and when family issues affected job performance.

The authors found that men whose wives worked full time reported more sleep disruption, and when jobs and family lives spilled into each other, but significantly less than women. "Overall, the results show that gendered reactions to work-family situations accounted for more than half of the gender gap in sleep disruption," state the authors.

Men who considered their work/family roles on equal footing with their partner were also more likely to report sleep disruption.

"To the extent that sleep, as a specific type of discretionary time, is an activity that may be fragmented, curtailed, or otherwise rescheduled in order to meet the often conflicting demands of jobs and loved ones, these results suggest that this is more characteristic of women's lives than men's," write the authors.

The sociologists conclude that sleep differences should continue to be examined in terms of gender inequality in contemporary society.

Funding for the research was supported by grants from the National Science Foundation as well as the Charles Phelps Taft Research Center at the University of Cincinnati.

Chapter 5

Women's Sleep Issues

Chapter Contents

Section 5.1

Women and Sleep: An Overview

"Women's Sleep Issues," © 2009 Illinois Neurological Institute
(www.ini.org). Reprinted with permission.

Just like healthy eating habits, healthy sleep habits are an important part of good overall health. But, unlike food, we often try to get by with as little sleep as possible to get through our days. That can lead to poor performance, irritability, excessive daytime sleepiness, and maybe even illness.

Most healthy adults require about eight hours of sleep a night, at about the same time each night. Like our food intake, we can manipulate how much and when we sleep, but we cannot change our actual sleep need. Sleep scientists continue to find more and more evidence that we do not perform well without it. While we might be able to "get by" on a few hours of sleep or even none at all for a night or two, continuous short nights of sleep (even six hours) leads to reduced daytime function.

Women versus Men

Sleep in women differs from sleep in men in a few important ways. Most women who have been pregnant know that sleepiness is common in the first trimester, while insomnia is common in the last. The physical changes that occur in the last few months make sleeping cumbersome. Of course, worry and excitement can make sleep difficult, too. Muscle cramps are also common in pregnancy and can cause abrupt awakening.

Restless Legs Syndrome

Restless legs syndrome is a sensation in the legs, and sometimes arms, that makes one have to move to get comfortable. It occurs in the evening, at rest, and gets better with movement or tensing of the muscles. It may cause difficulty falling asleep. Although it affects both men and women, it is more common in pregnancy. It is easily treated with medication, but this is usually not advised in pregnancy. Other strategies to control the symptoms include avoiding all caffeine and alcohol, and taking warm baths.

Pregnancy Can Disturb Sleep

While pregnancy can disturb sleep, there is nothing quite like the first few weeks of motherhood when it comes to sleep disruption. Awakening to a baby's hungry cry is natural, but getting enough sleep at other times is sometimes hard to accomplish. "Sleep when the baby sleeps" doesn't always happen for mothers with other children and busy schedules. The best strategy may be to sleep when one can, and try to get as many hours in a row as possible. Continuous sleep is more refreshing than the same amount of sleep broken up into shorter periods. It is reassuring to remember that this phase is only temporary, and most babies sleep through the night by about three months of age.

Menopause and Sleep

Menopause is known to cause sleep disruption in many women. Hot flashes are an obvious cause for some, but other causes of arousal from sleep may occur. Sleep apnea is more common in men than it is in women who have not gone through menopause. After menopause, however, the odds start to even out. While some have speculated that this is related to hormonal changes, there is some evidence to suggest it is more closely related to body weight and other factors.

Obstructive Sleep Apnea

Obstructive sleep apnea, due to collapse of the upper airway, is the most common type of apnea, and the most commonly diagnosed sleep disorder. It is typically associated with snoring, and often causes excessive daytime sleepiness. An episode of apnea often causes a lower oxygen level, increased blood pressure, and brief awakening.

Most apnea is easily treated. Continuous positive airway pressure (CPAP) provides pressurized air through a mask worn over the nose during sleep, and almost always controls apnea. Weight loss can also help, and sometimes cures apnea. Others may benefit from surgery to remove the uvula and some of the soft palate at the back of the throat, but this is only effective in fewer than half of patients. An oral appliance can be worn during sleep to reposition the jaw forward. This treats some people with mild to moderate sleep apnea, but is not generally effective in severe cases.

Insomnia

Insomnia refers to difficulty initiating sleep or difficulty maintaining sleep. In general, it is more common in women than in men, especially over the age of forty. In younger adults, it is equally common in both sexes. It is very important to think of insomnia as a symptom rather than a diagnosis. The underlying causes must therefore be recognized and treated. Our sleep habits, or "sleep hygiene," can play a major role in insomnia. Starting with good sleep hygiene is always a good idea when trying to overcome insomnia. If that is not effective, looking for other causes may be in order.

Sleep Hygiene

Good sleep hygiene is simple. The idea is to give yourself enough time to sleep, sleep in bed, be awake everywhere else, and don't do anything to interfere with any of those. But, like dieting, this may be easier said than done for some of us. Here are some ground rules to help you stay on track:

- Go to bed when you are sleepy, not earlier. Going to bed before you are sleepy will promote lying awake in bed, which can condition (teach) the brain to be awake in bed. Limiting your time in bed helps consolidate and deepen your sleep. Excessively long times in bed lead to fragmented and shallow sleep. When you wake up refreshed, get up. Don't linger in bed for long.

- Get up at the same time every day, seven days a week. A regular wake time will help you fall asleep more easily at night, and helps set your "internal clock."

- Sleep only in bed. Sleeping in other locations at home may make it more difficult to sleep in bed.

- Use the bedroom only for sleeping and sexual activity. Avoid reading, watching TV, eating, or talking on the phone in bed. Also avoid lying awake thinking in bed. If you need to problem-solve, make plans, or sort things out in your mind, do it elsewhere. Get up and sit in another room to "process" your thoughts. Do not take your problems to bed. It is often helpful to spend time earlier in the evening to work on your problems or plan the next day's activities. Some people find it helpful to designate "worry time" before bed to work through difficult issues that might otherwise keep them awake. All this should be done in a room other than the bedroom.

- Cover the clock or put it where you cannot see it. Looking at the clock when you either can't fall asleep or have awakened and can't get back to sleep only perpetuates the problem.

- Regular daily exercise may help deepen sleep. Exercise too close to bedtime may disturb sleep. Finish exercising at least three hours before bedtime.

- Insulate your bedroom against sounds. Carpeting, wearing earplugs, and closing the door may help. Noise may disturb your sleep even if you are not fully aware of it. This is especially problematic for third-shift workers who need to sleep during the day when most people are awake.

- Keep the room temperature moderate. Excessively warm rooms may disturb sleep, even more than you might be aware of.

- Don't go to bed hungry, as it may keep you from falling asleep. A light snack at bedtime may help sleep, but avoid having a big meal. Stomach and intestinal activity slow down and food is not well digested during sleep.

- Avoid excessive fluid intake in the evening to minimize the need for nighttime trips to the bathroom. While it is generally healthy to drink plenty of water during the day, limiting this for the last two to three hours before bedtime can help you sleep through the night.

- Avoid caffeine, especially in the afternoon or evening. A single cup of coffee in the morning can affect sleep at night, even if you are not aware of it. This doesn't mean caffeine should be avoided by everyone, but it does mean that anyone with trouble sleeping should stop it completely, at least until the insomnia is in control. Many people say "caffeine doesn't affect me," or "I stopped caffeine once and it didn't do any good." If a person has insomnia and uses any caffeine, there could be a relationship. And, stopping caffeine without following all the points of good sleep hygiene may not have been enough on its own. Use of caffeine to treat headaches may actually disrupt sleep. If sleep disruption is an issue for an individual, other treatments should be considered.

- Avoid alcohol, especially in the evening. Although alcohol may help some people fall asleep at the start of the night, the sleep through the night becomes fragmented. Occasional social use of alcohol in modest amounts is fine for most people, but regular use or drinking large quantities may be a significant problem for sleep.

- Avoid using tobacco in any form, especially at bedtime or if you awaken at night. Tobacco use disturbs sleep.

41

- If you cannot fall asleep, do not "try harder" to fall asleep. This often makes the problem worse. Instead, get out of bed, go to another room, and do something quietly (such as reading a book) until you become sleepy again. Avoid television, computer use, snacks, or tobacco use, as these can make you more alert. Return to bed only when you become sleepy again. Get up at your regular time in the morning, no matter how much you slept.

- Avoid naps. If you have an irresistible urge to sleep during the day, a single nap of thirty minutes or less may be taken in bed. Longer or more numerous naps can disturb sleep the following night.

Section 5.2

Menopause and Sleep

Reprinted from "Difficulty Sleeping Increases as Women Progress Through Menopause According to Study by Rush University Medical Center," © 2008 Rush University Medical Center (www.rush.edu). Reprinted with permission.

Difficulty falling asleep and staying asleep increases as women go through menopause, according to research by Rush University Medical Center. Waking up earlier than planned also increases through late perimenopause but decreases when women become postmenopausal. The study is published in the July 1, 2008, issue of the journal *Sleep*.

"Sleep difficulties, especially problems staying asleep, are relatively prevalent concerns among women going through the menopausal transition," said Dr. Howard Kravitz, associate professor of psychiatry and preventive medicine at Rush University Medical Center and a principal investigator of the study. "Approximately 16 percent of postmenopausal women report having difficulty falling asleep and 41 percent report waking up frequently during the night."

Compared with other ethnic groups, Caucasian women were more likely to report difficulty staying asleep, while Hispanic women were less likely than other ethnic groups to wake several times during the night. Hispanic women were also significantly less likely to report waking early than other ethnic groups. Compared with Hispanic,

Caucasian, African American, and Japanese women, Chinese women were more likely to report early morning awakening.

The study involved over three thousand women aged forty-two to fifty-two years and beginning menopausal transition at the time of their enrollment in the Study of Woman's Health Across the Nation (SWAN). Participants underwent annual assessments for up to seven years. At each visit, participants were asked about frequency of trouble falling asleep, waking up several times a night, and waking up earlier than planned and unable to fall asleep again. They were also asked about the frequency of vasomotor systems such as hot flashes, cold sweats, and night sweats. Transition status was determined using bleeding criteria.

Sleep changes can be attributed at least in part to changing hormone levels. The study found decreases in estradiol, the major form of estrogen in the body, were associated with trouble falling asleep and waking several times, and increases in follicle stimulating hormone (FSH), a reproductive hormone, associated with waking several times.

In naturally postmenopausal women, women who were on hormone therapy had less trouble falling asleep and waking several times during the night than naturally postmenopausal women not on hormone therapy. However, whether or not women were hormone users did not influence the effect of vasomotor systems or changing hormone levels on sleep symptoms.

"Although we found some evidence that hormonal therapy could benefit these menopausal sleep-related symptoms, this was not a consistent finding across all groups compared, so the role for this particular treatment needs more study," said Kravitz.

Among the eight menopausal status categories, women who were surgically menopausal without current hormone therapy treatment were most likely to report trouble falling asleep and waking several times. Women who reported vasomotor symptoms on more days in the preceding two weeks also were more likely to report difficulty sleeping.

"Women should feel comfortable discussing their sleep problems with their healthcare providers to sort out the many potential contributing factors," said Kravitz. "Undiagnosed and untreated sleep disturbances can contribute to decreased well-being and functioning in family, social, and occupational roles."

Section 5.3

Pregnancy and Sleep

Many expectant parents know how hard it might be to get a good night's sleep in the months that follow the birth of their child, but who would have guessed that catching some ZZZs during pregnancy would prove to be so difficult?

Actually, you may sleep more than usual during the first trimester of your pregnancy. It's normal to feel tired as your body works to protect and nurture the developing baby. The placenta (the organ that nourishes the fetus until birth) is just forming, your body is making more blood, and your heart is pumping faster.

It's usually later in pregnancy, though, that most women have trouble getting enough deep, uninterrupted sleep.

Why Can Sleeping Be Difficult during Pregnancy?

The first and most pressing reason behind sleep problems during pregnancy is the increasing size of the fetus, which can make it hard to find a comfortable sleeping position. If you've always been a back or stomach sleeper, you might have trouble getting used to sleeping on your side (as doctors recommend). Also, shifting around in bed becomes more difficult as the pregnancy progresses and your size increases.

Other common physical symptoms may interfere with sleep as well:

- **The frequent urge to urinate:** Your kidneys are working harder to filter the increased volume of blood (30 to 50 percent more than you had before pregnancy) moving through your body, and this filtering process results in more urine. Also, as your baby grows and the uterus gets bigger, the pressure on your bladder increases. This means more trips to the bathroom, day and night.

The number of nighttime trips may be greater if your baby is particularly active at night.

- **Increased heart rate:** Your heart rate increases during pregnancy to pump more blood, and as more of your blood supply goes to the uterus, your heart will be working harder to send sufficient blood to the rest of your body.

- **Shortness of breath:** At first, your breathing may be affected by the increase in pregnancy hormones, which will cause you to breathe in more deeply. This might make you feel as if you're working harder to get air. Later on, breathing may feel more difficult as your enlarging uterus takes up more space, resulting in pressure against your diaphragm (the muscle just below your lungs).

- **Leg cramps and backaches:** Pains in your legs or back are caused in part by the extra weight you're carrying. During pregnancy, the body also produces a hormone called relaxin, which helps prepare the body for childbirth. One of the effects of relaxin is the loosening of ligaments throughout the body, making pregnant women less stable and more prone to injury, especially in their backs.

- **Heartburn and constipation:** Many women experience heartburn, which occurs when the stomach contents reflux back up into the esophagus. During pregnancy, the entire digestive system slows down and food tends to remain in the stomach and intestines longer, which may cause heartburn or constipation. Heartburn and constipation can both get worse later on in the pregnancy when the growing uterus presses on the stomach or the large intestine.

Your sleep problems may have other causes as well. Many pregnant women report that their dreams become more vivid than usual, and some even experience nightmares. Stress can interfere with sleep, too. Maybe you're worried about your baby's health, anxious about your abilities as a parent, or feeling nervous about the delivery itself. All of these feelings are normal, but they might keep you (and your partner) up at night.

Finding a Good Sleeping Position

Early in your pregnancy, try to get into the habit of sleeping on your side. Lying on your side with your knees bent is likely to be the most comfortable position as your pregnancy progresses. It also makes your heart's job easier because it keeps the baby's weight from applying pressure to the large vein (called the inferior vena cava) that carries blood back to the heart from your feet and legs.

Some doctors specifically recommend that pregnant women sleep on the left side. Because your liver is on the right side of your abdomen, lying on your left side helps keep the uterus off that large organ. Sleeping on the left side also improves circulation to the heart and allows for the best blood flow to the fetus, uterus, and kidneys. Ask what your doctor recommends—in most cases, lying on either side should do the trick and help take some pressure off your back.

But don't drive yourself crazy worrying that you might roll over onto your back during the night. Shifting positions is a natural part of sleeping that you can't control. Most likely, during the third trimester of your pregnancy, your body won't shift into the back-sleeping position anyway because it will be too uncomfortable.

If you do shift onto your back and the baby's weight presses on your inferior vena cava, the discomfort will probably wake you up. See what your doctor recommends about this; he or she may suggest that you use a pillow to keep yourself propped up on one side.

Try experimenting with pillows to discover a comfortable sleeping position. Some women find that it helps to place a pillow under their abdomen or between their legs. Also, using a bunched-up pillow or rolled-up blanket at the small of your back may help to relieve some pressure. In fact, you'll find that there are many "pregnancy pillows" on the market. If you're thinking about purchasing one, talk with your doctor first about which one might work for you.

Tips for Sleeping Success

Although they might seem appealing when you're feeling desperate to get some ZZZs, remember that over-the-counter sleep aids, including herbal remedies, are not recommended for pregnant women. Instead, the following pointers may safely improve your chances of getting a good night's sleep:

- Cut out caffeinated drinks like soda, coffee, and tea from your diet as much as possible. Restrict any intake of them to the morning or early afternoon.

- Avoid drinking a lot of fluids or eating a full meal within a few hours of going to bed at night. (But make sure that you also get plenty of nutrients and liquids throughout the day.) Some women find it helpful to eat more at breakfast and lunch and then have a smaller dinner. If nausea is keeping you up, you may want to eat a few crackers before you go to bed.

- Get into a routine of going to bed and waking up at the same time each day.

- Avoid rigorous exercise right before you go to bed. Instead, do something relaxing, like soaking in a warm bath for fifteen minutes or having a warm, caffeine-free drink, such as milk with honey or a cup of herbal tea.

- If a leg cramp awakens you, it may help to press your feet hard against the wall or to stand on the leg. Also, make sure that you're getting enough calcium in your diet, which can help reduce leg cramps.

- Take a class in yoga or learn other relaxation techniques to help you unwind after a busy day. (Be sure to discuss any new activity or fitness regimen with your doctor first.)

- If fear and anxiety are keeping you awake, consider enrolling in a childbirth or parenting class. More knowledge and the company of other pregnant women may help to ease the fears that are keeping you awake at night.

What to Do When You Can't Sleep

Of course, there are bound to be times when you just can't sleep. Instead of tossing and turning, worrying that you're not asleep, and counting the hours until your alarm clock will go off, get up and do something: read a book, listen to music, watch TV, catch up on letters or e-mail, or pursue some other activity you enjoy. Eventually, you'll probably feel tired enough to get back to sleep.

And if possible, take short naps (thirty to sixty minutes) during the day to make up for lost sleep. It won't be long before your baby will be setting the sleep rules in your house, so you might as well get used to sleeping in spurts!

Chapter 6

Men's Sleep Issues

Chapter Contents

Section 6.1

Trouble in the Bedroom: Men and Sleep Disorders

"Trouble in the Bedroom: Men and Sleep Disorders,"
by David A. Cooke, MD, FACP, © 2010 Omnigraphics.

We all sleep, but it's something most give little thought. Early in life, we learn that we don't feel well unless we sleep, but we don't really appreciate the importance of sleep in our lives. Indeed, while sleep research has made great advances in recent decades, even sleep specialists admit there is a great deal that is not known about why we need to sleep at all.

It seems obvious that sleep gives muscles and organs opportunities to grow and repair themselves. However, scientific evidence increasingly indicates that sleep is critical for proper brain function, particularly for memory and learning. While many details are not understood, it appears that sleep is a time for the brain to "weed" through memories of recent events and experiences. Connections between nerve cells that hold the imprints of new information and important experiences are strengthened, organized, and made permanent. Memories of trivial events are removed, leaving the brain prepared for the next day's happenings.

Inadequate sleep and disturbed sleep are increasingly being recognized to have a major impact on health. Poor sleep can do far more than cause sleepiness; it can raise blood pressure, affect heart function, and create complex hormonal changes that predispose to obesity, diabetes, sexual dysfunction, and depression. Getting adequate sleep, and treating conditions that disrupt sleep, is important to maintaining health and achieving longevity.

This section will review common conditions that may lead men to sleep poorly. Many of these disorders are not unique to men, but may affect them disproportionately.

Work Schedules

The traditional role of men as primary wage earners has changed as women have increasingly entered the workforce. However, many, if not most, men still work full time to support for their families. Often, this can mean long hours, and increasingly, bringing work home.

Work responsibilities can affect sleep several different ways. Often, men will sacrifice sleep to finish work, or to compensate for lost leisure time. Stress, anxiety, or frustration over work issues may lead to difficulty falling asleep, or middle-of-the-night awakenings to ruminate over problems.

Men who work nights also frequently suffer significant sleep disruption. Men's brains maintain an internal clock timed to the normal day-night cycle. Departures from this schedule are disruptive. While adjustments to an altered schedule are made with time, compensation is rarely complete. The situation is even worse for men who work rotating shifts, because frequent changes in schedules do not allow for establishing stable rhythms.

Several approaches can help these problems. Simple recognition that sleep has to be given priority on par with other activities often makes a difference. Avoiding working right before bedtime allows the brain to "cool down" and prepare for sleep to start. In cases where work stress is seriously impacting sleep, working with a psychologist or psychiatrist may be helpful.

For men who work at unusual times, keeping a consistent schedule on both work days and days off can help a great deal. Minimizing the frequency of shift changes is also important. In selected cases, medications can also be helpful.

Alcohol and Sedatives

Excessive alcohol use is common among men, and occurs for a variety of reasons. While physical, emotional, social, and legal hazards of alcohol are generally known, many do not realize that alcohol can also negatively affect sleep. Alcohol intoxication tends to cause drowsiness, and some men will use alcohol to help themselves fall asleep. However, alcohol-induced sleep is not normal sleep, and does not provide the full benefits of natural sleep. Early-morning awakening from sleep often occurs as the body processes alcohol and removes it from the bloodstream overnight. Heavy drinkers may also suffer from degrees of alcohol withdrawal.

Over-the-counter and prescription medications are commonly used for difficulty sleeping. While they can be appropriate in some situations, prolonged or nightly use can lead to sleep abnormalities and dependence upon medication to fall asleep. Men in this situation may feel trapped, as they feel they cannot sleep without medication, yet sleep poorly with them.

Reducing alcohol use and avoiding drinking before bed tend to significantly improve sleep quality. Avoiding regular use of sleep medications is important, but significant medical support and treatment may be necessary to break cycles of dependence.

Sleep Apnea

Sleep apnea is among the most common sleep disorders, and is more common in men than women. While it may occur in young men, it becomes progressively more common as men enter their thirties, forties, and beyond. Typically, this is related to weight gain and obesity that tend to accompany aging.

Excess fat and redundant tissue around the throat predispose to airway closure during sleep, and interruptions in breathing. This forces an affected person to awaken frequently from sleep in order to breathe and prevents sustained, deep sleep. Men with sleep apnea often find themselves sleepy during the day and have trouble maintaining their concentration due to fatigue. Frequently, they also complain that they never feel rested, regardless of how much time they stay in bed.

In addition to constant tiredness, sleep apnea can impact on men's lives in other ways. High blood pressure is strongly associated with sleep apnea, and sleep apnea can also lead to heart failure and stroke. Many men with sleep apnea complain of sexual difficulty. It can also affect relationships with a bed partner. Sleep apnea sufferers are almost invariably loud snorers, and this may quite literally drive partners out of the bedroom. It's not uncommon for couples to sleep in different bedrooms when one of them is affected by sleep apnea.

Despite these issues, many men with sleep apnea are undiagnosed. Surprisingly, sufferers often fail to recognize their own problems with sleep, and do not seek evaluation. As a group, men are less likely to make preventative care appointments, when their physicians would be more likely to identify the problem.

Fortunately, sleep apnea can be treated quite effectively. Weight loss will greatly improve or resolve the problem in most cases. Continuous positive airway pressure (CPAP) devices worn during sleep prevent airway closure and restore normal breathing during sleep. Specialized dental appliances and surgical procedures can also help in selected cases.

Sleep Movement Disorders and Parasomnias

During normal sleep, men remain relatively still, with occasional changes in position. However, some people move quite frequently and vigorously during sleep, which can cause awakenings.

Periodic limb movements of sleep (PLMS) are bursts of involuntary twitching of the legs during sleep. Such movements are common upon initially falling asleep and occasionally during the night. However, in some people, the frequency of these movements may be much higher, and they may lead to partial or complete awakenings from sleep. In some cases, movements can be quite violent, and may lead to falling out of bed. Restless leg syndrome is another common disorder that resembles PLMS, but is associated with a strong sense of needing to move the legs, and this may occur while awake.

Men may also suffer from parasomnias, in which they perform unusual activities in a semi-conscious state during sleep. Sleep talking, sleep-walking, and other complex behaviors may occur during sleep, and these can lead not only to sleep disruption, but even physical injury. Cooking, eating, and even driving while asleep are have been reported.

The causes of these disorders are unknown, although iron deficiency, caffeine intake, and certain medications may play roles. Once recognized, these unusual sleep behaviors can usually be controlled with medications.

Benign Prostatic Hypertrophy

As men grow older, many begin to develop a disorder, benign prostatic hypertrophy (BPH), which can significantly impact upon their sleep. An enlarged prostate may obstruct urine flow as it passes through the gland, and make it difficult to fully empty the bladder. If the bladder is not completely emptied during urination, it will take much less time until it is filled to capacity again.

As a result of urinary retention from BPH, men often wake up at night to urinate. While waking up once per night is not unusual for healthy individuals, men with BPH may be waking up four, six, or more times per night to urinate. This can be severely disruptive, and may not allow for more than an hour of sleep at a time.

Several approaches can help sleep problems related to BPH. For milder cases, simply restricting fluids in the hours before bed may help considerably. Medications known as alpha-adrenergic blockers relax muscles around the urethra and improve urinary flow. Drugs known as 5-alpha-reductase inhibitors block the effects of testosterone on the prostate and may lead to gradual shrinkage of the gland. A surgical procedure known as transurethral resection of the prostate (TURP) enlarges the urinary passage through the prostate. In recent years, a number of variations on the TURP procedure involving microwave radiation, freezing, and other methods have also become widespread.

Summary

Sleep is an underappreciated but critical element of our lives, and lack of good quality sleep causes serious problems. A wide variety of problems can impact sleep, but most are treatable. If you suffer from excessive drowsiness or are told of unusual behaviors by others, speak to your physician. There may be testing or treatments that can solve your sleep problems.

Section 6.2

Men at Higher Risk from Sleep-Disordered Breathing

Excerpted from Punjabi, N.M., Caffo, B.S., Goodwin, J.L., Gottlieb, D.J., Newman, A.B., et al. (2009) Sleep-Disordered Breathing and Mortality: A Prospective Cohort Study. *PLoS Med* 6(8): e1000132. doi:10.1371/journal .pmed.1000132. Reprinted under terms of the Creative Commons Attribution License.

Background

About one in ten women and one in four men have a chronic condition called sleep-disordered breathing although most are unaware of their problem. Sleep-disordered breathing, which is commonest in middle-aged and elderly people, is characterized by numerous, brief (ten second or so) interruptions of breathing during sleep. These interruptions, which usually occur when relaxation of the upper airway muscles decreases airflow, lower the level of oxygen in the blood and, as a result, affected individuals are frequently aroused from deep sleep as they struggle to breathe. Symptoms of sleep-disordered breathing include loud snoring and daytime sleepiness. Treatments include lifestyle changes such as losing weight (excess fat around the neck increases airway collapse) and smoking cessation. Affected people can also use special devices to prevent them sleeping on their backs, but for severe sleep-disordered breathing, doctors often recommend continuous positive airway pressure (CPAP), a machine that pressurizes the upper airway through a face mask to keep it open.

Why Was This Study Done?

Sleep-disordered breathing is a serious condition. It is associated with several adverse health conditions, including coronary artery disease (narrowing of the blood vessels that supply the heart, a condition that can cause a heart attack) and daytime sleepiness that can affect an individual's driving ability. In addition, several clinic- and community-based studies suggest that sleep-disordered sleeping may increase a person's risk of dying. In this prospective cohort study (part of the Sleep Heart Health Study, which is researching the effects of sleep-disordered breathing on cardiovascular health), the researchers examine whether sleep-disordered breathing is associated with all-cause mortality (death from any cause) in a large community sample of adults.

What Did the Researchers Do and Find?

At enrollment, the study participants—more than 6,000 people aged forty years or older, none of whom were being treated for sleep-disordered breathing—had a health examination. Their nighttime breathing, sleep patterns, and blood oxygen levels were also assessed and these data used to calculate each participant's apnea-hypopnea index (AHI)—the number of apneas and hypopneas per hour. During the study follow-up period, 1,047 participants died. Compared to participants without sleep-disordered sleeping, participants with severe sleep-disordered breathing (an AHI of 30 or more) were about one and a half times as likely to die from any cause after adjustment for potential confounding factors. People with milder sleep-disordered breathing did not have a statistically significant increased risk of dying. After dividing the participants into subgroups according to their age and sex, men aged forty to seventy years with severe sleep-disordered breathing had a statistically increased risk of dying from any cause (twice the risk of men of a similar age without sleep-disordered breathing). Finally, death from coronary artery disease was also associated with sleep-disordered breathing in men but not in women.

What Do These Findings Mean?

These findings indicate that sleep-disordered breathing is associated with an increased risk of all-cause mortality, particularly in men aged forty to seventy years, even after allowing for known confounding factors. They also suggest that the increased risk of death is specifically associated with coronary artery disease although further studies are needed to confirm this finding.

Section 6.3

Do Abnormal Sleep Patterns Affect Testosterone Levels?

Barrett-Connor, E., et. al. "The Association of Testosterone Levels with Overall Sleep Quality, Sleep Architecture, and Sleep-Disordered Breathing" *Journal of Clinical Endocrinology & Metabolism*. July 2008. © 2008 The Endocrine Society. Reprinted with permission.

Context

Little is known about the association of low endogenous testosterone levels and abnormal sleep patterns in older men, although pharmacological doses of testosterone are associated with increased severity of sleep apnea and other sleep disturbances.

Objective

The objective of the study was to examine the association between serum testosterone levels with objectively measured sleep characteristics.

Design

This was a cohort study.

Setting

Community-dwelling men aged sixty-five years or older from six clinical centers in the United States participated in the study.

Participants and Main Outcome Measures

A total of 1,312 men had baseline total testosterone levels measured in 2000–2002, followed 3.4 years later by seventy-two-hour (minimum) actigraphy and one-night in-home polysomnography to assess sleep duration, sleep fragmentation, and sleep apnea. Analyses were performed by quartile of total testosterone and categorically defined low vs. higher total testosterone (<250 ng/dl vs. 250 ng/dl). Lifestyle and body size were covariates.

Results

Total testosterone levels were unrelated to age or duration of sleep. Men with lower testosterone levels had lower sleep efficiency, with increased nocturnal awakenings and less time in slow-wave sleep as well as a higher apnea-hypopnea index and more sleep time with O_2 saturation levels below 90 percent. Low testosterone levels were associated with overweight, and all significant associations were attenuated or absent after adjusting for body mass index or waist circumference. In a post hoc analysis in men with higher body mass index (>27 kg/m^2), testosterone was significantly associated with more periods awake after sleep onset and lower sleep efficiency.

Conclusion

Low total testosterone levels are associated with less healthy sleep in older men. This association is largely explained by adiposity. Clinical trials are necessary to determine whether body weight acts directly or indirectly (via low testosterone) in the causal pathway for sleep-disordered breathing in older men.

Section 6.4

Disturbed Rest Linked to Mortality in Older Men

"Disturbed Rest, Activity Linked to Mortality in Older Men," June 11, 2008, University of Minnesota Academic Health Center. © 2008 Regents of the University of Minnesota. Reprinted with permission.

It appears that disrupted rest and activity rhythms are associated with increased mortality rates among older men, according to new University of Minnesota research.

A group of about three thousand men older than sixty-seven, were tested for rest and activity biological rhythms via a wrist device called an Actigraph. The device tracked participants' movement, including the peak times of rest and activity, as well as the robustness of the activity for twenty-four hours a day for an average of about a week between December 2003 and March 2005. As of January 2008, there were 180 deaths in the group, and men who had peak activity times that were the earliest or latest, in comparison with the groups' average, had a much greater risk of death.

"It's important to have a regular routine of waking and going to sleep," said Misti Paudel, M.P.H., principal investigator of the study and a member of the School of Public Health. "Waking early, staying up late, and severely disturbed sleep patterns may have a detrimental impact on health in older men, especially since this group was generally in good health. A good night sleep is important."

This is the first study to report strong associations between disturbed rest and activity rhythms and mortality rates in older men, who are still living in their homes (not institutionalized)—however, studies in cancer patients as well as institutionalized Alzheimer patients have reported similar findings.

Paudel presented information from the study during the Associated Professional Sleep Societies Conference on June 11, 2008, in Baltimore, Maryland.

Lack of sleep can lead to a number of problems in older adults including depression, memory problems, and decreased attentiveness, and also can lead to serious health problems such as an increased risk of obesity, cardiovascular disease, and diabetes, Paudel said.

Another key study finding is that men with more robust rest/activity rhythms had much lower mortality rates. Having greater levels of activity during the day and/or lower levels of activity during the night (better sleep quality) are characteristics of robust rhythms.

"From a sleep standpoint, getting a good night's sleep appears to be important factor for health and longevity for people of all ages, and especially for older adults—where complaints of insomnia and other sleep disturbances are much more common than in younger cohorts," she said. "It is important that anyone who has concerns about their sleep quality should consult their physician."

Future research should examine association with specific causes of death and with health related outcomes, Paudel said. The study was funded by the National Institute on Aging.

Chapter 7

Sleep and Aging

Older adults need about the same amount of sleep as young adults—seven to nine hours each night. But seniors tend to go to sleep earlier and get up earlier than when they were younger. Older people may nap more during the day, which can sometimes make it hard to fall asleep at night.

There are two kinds of sleep—REM (rapid eye movement) sleep and non-REM sleep. We dream mostly during REM sleep and have the deepest sleep during non-REM sleep. As people get older, they spend less time in deep sleep, which may be why older people are often light sleepers.

Sleep Problems

There are many reasons why older people may not get enough sleep at night. Feeling sick or being in pain can make it hard to sleep. Napping during the day can disrupt sleep at night. Some medicines can keep you awake. No matter the reason, if you don't get a good night's sleep, the next day you may:

- be irritable;
- have memory problems or be forgetful;
- feel depressed;
- have more falls or accidents;
- feel very sleepy during the day.

"A Good Night's Sleep," National Institute on Aging, National Institutes of Health, August 13, 2009.

Insomnia

Insomnia is the most common sleep problem in adults age sixty and older. People with insomnia have trouble falling and staying asleep. Insomnia can last for days, months, or even years. If you're having trouble sleeping, you may:

- take a long time to fall asleep;
- wake up many times in the night;
- wake up early and be unable to get back to sleep;
- wake up tired;
- feel very sleepy during the day.

There are many causes of insomnia. Some of them you can control, but others you can't. For example, if you are excited about a new activity or worrying over your bills, you may have trouble sleeping. Sometimes insomnia may be a sign of other problems. Or it could be a side effect of a medication or an illness.

Often, being unable to sleep becomes a habit. Some people worry about not sleeping even before they get into bed. This may even make insomnia worse.

Older adults who have trouble sleeping may use more over-the-counter sleep aids. Using prescription medicines for a short time might help. But remember, medicines aren't a cure for insomnia. Developing healthy habits at bedtime may help you get a good night's sleep.

Sleep Apnea

Sleep apnea is another serious sleep disorder. A person with sleep apnea has short pauses in breathing while sleeping. These pauses may happen many times during the night. If not treated, sleep apnea can lead to other problems such as high blood pressure, stroke, or memory loss.

You can have sleep apnea and not even know it. But your loud snoring and gasping for air can keep other people awake. Feeling sleepy during the day and being told you are snoring loudly at night could be signs that you have sleep apnea.

If you think you have sleep apnea, see a doctor who knows about this sleep problem. You may need to learn to sleep in a position that keeps your airways open. Sometimes a medical device called continuous positive air pressure (CPAP), a dental device, or surgery can help.

Movement Disorders

Restless legs syndrome, periodic limb movement disorder, and rapid eye movement sleep behavior disorder are common in older adults. These movement disorders can rob you of needed sleep.

People with restless legs syndrome, or RLS, feel like there is tingling, crawling, or pins and needles in one or both legs. It's worse at night. Moving the legs brings some relief, at least for a short time. RLS tends to run in families. See your doctor for more information about medicines to treat RLS.

Periodic limb movement disorder, or PLMD, causes people to jerk and kick their legs every twenty to forty seconds during sleep. Some people have hundreds of these movements each night, which may result in loss of sleep and feeling tired and sleepy the next day. Medication, warm baths, exercise, and learning ways to relax can help.

Rapid eye movement sleep behavior disorder, also known as REM sleep behavior disorder, is another condition that may make it harder to get a good night's sleep. REM sleep, or rapid eye movement sleep, is the most active stage of sleep, when dreaming often occurs. During normal REM sleep, your muscles cannot move, so your body stays still. But if you have REM sleep behavior disorder, your muscles can move, and your sleep is disrupted.

Alzheimer Disease and Sleep—A Special Problem

Alzheimer disease often changes a person's sleeping habits. For example, some people with Alzheimer disease sleep too much; others don't sleep enough. Some people wake up many times during the night; others wander or yell at night. The person with Alzheimer disease isn't the only one who loses sleep. Caregivers may have sleepless nights, leaving them tired for the challenges they face.

If you're caring for someone with Alzheimer disease, there are steps you can take for his or her safety and that might help you sleep better at night. Try the following:

- Make sure the floor is clear of objects.

- Lock up any medicines.

- Attach grab bars in the bathroom.

- Place a gate across the stairs.

Getting a Good Night's Sleep

Being older doesn't mean you have to feel tired all the time. There are many things you can do to help you get a good night's sleep. Here are some ideas:

- Follow a regular sleep schedule. Go to sleep and get up at the same time each day, even on weekends. Try to avoid napping in the late afternoon or evening, as it may keep you awake at night.

- Develop a bedtime routine. Take time to relax before bedtime each night. Some people watch television, read a book, listen to soothing music, or soak in a warm bath.

- Keep your bedroom dark, not too hot or too cold, and as quiet as possible.

- Have a comfortable mattress, a pillow you like, and enough blankets for the season.

- Exercise at regular times each day but not within three hours of your bedtime.

- Make an effort to get outside in the sunlight each day.

- Be careful about when and how much you eat. Large meals close to bedtime may keep you awake, but a light snack in the evening can help you get a good night's sleep.

- Stay away from caffeine late in the day. Caffeine (found in coffee, tea, soda, and hot chocolate) can keep you awake.

- Drink fewer beverages in the evening. Waking up to go to the bathroom and turning on a bright light break up your sleep.

- Remember that alcohol won't help you sleep. Even small amounts make it harder to stay asleep.

- Use your bedroom only for sleeping. After turning off the light, give yourself about twenty minutes to fall asleep. If you're still awake and not drowsy, get out of bed. When you feel sleepy, go back to bed.

Safe Sleeping

Try to set up a safe and restful place to sleep. Make sure you have smoke alarms on each floor of your house or apartment. Lock the outside doors before going to bed. Other ideas for a safe night's sleep are as follows:

- Keep a telephone with emergency phone numbers by your bed.

- Have a good lamp within reach that turns on easily.

- Put a glass of water next to the bed in case you wake up thirsty.

- Use nightlights in the bathroom and hall.

- Don't smoke, especially in bed.

- Remove area rugs so you won't trip if you get out of bed in the middle of the night.

- Don't fall asleep with a heating pad on; it may burn.

Sweet Dreams

There are some tricks to help you fall asleep. You don't really have to count sheep—but you could try counting slowly to one hundred. Some people find that playing mental games makes them sleepy. For example, tell yourself it's five minutes before you have to get up, and you're just trying to get a few extra winks. Other people find that relaxing their body puts them to sleep. You might start by telling yourself that your toes feel light as feathers and then work your way up the rest of the body, saying the same words. You may drift off to sleep before getting to the top of your head.

If you feel tired and unable to do your activities for more than two or three weeks, you may have a sleep problem. Talk to your doctor about changes you can make to get a better night's sleep.

Part Two

The Causes and Consequences of Sleep Deprivation

Chapter 8

Are You Sleep Deprived?

Chapter Contents

Section 8.1

The Causes and Effects of Sleep Deprivation

Sleep is not the simple thing it appears to be. Most of us think that sleep is simply restorative: we go about our day, become tired and then fall asleep at night, during which we recover our energies for the coming day, similar to a battery being recharged.

In fact, sleep is far more complex. Sleep is regulated by two different systems—the circadian (twenty-four-hour) system and the sleep-wake system—which, together, determine alertness, performance and the timing of sleep.[1]

Circadian Rhythms and Sleep-Wake Cycles

The circadian system is controlled by an internal biological mechanism called the circadian pacemaker.[2] Located in the brain above the optic chiasm, the circadian pacemaker is responsible for the fact that in a normal twenty-four-hour cycle, we will sleep at night and performance and alertness will reach low points between 3:00 a.m. and 5:00 a.m.—a time when almost all of us, even confirmed night owls, tend to be asleep—and between 3:00 p.m. and 5:00 p.m.—classic siesta time in many cultures.[3,4]

We experience these low points in performance and body temperature, along with a decline in arousal, alertness, and motivation, as fatigue.[5,6] As part of the sleep/wake system, the sleep drive is primarily responsible for the timing of sleep. The drive to sleep reaches its lowest point in the morning, at awakening, but as the day progresses the drive to sleep increases. Once we fall asleep, the sleep drive gradually decreases until we wake up.[7]

Fatigue, alertness, and performance levels are influenced by factors other than our internal circadian rhythms and sleep drive; they are affected by external factors such as the light/dark cycle, social interaction, and work demands. Although the inherent rhythm of the circadian pacemaker is actually about 24.2 hours,[8] the light/dark cycle entrains circadian rhythms to adopt a twenty-four-hour day.

Light dramatically affects circadian rhythms, bringing them into to a stable relationship with the sleep/wake cycle. Light is also able to adjust circadian rhythms to an earlier or later time within the biological day. Aging causes changes in the regulation of circadian rhythms which disrupt sleeping patterns and impair alertness and performance.[9]

Types of Sleep Loss

Sleep experts define sleep deprivation as either partial or total lack of sleep, whether voluntary or involuntary. Sleep deprivation can be either an acute (occasional) or a chronic lack of sleep. Partial sleep deprivation is the term used when an individual gets some, but not all, of the sleep necessary for waking alertness during the day. Partial sleep deprivation can be caused by medical conditions, sleep disorders, as well as lifestyle (e.g., shiftwork, jet lag, or working overtime).

Total sleep deprivation is defined as a complete lack of sleep lasting for sixteen hours or more in a healthy adult. When total sleep deprivation lasts longer than twenty-four hours, a divergence occurs between the sleep/wake cycle, which begins to build an escalating sleep debt, and the circadian clock, which maintains its normal cycle. The result is counterintuitive—when we remain awake for forty hours, we will feel less sleepy at the thirty-six- to thirty-eight-hour point than at the twenty-two- twenty-four-hour point.[10]

Fragmented Sleep

As many people know, sleep is not a continuous state; it follows a series of stages, including rapid eye movement (REM) and other types of sleep. Sleep fragmentation, a form of partial sleep deprivation, occurs when the normal progression and sequencing of sleep stages is disrupted. If sleep fragmentation is limited to a specific sleep stage, (e.g., when sleep apnea or medications disrupt a particular stage of sleep), this is called selective sleep stage deprivation.

The elderly are particularly prone to this kind of fragmentation and subsequent loss of sleep quality. Selective sleep stage deprivation is characterized by waking up frequently at night, difficulties falling asleep, and waking up unusually early in the morning.

Sleep fragmentation is also a symptom of sleep disorders such as obstructive sleep apnea, in which patients experience repetitive nocturnal respiratory pauses that produce chronic sleep deprivation and excessive sleepiness. Narcolepsy, in which patients show recurrent episodes of irresistible sleep (or sleep attacks), cataplexy (sudden, brief, loss of muscle control in response to strong emotions such as laughter or anger), hallucinations, and sleep paralysis (the inability to move while falling asleep or awakening), also produces excessive daytime sleepiness.[11]

Parkinson disease can also cause daytime sleepiness (up to 45 percent of cases); roughly 1 percent of those with Parkinson are at risk for sleep attacks.[12,13,14]

Chronic Sleep Debt

Sleep debt, or sleep restriction,[15] is a common form of partial sleep deprivation. Researchers have studied the changes that occur when sleep is steadily reduced in duration from eight to four hours each day, and the effects of these changes on sleep and waking functions.

Measuring Sleep

The effects of chronic sleep restriction are evaluated using one of two tests.[16,17,18] In one test, subjects are instructed to close their eyes and try to fall asleep while lying down, during which their sleep patterns are evaluated with a specially designed instrument called a polysomnograph (PSG). In the other type of test, subjects are seated upright and instructed to try and remain awake. For both tests, sleep propensity is measured as the time it takes to fall asleep.[19,20] Unsurprisingly, chronic shortening of nocturnal sleep increases daytime sleep propensity.[21]

Changes in the Structure of Sleep

Sleep restriction does not affect all sleep stages equally. For example, healthy adults fell asleep more quickly and had decreased time in non-rapid eye movement (NREM) and REM sleep when restricted to four hours of nocturnal sleep for multiple nights, but did not show any change in NREM slow wave sleep (SWS).[22,23,24,25]

How a Lack of Sleep Affects Us

More recent experiments have found clear evidence that behavioral alertness and a range of cognitive functions—including sustained attention and working memory—deteriorate when nightly sleep duration is limited to between four and seven hours.[26]

Decision-making skills—such as our ability to assess risk, assimilate changing information, and revise our strategies for solving problems based on new information, among other thinking and memory skills—are negatively affected by sleep loss. In addition, fatigue and deficits from sleep loss compromise certain memory and attention functions. These include assessment of the scope of a problem based on changing or distracting information, remembering the time order of information, maintaining focus, avoiding inappropriate risks, having insight into performance deficits, avoiding dwelling on ineffective thoughts and actions, and changing behavior based on new information.[27]

While the effects of chronic sleep restriction seem to be similar to those of total sleep deprivation, tests show a more muted response to chronic sleep restriction, suggesting that a different mechanism may be involved.

Sleepiness, as reported and described by research subjects, is quite different during chronic sleep debt than during total sleep deprivation. While total sleep deprivation immediately increases feelings of sleepiness, fatigue, and cognitive confusion, with decreases in energy and alertness,[28,29,30,31] chronic sleep debt or restriction causes much subtler changes that are more likely to escape notice. After a week or more of sleep restriction, subjects were markedly impaired and less alert but rated themselves as only moderately sleepy. People frequently underestimate the impact a lack of sleep has on their ability to function and overestimate their performance readiness when sleep restricted.[32]

Overall, these studies suggest that when people are only getting seven hours or less sleep a night, most healthy adults' mental abilities—to make decisions or solve problems or be able to recall information—suffer. These cognitive impairments also get worse over time. Improvement only comes when adults experience a longer recovery sleep period.

Eight hours rest between work periods is inadequate. This is because people tend to use only 50 to 75 percent of rest periods to sleep. Thus, it is advisable for individuals to take longer rest breaks (e.g., ten to fourteen hours), so that they can get adequate recovery sleep.

Sleep Restriction: Individual Differences

Each of us differs to some degree in our sleep and circadian patterns; the same is true for our responses to sleep deprivation.[33,34,35] In studies, sleep loss uncovers marked differences between subjects and, as sleep loss continues over time, individual differences in the degree of cognitive deficits increase markedly. Some people experience very severe impairments even with modest sleep restriction, while others show few, if any, impairments until sleep restriction reaches severe levels. This is also true of chronic partial sleep restriction.[36]

While there is no question that responses to sleep deprivation are stable and reliable within individuals, the reasons for this are not known.[37,38,39,40]

Chronic Sleep Deprivation in the "Real World"

Some jobs require shifting work schedules and irregular sleep/wake cycles. These shifts cause misalignment between circadian rhythms and the sleep/wake cycle. The results can include increased sleep disruption, feelings of malaise, performance errors, uncontrollable falling asleep during waking hours, negative moods and problems with social interaction, inefficient communication, and accidents.[41] Any occupation that requires workers to maintain high levels of alertness over extended periods of time is vulnerable to the consequences of sleep loss and circadian disruption. For obvious reasons, this can compromise safety.[42]

Driving

Driving is a prime example of how a lack of sleep affects real-world functioning. Studies have primarily focused on the effects of short-term sleep restriction on driving ability and the risk of accidents.[43,44] One study found that sleep-related crashes rose in drivers reporting an average of less than seven hours of sleep per night. Other factors that contributed to crashes included poor sleep quality or duration, daytime sleepiness, previous episodes of driving while drowsy, long periods of driving, and driving late at night. Individuals who work irregular schedules are also more likely to drive at night, thus increasing the chances of drowsy driving and decreasing their ability to respond correctly to emergency situations; both factors result in an increase in sleep-related crashes.[45]

Sleep deprivation affects physical coordination and reaction time in a way that is very similar to excessive alcohol consumption. Sleepiness-related motor vehicle crashes are on par with alcohol-related crashes in terms of their fatality rate and likelihood of injury. Drowsy driving is a particular problem for truck drivers. Fatigue is considered to be a factor in 20 to 40 percent of heavy truck crashes.

The Night Shift: What 24/7 Means to Your Sleep

Night work, irregular or prolonged work schedules, and shift work disrupt a person's internal, natural circadian clock and, consequently, their sleep and waking cycles. People who work at night come home and are faced with competing time cues: they are tired and ready to start winding down, but most other members are just getting started with the day. Thus, they often have trouble adapting to their work-rest schedule.

Night shift work is particularly disruptive to sleep. Many of the six million full-time employees in the United States who work at night on a permanent or rotating basis experience daytime sleep disruption leading to sleep loss and nighttime sleepiness on the job. More than 50 percent of shift workers complain of shortened or disrupted sleep and overall tiredness, with total amounts of sleep loss ranging from two to four hours per night.[46] This kind of sleep loss affects the productivity and performance of shift workers.

Jet Lag

Most of us have experienced the disruption of our sleep-wake cycles that is known as jet lag. Fatigue associated with jet lag is a major concern in aviation, particularly with travel across time zones. Flight crews often experience disrupted circadian rhythms and sleep loss. Studies have documented episodes of fatigue and uncontrolled sleep (microsleeps) in pilots. Flight crew members tend to remain at their destination for a short period of time and therefore do not adjust physiologically to a new time zone and altered work schedule before they embark upon another assignment, further compounding their risk for fatigue.

Although remaining at the new destination for a while after crossing time zones is beneficial, it does not guarantee that a person's sleep-wake cycle and circadian system will adapt quickly to a new time zone and light-dark cycle. Usually, passengers, pilots, and flight crew arrive at a new destination with an accumulated sleep debt. As a result, the first night of sleep in the new time zone will occur without incident—even if it is cut short by a wake-up signal from the circadian clock. However, on subsequent nights, most people will find it more difficult to stay asleep as a result of circadian rhythm disruption. As a consequence, individuals have increasing difficulty maintaining alertness during the daytime. These cumulative effects are incapacitating and often take more than a week to go away.

The severity of jet lag also depends on the direction of travel. Normally, eastward travel is more difficult to adjust to than westward travel because it advances the circadian clock, while westward transit causes a delay. Since the human internal clock is slightly longer than twenty-four hours, lengthening a day is easier to adjust to physiologically and behaviorally than shortening a day by the same amount of time.[47] Adjustment to either eastward or westward phase shifts often requires at least a twenty-four-hour period for each time zone crossed (e.g., crossing six time zones can require five to seven days), assuming proper daily exposure to the new light-dark cycle. Regardless of the direction individuals fly, if there is inadequate time to adjust physiologically to the new time zone, the cumulative sleep debt of flight crews and passengers will develop across days and waking performance deficits will accumulate.

The Case of Medical Professionals

Our modern healthcare system requires that physicians, nurses, and other healthcare providers often need to be awake at night and work for durations well in excess of twelve hours. Chronic partial sleep deprivation is an inherent consequence of such schedules.[48] Not surprisingly, human error increases with such prolonged work schedules. Studies have also shown that such schedules are tied to an increased likelihood of motor vehicle accidents for healthcare providers driving home from their shifts.[49]

In 2003, the Accreditation Council for Graduate Medical Education (ACGME) imposed duty hour limits for residents. These limited residents to an eighty-hour workweek and limited continuous duty periods to twenty-four to thirty hours. The ACGME also mandated that one out of every seven days be free from duty, averaged over a four-week period, and mandated ten-hour rest breaks between duty periods.[50,51]

Treatments for Sleep Deprivation

Clearly, travel across time zones, prolonged work hours, and work environments with irregular schedules contribute to performance problems, fatigue, and safety risks. What can a person do to counteract sleep deprivation? The obvious best countermeasure for sleep deprivation is to get adequate sleep. Research suggests that the definition of what constitutes "adequate" varies from person to person.

Individuals who are sleep-deprived because of their work or travel schedules should make sure they give themselves prolonged, restorative sleep in the form of ten to fourteen hours of recovery sleep whenever they can.

A number of treatments are available for individuals who are unable to obtain adequate sleep because of medical or sleep-related conditions (e.g., narcolepsy, obstructive sleep apnea). These include continuous positive airway pressure, modafinil, caffeine, and bright light.

Continuous Positive Airway Pressure

Continuous positive airway pressure (CPAP) uses a machine to increase air pressure in your throat so that your airway does not collapse when you breathe in. It is considered the most effective treatment for obstructive sleep apnea in both middle-aged and older adults.[52] CPAP increases alertness and improves cognitive processing, memory, and executive function.

Modafinil

In some patients, CPAP does not completely eliminate excessive sleepiness. For them, the stimulant drug modafinil[53,54] improves vigilance, general productivity, and activity level. In addition, modafinil is effective in the treatment of narcolepsy[55] and excessive daytime sleepiness caused by Parkinson disease.[56]

Caffeine

Caffeine improves alertness and vigilance, with the size of the effects increasing with caffeine dose,[57] and is as effective as modafinil.[58] Caffeine can block sleep inertia—the grogginess and disorientation that a person experiences after awakening from sleep—a fact which may explain why this common stimulant is so often used in the morning, after a night of sleep.

Bright Light

Exposure to bright light produces significant improvement in performance and alertness levels.[59] Light wavelength appears to play a role in such improvements. For example, in one experiment, people exposed to lower-frequency (460-nm) light had significantly lower subjective sleepiness ratings and fewer attention failures than people exposed to higher-frequency (555-nm) light.[60] In addition, light enhanced recovery from the circadian and sleep misalignments that result from jet lag, shiftwork, and aging.[61]

Conclusion

Fatigue, sleepiness, and general performance decline—including attention lapses, increased reaction times, cognitive slowing, and memory difficulties—are caused by acute and chronic sleep loss and circadian displacement of sleep-wake schedules. These are common occurrences in cases where people work unusual schedules or have sleep disorders, jet lag, or certain medical conditions. They increase the likelihood of cognitive errors and the risk of mistakes or accidents, although the degree of these effects varies from one person to another. Neurobehavioral and neurobiological research have demonstrated that waking functions depend upon stable alertness and that alertness, in turn, depends on adequate daily recovery sleep. Understanding and mitigating the risks imposed by physiologically based variations in fatigue and alertness are essential for making jobs such as driving trucks, flying airplanes, or practicing medicine safer, as well as for the development of effective countermeasures.

References

1. Van Dongen HPA, Dinges DF. Circadian rhythms in fatigue, alertness, and performance. In: Kyyger MH, Roth T, Dement WC, eds. Philadelphia: W.B. Saunders, *Principles and practice of sleep medicine* (3rd ed.), 2000; 391–99.

2. Klein DC, Moore RY, Reppert SM. *Suprachiasmatic nucleus: the Mind's Clock*. New York: Oxford University Press; 1991.

3. Bjerner B, Holm A, Swensson A. Diurnal variation in mental performance: a study of three-shift workers. *Br J Ind Med*. 1955; 12:103–10.

4. Monk TH, Buysse DJ, Reynolds III CF, Kupfer DJ. Circadian determinants of the postlunch dip in performance. *Chronobiol Int*. 1996; 13:123–33.

5. Frazier TW, Rummel JA, Lipscomb HS. Circadian variability in vigilance performance. *Aerospace Med*. 1968; 39:383–95.

6. Waterhouse JM, Minors DS, Akerstedt T, Reilly T, Atkinson G. Rhythms of human performance. In: Takahashi J, Turek F, Moore R, eds. New York: Kluver Academic, *Handbook of behavioral neurobiology: circadian clocks*, 2001; 571–601.

7. Borbély AA. A two process model of sleep regulation. *Hum Neurobiol* 1982; 1:195–204.

8. Czeisler CA, Duffy JF, Shanahan TL, Brown EN, Mitchell JF, et al. Stability, precision and the near 24-hr period of the human circadian pacemaker. *Science*. 1999; 284:2177–81.

9. Van Someren EJW. Circadian rhythms and sleep in human aging. *Chronobiol Int*. 2000; 17:233–43.

10. Walsh JK, Dement WC, Dinges DF. Sleep medicine, public policy, and public health. In: Kryger MH, Roth T, Dement WC, eds. Philadelphia: W.B. Saunders, *Principles and practice of sleep medicine* (4th ed.), 2005; 648–56.

11. Taheri S, Zeitzer JM, Mignot E. The role of hypocretins (orexins) in sleep regulation and narcolepsy. *Annu Rev Neurosci.* 2002; 25:283–313.

12. Paus S, Brecht HM, Koster J, et al. Sleep attacks, daytime sleepiness, and dopamine agonists in Parkinson's disease. *Mov Disord.* 2003;1 8:659–67.

13. Arnulf I, Konofal E, Merino-Andreu M, et al. Parkinson's disease and sleepiness: an integral part of PD. *Neurology.* 2002; 58:1019–24.

14. Dhawan V, Healy DG, Pal S, Chaudhuri KR. Sleep-related problems of Parkinson's disease. *Age Ageing.* 2006; 35:220–28.

15. Van Dongen HPA, Rogers NL, Dinges DF. Understanding sleep debt: Theoretical and empirical issues. *Sleep Biol Rhythms.* 2003; 1:4–12.

16. Roehrs T, Carskadon MA, Dement WC, Roth T. Daytime sleepiness and alertness. In: Kryger MH, Roth T, Dement WC, eds. Philadelphia: W.B. Saunders, *Principles and practice of sleep medicine* (3rd ed.), 2000; 1197–1216.

17. Carskadon MA, Dement WC. Nocturnal determinants of daytime sleepiness. *Sleep.* 1982; 5:S73–S81.

18. Mitler MM, Gujavarty KS, Browman CP. Maintenance of wakefulness test: a polysomnographic technique for evaluation treatment efficacy in patients with excessive somnolence. *Electroencephalogr Clin Neurophysiol.* 1982; 53:658–61.

19. Carskadon MA, Dement WC. Cumulative effects of sleep restriction on daytime sleepiness. *Psychophysiology.* 1981; 18:107–13.

20. Dinges DF, Pack F, Williams K, et al. Cumulative sleepiness, mood disturbance, and psychomotor vigilance performance decrements during a week of sleep restricted to 4-5 hours per night. *Sleep.* 1997; 20:267–77.

21. Punjabi NM, Bandeen-Roche K, Young T. Predictors of objective sleep tendency in the general population. *Sleep.* 2003; 26:678–83.

22. Belenky G, Wesensten NJ, Thorne DR, et al. Patterns of performance degradation and restoration during sleep restriction and subsequent recovery: A sleep dose-response study. *J Sleep Res.* 2003; 12:1–12.

23. Brunner DP, Dijk DJ, Borbély AA. Repeated partial sleep deprivation progressively changes in EEG during sleep and wakefulness. *Sleep.* 1993; 16:100–113.

24. Van Dongen HP, Maislin G, Mullington JM, Dinges DF. The cumulative cost of additional wakefulness: dose-response effects on neurobehavioral functions and sleep physiology from chronic sleep restriction and total sleep deprivation. *Sleep.* 2003; 26:117–26.

25. Guilleminault C, Powell NB, Martinez S, et al. Preliminary observations on the effects of sleep time in a sleep restriction paradigm. *Sleep Med.* 2003; 4:177–84.

26. Banks S, Dinges DF. Is the maintenance of wakefulness test sensitive to varying amounts of recovery sleep after chronic sleep restriction? *Sleep.* 2005; 28:A136.

27. Durmer JS, Dinges DF. Neurocognitive consequences of sleep deprivation. *Semin Neurol.* 2005; 25:117–29.

28. Dinges DF, Kribbs NB. Performing while sleepy: Effects of experimentally induced sleepiness. In: Monk TH, ed. Winchester, UK: John Wiley, *Sleep, sleepiness and performance*, 1991; 97–128.

29. Dorrian J, Dinges DF. Sleep deprivation and its effects on cognitive performance. In: Lee-Chiong T, ed. Hoboken, NJ: John Wiley and Sons, *Sleep: a comprehensive handbook*, 2006; 139–43.

30. Kleitman N. *Sleep and Wakefulness.* Second ed. Chicago: University of Chicago Press; 1963.

31. Harrison Y, Horne JA. The impact of sleep deprivation on decision making: A review. *J Exp Psychol Appl.* 2000; 6:236–49.

32. Banks S, Catcheside P, Lack L, et al. Low levels of alcohol impair driving simulator performance and reduce perception of crash risk in partially sleep deprived subjects. *Sleep.* 2004; 27:1063–67.

33. Van Dongen HP, Baynard MD, Maislin G, Dinges DF. Systematic interindividual differences in neurobehavioral impairment from sleep loss: evidence of trait-like differential vulnerability. *Sleep.* 2004; 27:423–33.

34. Russo M, Thomas M, Thorne D, et al. Oculomotor impairment during chronic partial sleep deprivation. *Clin Neurophysiol.* 2003; 114:723–36.

35. Doran SM, Van Dongen HPA, Dinges DF. Sustained attention performance during sleep deprivation: evidence of state instability. *Arch Ital Biol.* 2001; 139:253–67.

36. Goel N, Lakhtman L, Basner M, Banks S, Dinges DF. Phenotyping neurobehavioral and cognitive responses to partial sleep deprivation. *Sleep Res.* 2007; 30:A130.

37. Van Dongen HP, Maislin G, Dinges DF. Dealing with inter-individual differences in the temporal dynamics of fatigue and performance: importance and techniques. *Aviat Space Environ Med.* 2004; 75:A147–54.

38. Chee MWL, Chuah LYM, Venkatraman V, Chan WY, Philip P, Dinges DF. Functional imaging of working memory following normal sleep and after 24 and 35 h of sleep deprivation: Correlations of fronto-parietal activation with performance. *Neuroimage.* 2006; 31:419–28.

39. Caldwell JA, Mu Q, Smith JK, et al. Are individual differences in fatigue vulnerability related to baseline differences in cortical activation? *Behav Neurosci.* 2005; 119:694–707.

40. Mu Q, Mishory A, Johnson KA, et al. Decreased brain activation during a working memory task at rested baseline is associated with vulnerability to sleep deprivation. *Sleep.* 2005; 28:433–46.

41. Winget CM, DeRoshia CW, Markley CL, Holley DC. A review of human physiological and performance changes associated with desynchronosis of biological rhythms. *Aviat Space Environ Med.* 1984; 55:1085–96.

42. Dinges DF. An overview of sleepiness and accidents. *J Sleep Res.* 1995; 4:4–14.

43. Philip P, Ghorayeb I, Stoohs R, et al. Determinants of sleepiness in automobile drivers. *J Psychosom Res.* 1996; 41:279–88.

44. Philip P, Taillard J, Guilleminault C, Quera Salva MA, Bioulac B, Ohayon M. Long distance driving and self-induced sleep deprivation among automobile drivers. *Sleep.* 1999; 22:475–80.

45. Stutts JC, Wilkins JW, Scott Osberg J, Vaughn BV. Driver risk factors for sleep-related crashes. *Accid Anal Prev.* 2003; 35:321–31.

81

46. Akerstedt T. Shift work and disturbed sleep/wakefulness. *Occup Med (Lond)*. 2003; 53:89–94.

47. Mallis MM, Banks S, Dinges DF. Sleep and circadian control of neurobehavioral function. In: Parasuraman R, Rizzo M, eds. Oxford: Oxford University Press, *Neuroergonomics: the brain at work*, 2007; 207–20.

48. Weinger MB, Ancoli-Israel S. Sleep deprivation and clinical performance. *J Am Med Assoc*. 2002; 287:955–57.

49. Rogers AE, Hwang WT, Scott LD, Aiken LH, Dinges DF. The working hours of hospital staff nurses and patient safety. *Health Aff (Millwood)*. 2004; 23:202–12.

50. Landrigan CP, Rothschild JM, Cronin JW, et al. Effect of reducing interns' work hours on serious medical errors in intensive care units. *N Engl J Med*. 2004; 351:1838–48.

51. Barger LK, Cade BE, Ayas NT, et al. The Harvard Work Hours, Health, and Safety Group. Extended work shifts and the risk of motor vehicle crashes among interns. *N Engl J Med*. 2005; 352:125–34.

52. Weaver TE, Chasens ER. Continuous positive airway pressure treatment for sleep apnea in older adults. *Sleep Med Rev*. 2007; 11:99–111.

53. Black JE, Hirshkowitz M. Modafinil for treatment of residual excessive sleepiness in nasal continuous positive airway pressure-treated obstructive sleep apnea/hypopnea syndrome. *Sleep*. 2005; 28:464–71.

54. Pack AI, Black JE, Schwartz JR, Matheson JK. Modafinil as adjunct therapy for daytime sleepiness in obstructive sleep apnea. *Am J Respir Crit Care Med*. 2001; 164:1675–81.

55. Scammell TE, Matheson J. Modafinil: a novel stimulant for the treatment of narcolepsy. *Expert Opin Investig Drugs*. 1998; 7:99–112.

56. Hogl B, Saletu M, Brandauer E, et al. Modafinil for the treatment of daytime sleepiness in Parkinson's disease: a double-blind, randomized, crossover, placebo-controlled polygraphic trial. *Sleep*. 2002; 25:905–9.

57. Hewlett P, Smith A. Effects of repeated doses of caffeine on performance and alertness: new data and secondary analyses. *Hum Psychopharmacol*. 2007; 22:339–50.

58. Dagan Y, Doljansky JT. Cognitive performance during sustained wakefulness: A low dose of caffeine is equally effective as modafinil in alleviating the nocturnal decline. *Chronobiol Int*. 2006; 23:973–83.

59. Goel N, Etwaroo GR. Bright light, negative air ions and auditory stimuli produce rapid mood changes in a student population: A placebo-controlled study. *Psych Med*. 2006; 36:1253–64.

60. Lockley SW, Evans EE, Scheer FA, et al. Short-wavelength sensitivity for the direct effects of light on alertness, vigilance, and the waking electroencephalogram in humans. *Sleep*. 2006; 29:161–68.

61. Revell VL, Eastman CI. How to trick mother nature into letting you fly around or stay up all night. *J Biol Rhythms*. 2005; 20:353–65.

Section 8.2

Can the Effects of Sleep Deprivation Be Reversed?

"Researchers Reverse Effects of Sleep Deprivation," September 2006. © 2006 Wake Forest University Baptist Medical Center. Reprinted with permission.

Researchers at Wake Forest University School of Medicine have shown that the effects of sleep deprivation on cognitive performance can be reversed when the naturally occurring brain peptide, orexin-A, is administered in monkeys.

Their results are published in the December 26, 2007, *Journal of Neuroscience.*

"These findings are significant because of their potential applicability," said Samuel A. Deadwyler, Ph.D., professor of physiology and pharmacology at Wake Forest. "This could benefit patients suffering from narcolepsy and other serious sleep disorders. But it also has applicability to shift workers, the military, and many other occupations where sleep is often limited, yet cognitive demand remains high."

Orexin-A, also known as hypocretin-1, is a naturally occurring peptide produced in the brain that regulates sleep. It's secreted by a small number of neurons but affects many brain regions during the day and people who have normal amounts of orexin-A are able to maintain wakefulness. When people or animals are sleep-deprived, the brain attempts to produce more orexin-A, but often without enough success to achieve alertness past the normal day-night cycle.

The research team, consisting of Linda Porrino, Ph.D., and Robert Hampson, Ph.D, also of Wake Forest, and Jerome Siegel, Ph.D., of the University of California at Los Angeles, studied the effects of orexin-A on monkeys that were kept awake overnight for thirty to thirty-six hours with videos, music, treats, and interaction with technicians, until their normal testing time the next day. They were then allowed to perform their trained tasks with several cognitive problems that varied in difficulty, and their performance was significantly impaired.

However, if the sleep-deprived monkeys were administered orexin-A either intravenously or via a nasal spray immediately prior to testing, their cognitive skills improved to the normal, non-sleep-deprived, level. The researchers also noted that when the monkeys received the orexin-A via the intranasal spray they tested higher than when it was administered intravenously.

"Assessments of the monkeys' brain activity during testing through noninvasive imaging techniques also showed improvement by orexin-A which returned to its normal non-sleep-deprived pattern during performance of the task," said Deadwyler. "In addition, we observed that orexin-A at moderate dose levels had no effect on performance if the animals were not sleep-deprived."

Chapter 9

Why Your Body Needs Sleep

Chapter Contents

Section 9.1

Sleep Deprivation and Coronary Artery Disease

"Skipping Sleep May Signal Problems for Coronary Arteries," University of Chicago Medical Center Office of Communications, December 23, 2008. Reprinted with permission.

One extra hour of sleep per night appears to decrease the risk of coronary artery calcification, an early step down the path to cardiovascular disease, a research team based at the University of Chicago Medical Center reports in the December 24/31 issue of the *Journal of the American Medical Association (JAMA)*. The benefit of one hour of additional sleep was comparable to the gains from lowering systolic blood pressure by 17 mm Hg.

About 12 percent of those in the study, healthy volunteers in their forties, first developed coronary artery calcification over five years of follow-up. Calcified arteries, however, were found in 27 percent of those who slept less than five hours a night. That dropped to 11 percent for those who slept five to seven hours and fell to 6 percent for those who slept more than seven hours a night.

The benefits of sleep appeared to be greater for women. They did not vary according to race.

"The consistency and the magnitude of the difference came as a surprise," said study director Diane Lauderdale, PhD, associate professor of health studies at the University of Chicago Medical Center. "It's also something of a mystery. We can only speculate about why those with shorter average sleep duration were more likely to develop calcification of the coronary arteries."

Recent studies have suggested that chronic partial sleep deprivation may be a risk factor for an array of common medical problems, including weight gain, diabetes, and hypertension. One study found that both long and short self-reported sleep durations were independently associated with a modestly increased risk of coronary events. This is the first study to link objectively measured sleep duration to a pre-clinical marker for heart disease.

The research focused on 495 participants in the Coronary Artery Risk Development in Young Adults (CARDIA) study. An ongoing project begun in 1985, CARDIA was designed to assess the long-term impact of various factors on the development of coronary artery disease.

Participants underwent two electron beam computed tomography scans, designed to assess the buildup of calcium within the arteries that deliver blood to the heart muscle, five years apart.

They also filled out sleep questionnaires, kept a log of their hours in bed, and participated in six nights of sleep studies with a technique called wrist actigraphy that uses a motion sensor—worn like a watch—to estimate actual sleep duration. This approach provides the most accurate measure of routine sleep behavior without subjecting the volunteers to the unfamiliarity of multiple sensors that determine sleep by monitoring brain activity.

In a previous study, Lauderdale and colleagues used actigraphy and nightly logs to study, on average, how long people spent in bed (7.5 hours), how long it took them to fall asleep (22 minutes), how long they slept (6.1 hours), and their total sleep efficiency—time asleep divided by time trying to sleep in bed (81 percent).

This time they looked at the connections between sleep duration and coronary artery calcification. They found more than they anticipated.

Previous studies have correlated decreased sleep times with established risk factors for calcification, including high blood pressure, excess weight, and poor glucose regulation. But in this study, "after adjusting for age, sex, race, education, smoking, and apnea risk," the authors note, "longer measured sleep duration was associated with reduced calcification incidence."

The authors suggest three possible ways that shorter sleep could connect to calcification. First, there may be some factor not yet identified that can both reduce sleep duration and increase calcification. Second, although blood pressure measured during examinations did not seem to explain the association, blood pressure generally declines during sleep, so the twenty-four-hour average blood pressure of those who sleep less may be higher, and that could lead to calcification. Finally, stress or a stress hormone like cortisol, which has been tied to decreased sleep and increased calcification, may play a role. Cortisol data were not available for all study participants.

"This was a small study and a new finding, so we would love to see it duplicated in another study population," Lauderdale said. "But there is enough here to make a point. Although there are constant temptations to sleep less, there is a growing body of evidence that short sleep may have subtle health consequences. Although this single study does not prove that short sleep leads to coronary artery disease, it is safe to recommend at least six hours of sleep a night."

Additional authors of the paper include Christopher King, Kristen Knutson, and Paul Rathouz from the University of Chicago; Kiang Liu from Northwestern University; and Steve Sidney from Kaiser Permanente, Oakland, California. The study was supported by grants from the National Heart, Lung and Blood Institute and the National Institute on Aging.

Section 9.2

Sleep Deprivation and Diabetes

"Lack of Deep Sleep May Increase Risk of Type 2 Diabetes,"
University of Chicago Medical Center Office of Communications,
December 31, 2007. Reprinted with permission.

Suppression of slow-wave sleep in healthy young adults significantly decreases their ability to regulate blood-sugar levels and increases the risk of type 2 diabetes, report researchers at the University of Chicago Medical Center in the "Early Edition" of the *Proceedings of the National Academy of Science*, available online as soon as December 31, 2007.

Deep sleep, also called "slow-wave sleep," is thought to be the most restorative sleep stage, but its significance for physical well-being has not been demonstrated. This study found that after only three nights of selective slow-wave sleep suppression, young healthy subjects became less sensitive to insulin. Although they needed more insulin to dispose of the same amount of glucose, their insulin secretion did not increase to compensate for the reduced sensitivity, resulting in reduced tolerance to glucose and increased risk for type 2 diabetes. The decrease in insulin sensitivity was comparable to that caused by gaining twenty to thirty pounds.

Previous studies have demonstrated that reduced sleep quantity can impair glucose metabolism and appetite regulation resulting in increased risk of obesity and diabetes. This current study provides the first evidence linking poor sleep quality to increased diabetes risk.

"These findings demonstrate a clear role for slow-wave sleep in maintaining normal glucose control," said the study's lead author, Esra Tasali, MD, assistant professor of medicine at the University of Chicago Medical Center. "A profound decrease in slow-wave sleep had an immediate and significant adverse effect on insulin sensitivity and glucose tolerance."

"Since reduced amounts of deep sleep are typical of aging and of common obesity-related sleep disorders, such as obstructive sleep apnea, these results suggest that strategies to improve sleep quality, as well as quantity, may help to prevent or delay the onset of type 2 diabetes in populations at risk," said Eve Van Cauter, PhD, professor of medicine at the University of Chicago and senior author of the study.

"These findings shed light on a problem faced by many elderly, that of fragmented sleep and less time spent in restorative sleep," said Dr. Andrew Monjan, PhD, MPH, chief of the Neurobiology of Aging Branch at the National Institute on Aging, which partially funded the research. "More research is needed into the link between insufficient sleep and common metabolic disturbances of later life, such as type 2 diabetes and obesity."

The researchers studied nine lean, healthy volunteers, five men and four women between the ages of twenty and thirty-one. The subjects spent two consecutive nights in the sleep laboratory, where they went to bed at 11 p.m., slept undisturbed but carefully monitored, and got out of bed 8.5 hours later, at 7:30 a.m.

The same subjects were also studied for three consecutive nights during which they followed identical nighttime routines. During this session, however, when their brain waves indicated that they were drifting into slow-wave sleep they were subtly disturbed by sounds administered through speakers beside the bed.

These sounds were loud enough to disrupt deep sleep but not so loud as to cause a full awakening. This technique enabled the researchers to decrease slow-wave sleep by about 90 percent, shifting the subjects from the onset of deep sleep (stage 3 or 4) to a lighter sleep (stage 2) without altering total sleep time.

"Our system proved quite effective," Tasali said. When asked about the sounds the next morning, study subjects vaguely recalled hearing a noise "three or four times," during the night. Some recalled as many as 10 to 15. On average, however, subjects required about 250 to 300 interventions each night, fewer the first night but more on subsequent nights as "slow-wave pressure," the body's need for deep sleep, accumulated night after night.

"This decrease in slow-wave sleep resembles the changes in sleep patterns caused by forty years of aging," Tasali said. Young adults spend eighty to one hundred minutes per night in slow-wave sleep, while people over age sixty generally have less than twenty minutes. "In this experiment," she said, "we gave people in their twenties the sleep of those in their sixties."

At the end of each study, the researchers gave intravenous glucose (a sugar solution) to each subject, then took blood samples every few minutes to measure the levels of glucose and insulin, the hormone that controls glucose uptake.

They found that when slow-wave sleep was suppressed for only three nights, young healthy subjects became about 25 percent less sensitive to insulin. As insulin sensitivity decreased, subjects needed more insulin to dispose of the same amount of glucose. But for eight of the nine subjects, insulin secretion did not go up to compensate for reduced effects. The result was a 23 percent increase in blood-glucose levels, comparable to older adults with impaired glucose tolerance.

Those with low baseline levels of slow-wave sleep had the lowest levels after having their sleep patterns disrupted and the greatest decrease in insulin sensitivity.

The alarming rise in the prevalence of type 2 diabetes is generally attributed to the epidemic of obesity combined with the aging of the population. "Previous studies from our lab have demonstrated many connections between chronic, partial, sleep deprivation, changes in appetite, metabolic abnormalities, obesity, and diabetes risk," said Van Cauter. "These results solidify those links and add a new wrinkle, the role of poor sleep quality, which is also associated with aging."

"Chronic shallow non-REM sleep, decreased insulin sensitivity, and elevated diabetes risk are typical of aging," the authors conclude. "Our findings raise the question of whether age-related changes in sleep quality contribute to the development of these metabolic alterations."

The National Institutes of Health funded this research. Additional authors include Rachel Leproult and David Ehrmann of the University of Chicago Medical Center.

Section 9.3

Sleep Deprivation and Hypertension

If you're middle age and sleep five or fewer hours a night, you may be increasing your risk of developing high blood pressure, according to a study released by Columbia University's Mailman School of Public Health and the College of Physicians and Surgeons, and reported in *Hypertension: Journal of the American Heart Association.*

"Sleep allows the heart to slow down and blood pressure to drop for a significant part of the day," said James E. Gangwisch, PhD, lead author of the study and post-doctoral fellow in the psychiatric epidemiology training (PET) program at the Mailman School. "However, people who sleep for only short durations raise their average twenty-four-hour blood pressure and heart rate. This may set up the cardiovascular system to operate at an elevated pressure."

Dr. Gangwisch said that 24 percent of people ages thirty-two to fifty-nine who slept for five or fewer hours a night developed hypertension versus 12 percent of those who got seven or eight hours of sleep. Subjects who slept five or fewer hours per night continued to be significantly more likely to be diagnosed with hypertension after controlling for factors such as obesity, diabetes, physical activity, salt and alcohol consumption, smoking, depression, age, education, gender, and ethnicity.

The researchers conducted a longitudinal analysis of data from the Epidemiologic Follow-up Studies of the first National Health and Nutrition Examination Study (NHANES I). The analysis is based on NHANES I data from 4,810 people ages thirty-two to eighty-six who did not have high blood pressure at baseline. The 1982–84 follow-up survey asked participants how many hours they slept at night. During eight to ten years of follow-up, 647 of the 4,810 participants were diagnosed with hypertension.

Compared to people who slept seven or eight hours a night, people who slept five or fewer hours a night also exercised less and were more likely to have a higher body mass index. (BMI is a measurement used

93

to assess body fatness). They were also more likely to have diabetes and depression, and to report daytime sleepiness.

"We had hypothesized that both BMI and a history of diabetes would mediate the relationship between sleep and blood pressure, and the results were consistent with this," Dr. Gangwisch said.

Sleep deprivation has been shown previously to increase appetite and compromise insulin sensitivity.

Short sleep duration was linked to a new diagnosis of high blood pressure among middle-aged participants, but the association was not observed among people age sixty or older, he said. Dr. Gangwisch said the differences between the younger and older subjects might be explained by the fact that advanced age is associated with difficulties falling and staying asleep. Another factor could be that subjects suffering from hypertension, diabetes, and obesity would be less likely to survive into their later years.

Among study limitations, researchers found that high blood pressure often goes undetected. An analysis of NHANES III data showed that over 30 percent of people who had high blood pressure didn't know they had it.

Since the study is based on observational data, Dr. Gangwisch said more research is needed to confirm the association between short sleep duration and high blood pressure. "We need to investigate the biological mechanisms and, if confirmed, design interventions that will help people modify sleep behavior," he said.

Dr. Gangwisch said the study's main message is clear: "A good night's sleep is very important for good health."

Co-authors of the study include Andrew G. Rundle, DrPH, assistant professor of Epidemiology at the Mailman School of Public Health; and Columbia University Medical Center's Steven B. Heymsfield, MD; Bernadette Boden-Albala, DrPH; Ruud M. Buijs, PhD; Felix Kreier, PhD; Thomas G. Pickering, MD, DPhil; Gary K. Zammit, PhD; and Dolores Malaspina, MD.

Support for the study was provided by a National Research Service Award by the National Institute of Mental Health.

Section 9.4

Sleep Deprivation and the Immune System

Reprinted from ABC Health & Wellbeing—"The Pulse: Insomnia and Your Immune System," by Peter Levelle, first published by ABC Online, February 26, 2009. Reproduced by permission of the Australian Broadcasting Corporation and ABC Online. © 2009 ABC. All rights reserved.

One of the greatest mysteries about the human body is why it needs to sleep.

From the perspective of evolution, it's hard to see why we need sleep as an adaptation to help survival.

While asleep a creature can't eat, can't search for food, can't reproduce, and—being immobile and unconscious—is a sitting duck for a predator. And yet almost all animals sleep, even simple invertebrates.

The traditional theories state we need sleep to conserve energy to lay down new memories and consolidate learning, but these have never been backed by much scientific evidence.

However, the latest evidence suggests sleep is the body's way of recharging its immune system, which is bad news if you suffer insomnia.

A large body of evidence that suggests insomnia and poor sleep contribute to a range of diseases—from acute conditions, like the common cold, to chronic diseases like rheumatoid arthritis and heart disease.

Susceptibility to Infections

In January 2009, researchers from Carnegie Mellon University in Pittsburgh, Pennsylvania, published a study on a group of about 150 poor sleepers. The subjects' sleep patterns were monitored over two weeks and they were then inoculated with nasal drops containing a common cold virus (a rhinovirus called RV-39). Five days later, the researchers took nasal secretions from the subjects to see if the virus was in their nasal secretions, then twenty-eight days later the researchers tested subjects' blood for antibodies to the virus.

Most of the subjects (almost 90 percent) exposed to the virus became infected; that is, the virus was isolated from their nasal secretions and/or they developed neutralizing antibodies. But only 35 percent actually developed cold symptoms like cough, runny nose, tiredness, and fever. Those who did develop symptoms were statistically more likely to have recorded poor sleeping patterns.

People who slept less than seven hours a night were especially susceptible—almost three times more likely to get the clinical symptoms. Also susceptible were "inefficient sleepers," that is, people who spent more than 8 percent of the time actually awake while they were supposed to be asleep. These people were 5.5 times more likely to develop the clinical symptoms of a cold.

What this suggests is that lack of sleep blocks the immune system's ability to fight off an acute infection, the researchers concluded.

Chronic Illness

Studies have also linked insomnia with worsening of many chronic conditions.

In a study published in the *Journal of the American Medical Association* in December 2008, researchers from the University of Chicago monitored a group of nearly five hundred healthy, middle-aged Americans, who had no heart disease at the beginning of the study. After five years, the participants were given computed tomography (CT) scans of the heart; 12 percent had developed calcification of the coronary arteries (a sign of advanced coronary artery disease).

Researchers also gathered information about the subjects' sleeping patterns—subjects had to keep sleep diaries and were given a special device that monitored their sleep patterns.

Those who got a good night's sleep had a reduced risk of coronary artery calcification. One hour's regular lost sleep raised the risk of calcification by 33 percent, the researchers calculated.

Other research has linked poor sleep patterns with abnormalities of glucose metabolism, hypertension, inflammation, and obesity, say the researchers.

People who are sleep deprived have abnormalities of their immune function (this shows up in blood tests). They have also reduced amounts of certain "killer" white blood cells, poorer production of chemicals that reduce inflammation (such as interleukins), and increased levels of chemicals that promote inflammation called cytokines. Just how these changes cause disease, we still don't know.

We do know animals—all animals, not just humans—spend more time asleep when they're sick. And we know laboratory animals totally deprived of sleep tend to die from overwhelming bacterial infections. We also know people with poor sleep patterns show a reduced response to vaccinations—they don't develop high levels of antibodies after a vaccine booster, for example.

Researchers from the Max Planck Institute for Evolutionary Anthropology propose that one of the functions of sleep is to give the body time and energy to "recharge" the immune system.

They studied and compared the length of time different species of mammals sleep, with their resistance to various infections and found the longer a species sleeps, the better its resistance to infection.

They theorized that while awake, animals use the energy from their dietary intake to search for food, reproduce, defend territory, and look after offspring. When asleep, this demand for energy falls away, and the body can use available energy for recharging the immune system (replacing white cells that have been killed, for example). Large amounts of energy are needed—the body only gets a chance to do it while asleep.

It's a fascinating theory (published in the January 2009 edition of *BMC Evolutionary Biology*)—and more studies are needed to find out if it's true. But in the meantime there's enough scientific evidence to be reasonably sure there's a link between poor sleep and disease.

There are many reasons for getting a good night's sleep, and fighting off disease could well be one of them.

Section 9.5

Sleep Deprivation and Obesity

Millions of Americans only get five to six hours of sleep each night, not knowing that maintaining such sleep patterns can cause them to be dangerously overweight, resulting in many medical and health issues.

If you're sleep deprived, you're more likely to be overweight, and if you're both, you're more likely to be at risk for type 2 diabetes, hypertension, elevated cholesterol, and cardiovascular complications.

But it doesn't end there. "If you sleep less than six hours a night, you are 15 to 20 percent more likely to be overweight or obese," says Pete Bils, director of clinical research for Select Comfort, who has conducted fifteen sleep studies on quality of sleep. A healthy sleeping pattern means going to bed at the same time each night and waking up at the same time each morning, without an alarm clock, approximately seven to eight hours later.

"If you can lie down in a quiet, cool dark room anytime during daytime and fall asleep, especially within five to eight minutes, you are sleep deprived," says Bils.

And if you're already significantly overweight, you may be at higher risk for sleep deprivation, according to Dr. Carol Ash, medical director of the Sleep for Life Program at Somerset Medical Center in Somerville, New Jersey. "Obese people tend to be too warm [body temperature] and that can interfere with restful sleep."

Moreover, Ash says people who are continuously tired may tend to eat more to try to stay energized or eat more simply because they are awake more hours of the day, which can lead to weight gain. But there is also a growing area of research to suggest that being sleep deprived affects your weight issues on a hormonal level. "Without sufficient sleep, leptin, a hormone that suppresses appetite, is reduced in the body while ghrelin, a hormone that stimulates appetite, is increased," she says. Some studies have found that these hormonal changes may also increase cravings for high-carbohydrate sweets and salty foods.

Bils says often times society views people who sleep less and work more as more productive or successful, but that quite the opposite is true. "That's what I call societal sleep deprivation—sleep deprivation by choice," he says. "There's a state of denial, and people think it's normal until it gets to the point that it negatively affects your daytime functioning. And if that happens when they are behind the wheel, you don't know what could happen."

Ash says the United States is a "nation in a sleep crisis." She cites the primary social reasons for sleep deprivation as the advent of technology and increased time at work. "Before electricity was discovered, most people wound down their daily activities when darkness fell because they had no real choice," she says. "Today we live in a 24/7 society, and TVs, computers, and video games are competitors for our time."

There are also biological reasons for sleep deprivation including sleep disorders like sleep apnea and insomnia, both of which may need medical treatment.

The side effects of sleep deprivation can also translate into other kinds of problems in the bedroom—and we're not talking about sleep. It can have negative effects on your sex life. "A sleep deprived person does not have the energy to tend to the needs of his or her partner," says Dr. Joyce Walsleben, head of Behavioral Sleep Medicine at New York University. She says the mental stress that goes along with being sleep deprived should also not be overlooked and can lead to depression and mood changes.

Walsleben says that despite the numerous negative effects of sleep deprivation, it's something that can be changed with some minor life changes. "Sleep deprivation can be prevented by giving sleep as much importance as food and water," she says. "Start adding fifteen minutes of sleep each night for a week, then another fifteen minutes the following week until you feel better. Small nightly additions help over time without disrupting schedules."

Chapter 10

Why Your Brain Needs Sleep

Chapter Contents

Section 10.1

While You Sleep, Your Brain Keeps Working

You think when you go to sleep, you just, well, sleep?

Sleep, as it turns out, is far more complicated than we thought. And the brain not only doesn't turn off, but appears to help keep itself healthy.

We've all heard of REM—rapid eye movement—discovered by the late physiologists Eugene Aserinsky and Nathaniel Kleitman at the University of Chicago in 1953. *Scientific American* has the story:

> During REM sleep, our brain waves—the oscillating electro-magnetic signals that result from large-scale brain activity—look similar to those produced while we are awake. And in subsequent decades, the late Mircea Steriade of Laval University in Quebec and other neuroscientists discovered that individual collections of neurons were independently firing in between these REM phases, during periods known as slow-wave sleep, when large populations of brain cells fire synchronously in a steady rhythm of one to four beats each second. So it became clear that the sleeping brain was not merely "resting," either in REM sleep or in slow-wave sleep. Sleep was doing something different. Something active.

Discovering REM sleep was the first clue that sleep didn't just help keep our bodies healthy, but our minds as well. And while many studies have been conducted on sleep since 1953, it's only been in the last decade where we've begun to appreciate the complexity and importance of sleep for our minds. In 2000, researchers discovered that people that received more than six hours of sleep during an experiment helped improve their performance on tasks designed to tax the memory.

The key came in the discovery that participants didn't just require REM sleep to improve their performance—they needed all that other sleep time too (what scientists call "slow-wave" sleep).

The long article also provides a nice description of our current understanding of how memory works:

> To understand how that could be so, it helps to review a few memory basics. When we "encode" information in our brain, the newly minted memory is actually just beginning a long journey during which it will be stabilized, enhanced and qualitatively altered, until it bears only faint resemblance to its original form. Over the first few hours, a memory can become more stable, resistant to interference from competing memories. But over longer periods, the brain seems to decide what is important to remember and what is not—and a detailed memory evolves into something more like a story.

The researchers also discovered that sleep helps stabilize memories—sleep changes our memory, "making it robust and more resistant to interference in the coming day," as the article notes.

But wait, sleep does more! It may not just stabilize our memories, it may actually help our brains process the memories, keeping the bits we need for long-term memories (especially the emotional components), and dropping the extraneous details that would clog our limited storage capacity:

> Over just the past few years, a number of studies have demonstrated the sophistication of the memory processing that happens during slumber. In fact, it appears that as we sleep, the brain might even be dissecting our memories and retaining only the most salient details. [. . .] Instead of deteriorating, memories for the emotional objects actually seemed to improve by a few percent overnight, showing about a 15 percent improvement relative to the deteriorating backgrounds. After a few more nights, one could imagine that little but the emotional objects would be left. We know this culling happens over time with real-life events, but now it appears that sleep may play a crucial role in this evolution of emotional memories.

But wait, sleep does even more!

Even more recent research suggests that sleep helps our brain to process the information of the day and solve problems.

The upshot is that sleep is far, far more important than most of us realize and few of us appreciate. We miss it and think nothing of chopping off a few hours here or there. But the emerging research suggests that when we cut out sleep, we may be actually harming our formation of new memories for the recent past, and our ability to perform up to our usual standards. The researchers sum it up best:

103

As exciting findings such as these come in more and more rapidly, we are becoming sure of one thing: while we sleep, our brain is anything but inactive. It is now clear that sleep can consolidate memories by enhancing and stabilizing them and by finding patterns within studied material even when we do not know that patterns might be there. It is also obvious that skimping on sleep stymies these crucial cognitive processes: some aspects of memory consolidation only happen with more than six hours of sleep. Miss a night, and the day's memories might be compromised—an unsettling thought in our fast-paced, sleep-deprived society.

Section 10.2

Sleep as Healing Time for Your Brain

Sleep can be wonderfully restorative. After a long day of work you drag yourself to bed—and then you wake up seven or eight hours later, alert and recharged.

Now, researchers are finding that one reason we sleep may be that our brains, as well as our bodies, need time to rest and repair themselves. Recent studies have suggested that the brain, so active during the day, may use the downtime of sleep to repair damage caused by our busy metabolism, replenish dwindling energy stores, and even grow new neurons.

These studies, along with competing and complementary research on sleep and memory and the evolutionary forces driving sleep, are giving us a fuller picture of the biological imperatives behind this most basic need.

Messy Metabolism

One way that sleep may aid the brain is by reducing damage caused by oxidative stress. For years, researchers have known that molecules called free radicals can damage human cells, including brain cells. These molecules form naturally whenever the body metabolizes oxygen, so the damage they cause is called oxidative stress. Because free radicals are missing one electron, they're very unstable and bind to other molecules in nerve cells and elsewhere—and when they do they damage those cells.

The body combats free radicals with neutralizing enzymes, including one called superoxide dismutase (SOD) that can break down the damaging molecules into their component, and harmless, parts. But research has found that when a rat is sleep-deprived the level of SOD in its brain drops, suggesting that sleep may be crucial for minimizing the brain cell damage caused by oxidative stress, says study author Jerome Siegel, PhD, a psychologist at the University of California, Los Angeles.

In the 2002 study, published in the journal *Neuroreport* (Vol. 13, No. 11, pages 1387–90), Siegel and his colleagues kept rats awake for five to eleven days. At the end of the sleep deprivation period, they found that the level of SOD activity had decreased in the rats' hippocampus and brainstem.

In another 2002 study, this one in the journal *Brain Research* (Vol. 945, No. 1, pages 1–8), Siegel's team found some evidence of the effect that this reduced SOD activity might have—they discovered damage to cell membranes in the hypothalamus of rats kept awake for forty-five hours in a row.

Free radicals can also damage other cells in the body. But other types of tissue—like muscles—can rest any time we sit still, Siegel explains. The brain, on the other hand, is hard at work whenever we're awake.

"Putting these together, the message is that sleep deprivation causes oxidative stress in the brain, and in the regions where the stress is more severe, it causes damage," he says. On the other hand, he points out, the cells in his study were damaged but not dead—so some of the damage might be reversible with sleep. The results also fit with what we know about animal sleep, Siegel adds. In general, smaller animals require more sleep than larger ones. Smaller animals also generally have a higher metabolic rate—which would produce more free radicals, and thus necessitate more sleep to neutralize them.

The Brain's Battery

All that messy metabolism requires energy to keep running. And over the past decade or so, several researchers have suggested that another purpose of sleep might be to replenish the energy stores that we use up while awake.

Harvard Medical School neuroscientist Robert McCarley, MD, studies the link between sleep and a molecule called adenosine triphosphate (ATP), which provides energy to cells. ATP stores energy in the chemical bonds that hold it together, and when it breaks down into its component parts it releases that energy to the cell. One of those component parts is the neurotransmitter adenosine, which McCarley and others now think the brain may use as a signal to monitor its need for sleep.

In a 1997 study published in *Science* (Vol. 276, No. 5316, pages 1265–68), McCarley and his colleagues measured the level of adenosine in the brains of cats kept awake for six hours—much longer than a cat would naturally stay awake. The researchers found that the level of adenosine in the cat's basal forebrain—an important area for regulating sleep and wake—increased with each hour of sleep deprivation.

In a 2000 follow-up study, published in *Neuroscience* (Vol. 99, No. 3, pages 507–17), the researchers found that this was not true in other areas of the brain—such as the cerebral cortex—that were less important for regulating sleep.

The idea, then, is that this is a self-regulating cycle. As the level of ATP in brain cells drops, the level of adenosine rises. That rising level of adenosine sends a signal to the areas of the brain that regulate sleep that it's time to sleep.

"Adenosine is the messenger telling the cell to shut off—that you need some rest," McCarley says.

Other researchers have suggested other possible contenders for the substance linking energy to sleep. Neuroscientists Joel Benington, PhD, of St. Bonaventure University, and Craig Heller, PhD, of Stanford University, were among the first to suggest that energy restoration in the brain might be a function of sleep. They focused on glycogen, a form of glucose that provides energy to localized brain cells when they need a short-term boost.

Studies, though, have provided mixed results. While researchers have found that levels of glycogen dip in the brain after sleep deprivation in some strains of mice, other strains haven't shown that expected pattern.

"It's a mixed bag of results, with nothing conclusive yet," says Benington.

Neurogenesis

Other research suggests that sleep may contribute to neurogenesis, or the formation of new nerve cells in the brain.

For decades, scientists believed that animals and humans were born with all the brain cells they would ever have. Over the past thirty years, though, neuroscientists have chipped away at that theory, finding evidence of new brain cell growth first in adult rats, then in primates, and finally, in the late 1990s, in humans—particularly in an area of the hippocampus called the dentate gyrus.

But recent evidence shows that sleep deprivation can impede these new neurons' growth. In a 2003 study in the *Journal of Physiology* (Vol. 549, No. 2, pages 563–71), neuroscientist Dennis McGinty, PhD, and his colleagues at the University of California, Los Angeles, found that depriving rats of sleep for four days reduced the number of new cells in the dentate gyrus by more than 50 percent.

In a follow-up study published in October in the *European Journal of Neuroscience* (Vol. 22, No. 8, pages 2111–16), they found that many cells that formed during sleep-deprivation didn't mature normally.

"The nice thing about this model is that it's very concrete," McGinty says. "People have wanted for years to understand how sleep could play a role in brain development and growth, and this gives you a direct way to look at structural change."

Overall, McGinty points out, it's important to remember that most of the hypothesized functions of sleep—reducing oxidative stress, restoring energy levels, promoting neurogenesis, and others—are not mutually exclusive. In fact, many complement each other.

"Even something as simple as breathing has multiple functions," he says. "So it's quite likely that something as complex as sleep is in the same boat."

Section 10.3

Sleep and Memory

"Penn Study Shows Why Sleep Is Needed to Form Memories," Penn
Medicine News (www.uphs.upenn.edu/news), February 11, 2009,
© 2009 The Trustees of the University of Pennsylvania.

If you ever argued with your mother when she told you to get some
sleep after studying for an exam instead of pulling an all-nighter, you
owe her an apology, because it turns out she's right. And now, scientists
are beginning to understand why.

In research published in the February 12, 2009, edition of *Neuron*,
Marcos Frank, PhD, assistant professor of neuroscience, at the University of Pennsylvania School of Medicine, postdoctoral researcher
Sara Aton, PhD, and colleagues describe for the first time how cellular
changes in the sleeping brain promote the formation of memories.

"This is the first real direct insight into how the brain, on a cellular
level, changes the strength of its connections during sleep," Frank says.

The findings, says Frank, reveal that the brain during sleep is fundamentally different from the brain during wakefulness.

"We find that the biochemical changes are simply not happening
in the neurons of animals that are awake," Frank says. "And when
the animal goes to sleep it's like you've thrown a switch, and all of a
sudden, everything is turned on that's necessary for making synaptic
changes that form the basis of memory formation. It's very striking."

The team used an experimental model of cortical plasticity—the re-
arrangement of neural connections in response to life experiences. "That's
fundamentally what we think the machinery of memory is, the actual
making and breaking of connections between neurons," Frank explains.

In this case, the experience Frank and his team used was visual
stimulation. Animals that were young enough to still be establishing
neural networks in response to visual cues were deprived of stimulation through one eye by covering that eye with a patch. The team then
compared the electrophysiological and molecular changes that resulted
with control animals whose eyes were not covered. Some animals were
studied immediately following the visual block, while others were allowed to sleep first.

From earlier work, Frank's team already knew that sleep induced a stronger reorganization of the visual cortex in animals that had an eye patch versus those that were not allowed to sleep. Now they know why.

A molecular explanation is emerging. The key cellular player in this process is a molecule called N-methyl D-aspartate receptor (NMDAR), which acts like a combination listening post and gatekeeper. It both receives extracellular signals in the form of glutamate and regulates the flow of calcium ions into cells.

Essentially, once the brain is triggered to reorganize its neural networks in wakefulness (by visual deprivation, for instance), intra- and intercellular communication pathways engage, setting a series of enzymes into action within the reorganizing neurons during sleep.

To start the process, NMDAR is primed to open its ion channel after the neuron has been excited. The ion channel then opens when glutamate binds to the receptor, allowing calcium into the cell. In turn, calcium, an intracellular signaling molecule, turns other downstream enzymes on and off.

Some neural connections are strengthened as a result of this process, and the result is a reorganized visual cortex. And, this only happens during sleep.

"To our amazement, we found that these enzymes never really turned on until the animal had a chance to sleep," Frank explains, "As soon as the animal had a chance to sleep, we saw all the machinery of memory start to engage." Equally important was the demonstration that inhibition of these enzymes in the sleeping brain completely prevented the normal reorganization of the cortex.

Frank stresses that this study did not examine recalling memories. For example, these animals were not being asked to remember the location of their food bowl. "It's a mechanism that we think underlies the formation of memory." And not only memory; the same mechanism could play a role in all neurological plasticity processes.

As a result, this study could pave the way to understanding, on a molecular level, why humans need sleep, and why they are so affected by the lack of it. It could also conceivably lead to novel therapeutics that could compensate for the lack of sleep, by mimicking the molecular events that occur during sleep.

Finally, the study could lead to a deeper understanding of human memory. Though how and even where humans store long-lasting memories remains a mystery, Frank says, "we do know that changes in cortical connections is at the heart of the mystery. By understanding that in animal models, it will bring us close to understanding how it works in humans."

The research was funded by the National Institutes of Health, the National Sleep Foundation, and L'Oreal USA, and also involved researchers at the Penn's Center for Sleep and Respiratory Neurobiology and the School of Life Sciences, Jawaharlal Nehru University, New Delhi, India.

Section 10.4

Sleep and Problem Solving

"REM Sleep Enhances Creative Problem Solving," June 9, 2009, reprinted with permission from the University of California San Diego News Center. © 2009 Regents of the University of California.

Research led by a leading expert on the positive benefits of napping at the University of California, San Diego School of Medicine suggests that Rapid Eye Movement (REM) sleep enhances creative problem solving. The findings may have important implications for how sleep, specifically REM sleep, fosters the formation of associative networks in the brain.

The study by Sara Mednick, PhD, assistant professor of psychiatry at UC San Diego and the Veterans Affairs San Diego Healthcare System, and first author Denise Cai, graduate student in the UC San Diego Department of Psychology, shows that REM directly enhances creative processing more than any other sleep or wake state. Their findings were published in the June 8, 2009, online edition of the *Proceedings of the National Academy of Sciences (PNAS)*.

"We found that—for creative problems that you've already been working on—the passage of time is enough to find solutions," said Mednick. "However, for new problems, only REM sleep enhances creativity."

Mednick added that it appears REM sleep helps achieve such solutions by stimulating associative networks, allowing the brain to make new and useful associations between unrelated ideas. Importantly, the study showed that these improvements are not due to selective memory enhancements.

110

A critical issue in sleep and cognition is whether improvements in behavioral performance are the result of sleep-specific enhancement or simply reduction of interference—since experiences while awake have been shown to interfere with memory consolidation. The researchers controlled for such interference effects by comparing sleep periods to quiet rest periods without any verbal input.

While evidence for the role of sleep in creative problem solving has been looked at by prior research, underlying mechanisms such as different stages of sleep had not been explored. Using a creativity task called a remote associates test (RAT), study participants were shown multiple groups of three words (for example: cookie, heart, sixteen) and asked to find a fourth word that can be associated to all three words (sweet, in this instance). Participants were tested in the morning, and again in the afternoon, after either a nap with REM sleep, one without REM, or a quiet rest period. The researchers manipulated various conditions of prior exposure to elements of the creative problem, and controlled for memory.

"Participants grouped by REM sleep, non-REM sleep, and quiet rest were indistinguishable on measures of memory," said Cai. "Although the quiet rest and non-REM sleep groups received the same prior exposure to the task, they displayed no improvement on the RAT test. Strikingly, however, the REM sleep group improved by almost 40 percent over their morning performances."

The authors hypothesize that the formation of associative networks from previously unassociated information in the brain, leading to creative problem solving, is facilitated by changes to neurotransmitter systems during REM sleep.

Additional contributors to the study include Sarnoff A. Mednick, University of Southern California, Department of Psychology; Elizabeth M. Harrison, UCSD Department of Psychology; and Jennifer Kanady, UCSD Department of Psychiatry and Veterans Affairs San Diego Healthcare System, Research Service. Funding was provided by the National Institutes of Health.

Chapter 11

Sleep Deprivation Impacts Learning and Education

Chapter Contents

Section 11.1

Sleep and Learning

"Sleep Helps People Learn Complicated Tasks," University of Chicago
News Office, November 17, 2008. Reprinted with permission.

Sleep helps the mind learn complicated tasks and helps people
recover learning they otherwise thought they had forgotten over the
course of a day, research at the University of Chicago shows.

Using a test that involved learning to play video games, researchers showed for the first time that people who had "forgotten" how to
perform a complex task twelve hours after training found that those
abilities were restored after a night's sleep.

"Sleep consolidated learning by restoring what was lost over the
course of a day following training and by protecting what was learned
against subsequent loss," said Howard Nusbaum, professor of psychology at the University of Chicago and a researcher in the study. "These
findings suggest that sleep has an important role in learning generalized skills in stabilizing and protecting memory."

The results demonstrate that this consolidation may help in learning language processes such as reading and writing as well as eye-hand
skills such as tennis, he said.

For the study, researchers tested about two hundred college students, most of whom were women, who had little previous experience
playing video games. The team reported the findings in the paper, "Consolidation of Sensorimotor Learning During Sleep," in the November
2008 issue of *Learning and Memory*. Joining Nusbaum in the research
were lead author Timothy Brawn, a graduate student in psychology at
the university; Kimberly Fenn, now an assistant professor of psychology at Michigan State University; and Daniel Margoliash, professor in
the Departments of Organismal Biology and Anatomy and Psychology
at the university.

The team had students learn video games containing a rich, mul-
tisensory virtual environment in which players must use both hands
to deal with continually changing visual and auditory signals. The
first-person navigation games require learning maps of different environments.

For the study, researchers used first-person shooter games, with the goal of killing enemy bots (software avatars that play against the participant) while avoiding being killed.

The subjects were given a pre-test to determine their initial performance level on the games. Then they were trained to play the games and later tested on their performance. One group was trained in the morning and then tested twelve hours later after being awake for that time. A second group was trained in the morning and then tested the next day, twenty-four hours after being trained. Another group was trained in the evening, then tested twelve hours after a night's sleep, and a fourth group was trained in the evening and then also tested twenty-four hours after training.

When trained in the morning subjects showed an 8 percentage point improvement in accuracy immediately after training. However after twelve waking hours following training, subjects lost half of that improvement when tested in the evening. When subjects were tested the next morning twenty-four hours after training, they showed a 10 percentage point improvement over their pre-test performance.

"The students probably tested more poorly in the afternoon because following training, some of their waking experiences interfered with training. Those distractions went away when they slept and the brain was able to do its work," Nusbaum said.

Among the students who received evening training, scores improved by about 7 percentage points, and went to 10 percentage points the next morning and remained at that level throughout the day.

The study follows Fenn, Nusbaum, and Margoliash's earlier work, published in *Nature*, which showed for the first time that sleep consolidates perceptual learning of synthetic speech.

"In that study we showed that if after learning, by the end of the day, people 'forgot' some of what was learned, a night's sleep restored this memory loss," Nusbaum said. "Furthermore a night's sleep protected memory against loss over the course of the next day."

The latest study expanded that work to show that sleep benefits people learning complicated tasks as well, Nusbaum said.

Section 11.2

Sleep May Help Clear the Brain for New Learning

"Sleep May Help Clear the Brain for New Learning," by Michael Purdy, April 2, 2009. © Washington University in St. Louis. Reprinted with permission.

A new theory about sleep's benefits for the brain gets a boost from fruit flies in this week's (April 3, 2009) *Science*. Researchers at Washington University School of Medicine in St. Louis found evidence that sleep, already recognized as a promoter of long-term memories, also helps clear room in the brain for new learning.

The critical question: How many synapses, or junctures where nerve cells communicate with each other, are modified by sleep? Neurologists believe creation of new synapses is one key way the brain encodes memories and learning, but this cannot continue unabated and may be where sleep comes in.

"There are a number of reasons why the brain can't indefinitely add synapses, including the finite spatial constraints of the skull," says senior author Paul Shaw, Ph.D., assistant professor of neurobiology at Washington University School of Medicine in St. Louis. "We were able to track the creation of new synapses in fruit flies during learning experiences, and to show that sleep pushed that number back down."

Scientists don't yet know how the synapses are eliminated. According to theory, only the less important connections are trimmed back, while connections encoding important memories are maintained.

Many aspects of fly sleep are similar to human sleep; for example, flies and humans deprived of sleep one day will try to make up for the loss by sleeping more the next day. Because the human brain is much more complex, Shaw uses the flies as models for answering questions about sleep and memory.

Sleep is a recognized promoter of learning, but three years ago Shaw turned that association around and revealed that learning increases the need for sleep in the fruit fly. In a 2006 paper in *Science*, he and his colleagues found that two separate scenarios, each of which gave the fruit fly's brain a workout, increased the need for sleep.

The first scenario was inspired by human research linking an enriched environment to improved memory and other brain functions. Scientists found that flies raised in an enhanced social environment—a test tube full of other flies—slept approximately two to three hours longer than flies raised in isolation.

Researchers also gave male fruit flies their first exposure to female fruit flies, but with a catch—the females were either already mated or were actually male flies altered to emit female pheromones. Either fly rebuffed the test fly's attempts to mate. The test flies were then kept in isolation for two days and exposed to receptive female flies. Test flies that remembered their prior failures didn't try to mate again; they also slept more. Researchers concluded that these flies had encoded memories of their prior experience, more directly proving the connection between sleep and new memories.

Scientists repeated these tests for the new study, but this time they used flies genetically altered to make it possible to track the development of new synapses, the junctures at which brain cells communicate.

"The biggest surprise was that out of two hundred thousand fly brain cells, only sixteen were required for the formation of new memories, " says first author Jeffrey Donlea, a graduate student. "These sixteen are lateral ventral neurons, which are part of the circadian circuitry that let the fly brain perform certain behaviors at particular times of day."

When flies slept, the number of new synapses formed during social enrichment decreased. When researchers deprived them of their sleep, the decline did not occur.

Donlea identified three genes essential to the links between learning and increased need for sleep: rutabaga, period, and blistered. Flies lacking any of those genes did not have increased need for sleep after social enrichment or the mating test.

Blistered is the fruit fly equivalent to a human gene known as serum response factor (SRF). Scientists have previously linked SRF to plasticity, a term for brain change that includes both learning and memory and the general ability of the brain to rewire itself to adapt to injury or changing needs.

The new study shows that SRF could offer an important advantage for scientists hoping to study plasticity: unlike other genes connected to plasticity, it's not also associated with cell survival.

"That's going to be very helpful to our efforts to study plasticity, because it removes a large confounding factor," says co-author Naren Ramanan, Ph.D., assistant professor of neurobiology. "We can alter SRF activity and not have to worry about whether the resulting changes in brain function come from changes in plasticity or from dying cells."

Shaw plans further investigations of the connections between memory and sleep, including the question of how increased synapses induce the need for sleep.

"Right now a lot of people are worried about their jobs and the economy, and some are no doubt losing sleep over these concerns," Shaw says. "But these data suggest the best thing you can do to make sure you stay sharp and increase your chances of keeping your job is to make getting enough sleep a top priority."

Section 11.3

Sleep Deprivation and Attention Deficit Hyperactivity Disorder

Children with attention deficit-hyperactivity disorder (ADHD) are more likely to have sleep difficulties.

ADHD is a neurological condition characterized by inattention, hyperactivity, and impulsivity. Three subtypes of ADHD generally are recognized by professionals:

- hyperactive-impulsive (the child does not show significant inattention)

- inattentive (the child does not show significant hyperactive-impulsive behavior—previously called ADD); and

- combined (the child who displays both inattentive and hyperactive-impulsive behavior).

Children who are anxious or depressed, are sensitive to sugar, or are sleep-deprived also may display attention problems, poor impulse control, and hyperactivity. In the July/August 2003 issue of *Psychology Today*, a Brown University study suggests "sleep deprivation in normal children can lead to symptoms of attention-deficit hyperactivity disorder (ADHD)."

Researchers found that several days of sleep deprivation resulted in the development of ADHD symptoms, and that children's hyperactivity levels escalated with each additional night of poor sleep. The sleep deprivation may be due to sleep apnea, allergies, asthma, circadian rhythm disorder, or restless legs syndrome. Not only are children at serious risk of being misdiagnosed as ADHD, if their sleep or health problem remains undetected, their health can be jeopardized.

Research shows a clear link between sleep and school performance but many teachers and schools are slow to get the message. Teachers often are unaware that a lack of sleep is keeping many of their students from being able to concentrate at school and jump to the conclusion that a child has a learning problem or ADHD. Sleep deprivation generally is overlooked by school psychologists, who fail to take it into account when making their assessments.

Sleep problems associated with ADHD include:

- difficulty relaxing and falling asleep;

- restless legs syndrome;

- sensory processing deficits (may be overly sensitive to stimulation, sounds, light, clothing, blankets);

- motor restlessness;

- night awakenings;

- bed wetting;

- snoring;

- sleep apnea.

Children with ADHD usually respond well to relaxation techniques practiced at least twice a day. Adequate exercise also is important.

If you suspect that medication is interfering with your child's sleep, meet with your physician to discuss adjusting it. Be aware that stimulant medications such as Cylert®, Ritalin®, Dexedrine®, and Adderall® may make it difficult for a child to fall asleep at night, especially if they're taken in the late afternoon.

Section 11.4

Sleep Deprivation and Visual Perception

Neuroscience researchers at the Duke-NUS Graduate Medical School in Singapore have shown for the first time what happens to the visual perceptions of healthy but sleep-deprived volunteers who fight to stay awake, like people who try to drive through the night.

The scientists found that even after sleep deprivation, people had periods of near-normal brain function in which they could finish tasks quickly. However, this normalcy mixed with periods of slow response and severe drops in visual processing and attention, according to their paper, published in the *Journal of Neuroscience* on May 21, 2008.

"Interestingly, the team found that a sleep-deprived brain can normally process simple visuals, like flashing checkerboards. But the 'higher visual areas'—those that are responsible for making sense of what we see—didn't function well," said Dr. Michael Chee, lead author and professor at the Neurobehavioral Disorders Program at Duke-NUS. "Herein lies the peril of sleep deprivation."

The research team, including colleagues at the University of Michigan and University of Pennsylvania, used magnetic resonance imaging to measure blood flow in the brain during speedy normal responses and slow "lapse" responses. The study was funded by grants from the DSO National Laboratories in Singapore, the National Institutes of Health, the National Institute on Drug Abuse, the NASA Commercialization Center, and the Air Force Office of Scientific Research.

Study subjects were asked to identify letters flashing briefly in front of them. They saw either a large H or S, and each was made up of smaller Hs or Ss. Sometimes the large letter matched the smaller letters; sometimes they didn't. Scientists asked the volunteers to identify either the smaller or the larger letters by pushing one of two buttons.

During slow responses, sleep-deprived volunteers had dramatic decreases in their higher visual cortex activity. At the same time, as expected, their frontal and parietal "control regions" were less able to make their usual corrections.

Scientists also could see brief failures in the control regions during the rare lapses that volunteers had after a normal night's sleep. However, the failures in visual processing were specific only to lapses that occurred during sleep deprivation.

The scientists theorize that this sputtering along of cognition during sleep deprivation shows the competing effects of trying to stay awake while the brain is shutting things down for sleep. The brain ordinarily becomes less responsive to sensory stimuli during sleep, Chee said.

This study has implications for a whole range of people who have to struggle through night work, from truckers to on-call doctors. "The periods of apparently normal functioning could give a false sense of competency and security, when in fact, the brain's inconsistency could have dire consequences," Chee said.

"The study task appeared simple, but as we showed in previous work, you can't effectively memorize or process what you see if your brain isn't capturing that information," Chee said. "The next step in our work is to see what we might do to improve things, besides just offering coffee, now that we have a better idea where the weak links in the system are."

Other authors of the study include Jiat Chow Tan, Hui Zheng, and Sarayu Parimal of the Cognitive Neuroscience Lab at the Duke-NUS Graduate Medical School; Daniel Weissman of the University of Michigan Psychology Department; David Dinges of the University of Pennsylvania School of Medicine; and Vitali Zagorodnov of the Computer Engineering Department of the Nanyang Technological University in Singapore.

Section 10.2

Periodic Limb Movement Disorder

"Periodic Limb Movement Disorder," excerpted from Avidan, A.Y., and Zee, P.C., *A Handbook of Sleep Medicine and Management of Sleep Problems,* Philadelphia: Lippincott Williams & Wilkins, © 2006 Lippincott Williams and Wilkins; reprinted with permission. Reviewed by David A. Cooke, MD, FACP, March 2013.

What is periodic limb movement disorder?

Periodic limb movement disorder (PLMD) involves periodic episodes of repetitive movements, usually in the legs that occur approximately every twenty to forty seconds. The movements may appear as brief muscle twitches, jerking movements, or an upward flexing of the feet. These movements occur in clusters, lasting from a few minutes to a few hours. Most people with PLMD are not aware of the movements. PLMD can result in frequent brief arousals throughout the night, leading to daytime sleepiness. People with PLMD may also have restless legs syndrome, a movement disorder in which an individual experiences uncomfortable sensations in the legs during periods of rest or inactivity. The sensations are usually described as creepy, crawly, tingling, or painful, and can make it difficult to remain or stay at rest or fall asleep, or stay asleep.

What causes periodic limb movement disorder?

The cause of PLMD is not known, but it may be related to low iron content in midbrain cells. Also, individuals with conditions such as diabetes and kidney disease are at increased risk for developing PLMD. Pregnancy increases the incidence of ...

What are the symptoms of periodic limb movement disorder?

The symptoms of PLMD may include any of the following, although many with the condition do not report any symptoms:

- Leg movements: Leg movements or jerks are common in sleep characteristic of PLMD, but the person is usually not aware of these movements

Chapter 12

Sleep Deprivation and Medical Errors among Hospital Staff

The rate of serious medical errors committed by first-year doctors in training (interns) in two intensive care units (ICUs) at a Boston hospital fell significantly when traditional thirty-hour-in-a-row extended work shifts were eliminated and when interns' continuous work schedule was limited to sixteen hours, according to two complementary studies funded by the National Institute for Occupational Safety and Health (NIOSH) and the Agency for Healthcare Research and Quality (AHRQ).

The studies were published in the October 28, 2004, issue of the *New England Journal of Medicine*.

Interns made 36 percent more serious medical errors, including five times as many serious diagnostic errors, on the traditional schedule than on an intervention schedule that limited scheduled work shifts to sixteen hours and reduced scheduled weekly work from approximately eighty hours to sixty-three. The rate of serious medication errors was 21 percent greater on the traditional schedule than on the new schedule.

In the first research of its kind on the impact of lack of sleep on the safety of hospital care, researchers at Brigham and Women's Hospital in Boston eliminated the traditional schedule that required interns—doctors who have completed medical school and are finishing their medical training by working in the hospital—to work "extended duration work shifts" of approximately thirty consecutive hours every other shift.

"Medical Errors Decreased When Work Schedules for Interns Were Limited, NIOSH- and AHRQ-Funded Studies Find," Centers for Disease Control and Prevention, October 28, 2004. Editor's note added by David. A. Cooke MD, FACP, March 2010.

Under the traditional schedule, interns in hospital ICUs were scheduled to work approximately eighty hours per week. Under the intervention schedule that was tested in the studies, the "extended duration work shift" was eliminated and weekly scheduled work hours were decreased by approximately twenty hours. Interns also were encouraged to sleep on their time off and to take naps before night shifts.

"As NIOSH works with hospital administrators, physicians, nurses, and other partners to assess the impact of long working hours on health and performance, studies such as these will help us better identify steps to promote the health and well-being of health professionals, as well as the health and well-being of their patients," said John Howard, M.D., NIOSH director.

"The impact of sleep deprivation on performance has been well documented in other industries, but studies like these are providing evidence of its impact in health care," said Carolyn M. Clancy, M.D., AHRQ's director. "This research clearly demonstrates that changing the design and structure of the systems in which clinicians practice is essential to improving patient safety."

In this study, "Effect of Reducing Interns' Work Hours on Serious Medical Errors in Intensive Care Units," Christopher P. Landrigan, M.D., M.P.H., director of the Sleep and Patient Safety Program at Brigham and Women's Hospital, and his colleagues randomly assigned twenty-four interns to work either the traditional schedule in the cardiac care unit and the intervention schedule in the medical intensive care unit or the converse from July 2002 to June 2003.

The change in work schedule did not diminish interns' role in ICUs or shift the burden of work to more senior staff, according to the study authors. The number of medications ordered and tests interpreted by interns did not differ significantly. In addition, the error rates for more senior residents and other staff did not increase during the study.

The other study, "Effect of Reducing Interns' Weekly Work Hours on Sleep and Attentional Failures," examined the impact of the new work schedule on interns' sleep patterns and "attentional failures," characterized by nodding off while on duty, even while providing care to patients. Steven W. Lockley, Ph.D., and his colleagues studied twenty interns each in two three-week ICU rotations under both the traditional and intervention work schedules. Interns worked an average of 84.9 hours per week on the traditional schedule and 65.4 hours per week on the new schedule. They completed daily sleep and work logs that were validated through observation by study staff. In addition, interns were monitored using polysomnography, a device that can objectively document sleep and attentional failures.

The study found that under the new schedule interns worked 19.5 hours per week less, slept 5.8 hours per week more, and had typically slept more in the previous twenty-four hours when working. The percentage of work hours preceded by more than eight hours of sleep in the traditional schedule was 17 percent as compared with 33 percent for the new schedule. Overall, the rate of attentional failures was twice as high at night on the traditional schedule as on the intervention schedule.

The study concludes that interns who worked the intervention schedule were less sleep deprived at work and were able to sleep longer at home, which led to them having less cumulative and acute sleep deprivation. Interns on the new schedule were encouraged to take naps in the afternoon before overnight shifts to mitigate the effects of sleep deprivation on their ability to provide care.

Charles A. Czeisler, Ph.D., M.D., the senior author of both papers and professor of sleep medicine at Harvard Medical School, says, "While sleep experts advocate eight hours of sleep per twenty-four-hour period, it has historically been difficult to achieve in medicine, as patient care is an around-the-clock effort. These are the first studies to demonstrate clinically that reducing work shifts and tackling sleep deprivation will help increase attentiveness and reduce medical errors."

Editor's Note

Since the publication of the above articles, a number of additional studies have mostly, but not uniformly, confirmed that sleep deprivation among medical staff has negative impacts on patient safety and increased medical errors. The Accreditation Council on Graduate Medical Education (ACGME) instituted limits on resident work hours in 2003, in hopes of improving patient safety. Additional research is being conducted to better quantify the effects of sleep deprivation on medical errors and find better ways to protect patient safety.

Chapter 13

Sleep Deprivation among Public Safety Officers

When I speak to police officers about my research on sleep, job performance, and shift work, they always ask, "What's the best shift?"

I always answer, "That's the wrong question. Most shift arrangements have good and bad aspects." The right question is this: "What is the best way to manage shift work, keep our officers healthy, and maintain high performance in our organization?"

Scheduling and staffing around the clock requires finding a way to balance each organization's unique needs with those of its officers. Questions like "How many hours in a row should officers work?" and "How many officers are needed on which shift?" need to be balanced against "How much time off do officers need to rest and recuperate properly?" and "What's the best way to schedule those hours to keep employees safe and performing well?"

After all, shift work interferes with normal sleep and forces people to work at unnatural times of the day when their bodies are programmed to sleep. Sleep-loss-related fatigue degrades performance, productivity, and safety as well as health and well-being. Fatigue costs the U.S. economy $136 billion per year in health-related lost productivity alone.[1]

In the last decade, many managers in policing and corrections have begun to acknowledge—like their counterparts in other industries—that rotating shift work is inherently dangerous, especially when one works the graveyard shift. Managers in aviation, railroading, and trucking, for example, have had mandated hours-of-work laws for decades. And

Reprinted from "Sleep Deprivation: What Does It Mean for Public Safety Officers?" National Institute of Justice, U.S. Department of Justice, March 2009.

more recently they have begun to use complex mathematical models to manage fatigue-related risks.[2]

All of us experience the everyday stress associated with family life, health, and finances. Most of us also feel work-related stress associated with bad supervisors, long commutes, inadequate equipment, and difficult assignments. But police and corrections officers also must deal with the stresses of working shifts, witnessing or experiencing trauma, and managing dangerous confrontations.

My colleague, John Violanti, Ph.D., a twenty-three-year veteran of the New York State Police, is currently a professor in the Department of Social and Preventive Medicine at the University at Buffalo and an instructor with the Law Enforcement Wellness Association. His research shows that law enforcement officers are dying earlier than they should. The average age of death for police officers in his forty-year study was sixty-six years of age—a full ten years sooner than the norm.[3]

He and other researchers also found that police officers were much more likely than the general public to have higher-than-recommended cholesterol levels, higher-than-average pulse rates and diastolic blood pressure,[4] and much higher prevalence of sleep disorders.[5]

So what can we do to make police work healthier? Many things. One of the most effective strategies is to get enough sleep. It sounds simple, but it is not. More than half of police officers fail to get adequate rest, and they have 44 percent higher levels of obstructive sleep apnea than the general public.

More than 90 percent report being routinely fatigued, and 85 percent report driving while drowsy.[6]

Sleep deprivation is dangerous. Researchers have shown that being awake for nineteen hours produces impairments that are comparable to having a blood alcohol concentration (BAC) of .05 percent. Being awake for twenty-four hours is comparable to having a BAC of roughly .10 percent.[7] This means that in just five hours—the difference between going without sleep for nineteen hours versus twenty-four hours—the impact essentially doubles. (It should be noted that, in all fifty states and the District of Columbia, it is a crime to drive with a BAC of .08 percent or above.)

If you work a ten-hour shift, then attend court, then pick up your kids from school, drive home (hoping you do not fall asleep at the wheel), catch a couple hours of sleep, then get up and go back to work—and you do this for a week—you may be driving your patrol car while just as impaired as the last person you arrested for driving under the influence (DUI).

Bars and taverns are legally liable for serving too many drinks to people who then drive, have an accident, and kill someone. There is recent precedent for trucking companies and other employers being held responsible for drivers who cause accidents after working longer than permitted. It seems very likely that police departments eventually will be held responsible if an officer causes a death because he was too tired to drive home safely.

Sleep and fatigue are basic survival issues, just like patrol tactics, firearms safety, and pursuit driving. To reduce risks, stay alive, and keep healthy, officers and their managers have to work together to manage fatigue. Too-tired cops put themselves, their fellow officers, and the communities they serve at risk.

Accidental Deaths and Fatigue

The number of police officer deaths from both felonious assaults and accidents has decreased in recent years. Contrary to what most people might think, however, more officers die as a result of accidents than criminal assaults. Ninety-one percent of accidental deaths are caused by car crashes, being hit by vehicles while on foot, aircraft accidents, falls, or jumping.

We know that the rate of these accidents increases with lack of sleep and time of day. Researchers have shown that the risk increases considerably after a person has been on duty nine hours or more. After ten hours on duty, the risk increases by approximately 90 percent; after twelve hours, 110 percent.[8] The night shift has the greatest risk for accidents; they are almost three times more likely to happen during the night shift than the morning shift.

Countering Fatigue

Researchers who study officer stress, sleep, and performance have a number of techniques to counteract sleep deprivation and stress. They fall into two types:

- Things managers can do
- Things officers can do

The practices listed below have been well-received by departments that recognize that a tired cop is a danger both to himself and to the public.

Things Managers Can Do

- Review policies that affect overtime, moonlighting, and the number of consecutive hours a person can work. Make sure the policies keep shift rotation to a minimum and give officers adequate rest time. The Albuquerque (New Mexico) Police Department, for example, prohibits officers from working more than sixteen hours a day and limits overtime to twenty hours per week. This practice earned the Albuquerque team the Healthy Sleep Capital award from the National Sleep Foundation.

- Give officers a voice in decisions related to their work hours and shift scheduling. People's work hours affect every aspect of their lives. Increasing the amount of control and predictability in one's life improves a host of psychological and physical characteristics, including job satisfaction.

- Formally assess the level of fatigue officers experience, the quality of their sleep, and how tired they are while on the job, as well as their attitudes toward fatigue and work hours issues. Strategies include: administering sleep quality tests like those available on the National Sleep Foundation's Web site, and training supervisors to be alert for signs that officers are overly tired (for example, falling asleep during a watch briefing) and on how to deal with those who are too fatigued to work safely. Several Canadian police departments are including sleep screening in officers' annual assessments—something that every department should consider.

- Create a culture in which officers receive adequate information about the importance of good sleep habits, the hazards associated with fatigue and shift work, and strategies for managing them. For example, the Seattle Police Department has scheduled an all-day fatigue countermeasures training course for every sergeant, lieutenant, and captain. In the Calgary Police Service, management and union leaders are conducting a long-term, research-based program to find the best shift and scheduling arrangements and to change cultural attitudes about sleep and fatigue.

Things Officers Can Do

- Stay physically fit: Get enough exercise, maintain a healthy body weight, eat several fruits and vegetables a day, and stop smoking.

- Learn to use caffeine effectively by restricting routine intake to the equivalent of one or two eight-ounce cups of coffee a day. When you need to combat drowsiness, drink only one cup every hour or two; stop doses well before bedtime.[9]

- Exercise proper sleep hygiene. In other words, do everything possible to get seven or more hours of sleep every day. For example, go to sleep at the same time every day as much as possible; avoid alcohol just before bedtime; use room darkening curtains; make your bedroom a place for sleep, not for doing work or watching TV. Do not just doze off in an easy chair or on the sofa with the television on.

- If you have not been able to get enough sleep, try to take a nap before your shift. Done properly, a twenty-minute catnap is proven to improve performance, elevate mood, and increase creativity.

- If you are frequently fatigued, drowsy, snore, or have a large build, ask your doctor to check you for sleep apnea. Because many physicians have little training in sleep issues, it is a good idea to see someone who specializes in sleep medicine.

Notes

1. Ricci, J.A., E. Chee, A.L. Lorandeau, and J. Berger, "Fatigue in the U.S. Workforce: Prevalence and Implications for Lost Productive Work Time," *Journal of Occupational and Environmental Medicine* 49 (1) (2007): 1–10.

2. U.S. Department of Transportation/Federal Railroad Administration, Validation and Calibration of a Fatigue Assessment Tool for Railroad Work Schedules (pdf, 42 pages), Summary Report (2006) (DOT/FRA/ORD-06/21).

3. "Dying for the Job," in *Policing and Stress*, ed. H. Copes and M.L. Dantzker, Upper Saddle River, NJ: Pearson Prentice Hall, 2005: 87–102.

4. Merrill, M., "Cardiovascular Risk Among Police Officers" (master's thesis, State University of New York at Buffalo, n.d.).

5. Vila, B., and C. Samuels, "Sleep Problems in First Responders and the Military," in *Principles and Practice of Sleep Medicine*, 5th ed., ed. M.H. Kryger, T. Roth, and W.C. Dement, Philadelphia: Elsevier Saunders, 2010: Chapter 72.

6. National Law Enforcement and Corrections Technology Center, "No Rest for the Weary (pdf, 2 pages)," TechBeat (Winter 2008).

7. Dawson, D., and K. Reid, "Fatigue, Alcohol and Performance Impairment," *Nature* 388 (July 17, 1997): 235.

8. Folkard, S., and D.A. Lombardi, "Modeling the Impact of the Components of Long Work Hours on Injuries and 'Accidents,'" *American Journal of Industrial Medicine* 49 (11) (November 2006): 953–63.

9. Wesensten, N.J., "Pharmacological Management of Performance Deficits Resulting From Sleep Loss and Circadian Desynchrony," in *Principles and Practice of Sleep Medicine*, 5th ed., ed. M.H. Kryger, T. Roth, and W.C. Dement, Philadelphia: Elsevier Saunders, 2010: Chapter 73.

Chapter 14

Drowsy Driving

Introduction

The National Highway Traffic Safety Administration (NHTSA) conservatively estimates that 100,000 police-reported crashes are the direct result of driver fatigue each year, resulting in an estimated 1,500 deaths, 71,000 injuries, and $12.5 billion in monetary losses.

Definitions of drowsy driving generally involve varying uses and definitions of fatigue, sleepiness, and exhaustion. For the purpose of the discussion at hand, drowsy driving is simply driving in a physical state in which the driver's alertness is appreciably lower than it would be if the driver were "well rested" and "fully awake."

How serious of a problem is drowsy driving?

On the national level, the National Highway Traffic Safety Administration (NHTSA) conservatively estimates that 100,000 police-reported crashes are the direct result of driver fatigue each year, resulting in an estimated 1,500 deaths, 71,000 injuries, and $12.5 billion in monetary losses. However, it is very difficult to determine when fatigue causes or contributes to a traffic crash, and many experts believe these statistics understate the magnitude of the problem.

"FAQs: Drowsy Driving," © 2005 AAA Foundation for Traffic Safety (www .aaafoundation.org). Reprinted with permission. Although this document has an older date, the tips about drowsy driving are still pertinent to today's readers.

On the individual level, driving while tired is very dangerous, because a driver who falls asleep may crash head-on into another vehicle, a tree, or a wall, at full driving speed, without making any attempt to avoid the crash by steering or braking.

The inability of a sleeping driver to try to avoid crashing makes this type of crash especially severe. Some studies have found people's cognitive-psychomotor abilities to be as impaired after twenty-four hours without sleep as with a blood alcohol content (BAC) of 0.10 percent, which is higher than the legal limit for driving while under the influence (DWI) conviction in all U.S. states.

What are the warning signs of drowsy driving?

Some warning signs you may experience that signify drowsiness while driving are:

- the inability to recall the last few miles traveled;
- having disconnected or wandering thoughts;
- having difficulty focusing or keeping your eyes open;
- feeling as though your head is very heavy;
- drifting out of your driving lane, perhaps driving on the rumble strips;
- yawning repeatedly;
- accidentally tailgating other vehicles;
- missing traffic signs.

In fact, drowsy drivers sometimes drive so poorly that they might appear to be drunk. In a survey of police officers conducted by the AAA Foundation for Traffic Safety, nearly 90 percent of responding officers had at least once pulled over a driver who they expected to find intoxicated, but turned out to be sleepy (and not intoxicated).

What are the specific at-risk groups affected by drowsy driving?

The specific at-risk group for drowsy-driving-related crashes comprises people who drive after having not slept enough, qualitatively or quantitatively. If you're tired and you're driving, you are at risk. In general, individuals who are "most at-risk for being at-risk" of drowsy driving include:

- **Young people:** Sleep-related crashes are most common in young people, especially those who tend to stay up late, sleep too little, and drive at night—a dangerous combination. A study by the National Highway Traffic Safety Administration and the State of New York found that young drivers are more than four times more likely to have sleep-related crashes than are drivers over age thirty.

- **Shift workers and people with long work hours:** Shift workers and people who work long hours are at high risk of being involved in a sleep-related crash. The human body never fully adjusts to shift work, according to the National Sleep Foundation. The body's sleep and wake cycles are dictated by light and dark cycles, and generally will lead one to feel sleepy between midnight and 6 a.m.

- **People with undiagnosed or untreated sleep disorders:** Approximately forty million people are believed to have some kind of sleep disorder. Many different sleep disorders result in excessive daytime sleepiness, placing this group at high risk for sleep-related crashes. Common sleep disorders that often go unnoticed or undiagnosed include sleep apnea, narcolepsy, and restless leg syndrome.

- **Business travelers:** Business travelers struggle with jet lag, a common sleep disorder that causes sleepiness and negatively affects alertness. "Jet lag" as well as long work hours put these weary travelers at increased risk for sleep-related crashes.

Finally, it is important to realize that although these specific groups of people are statistically most likely to be involved in drowsy driving crashes, one who does not fall into any of these groups is by no means "immune" to drowsy driving. "Average drivers" who don't happen to be under age thirty, working the night shift, traveling for business, or suffering from sleep apnea are still at risk if they drive while fatigued.

Do people realize how dangerous it is to drive while drowsy?

According to AAA Foundation for Traffic Safety research, the public perceives drowsy driving to be an important cause of motor vehicle crashes. Three out of four non-crash-involved drivers, and four out of five of those in recent crashes, said that driver drowsiness was "very important" in causing crashes. These results place drowsy driving as being less of a contributor to crashes in the public's view than alcohol, but more important than poor weather conditions, speeding, or driver inexperience. Drowsy driving and aggressive driving, which have both received fairly widespread media attention, were rated about the same.

What can be done in advance to avoid drowsy driving altogether?

- **Get a good night's sleep:** The amount needed varies from individual to individual, but sleep experts recommend between seven and nine hours of sleep per night.

- **Plan to drive long trips with a companion:** Passengers can help look for early warning signs of fatigue, and switching drivers may be helpful. Passengers should stay awake and monitor the driver's condition.

- **Take regular breaks:** Schedule regular stops—every one hundred miles or two hours, even if you don't feel tired, and more often if you feel like you need it.

- **Avoid alcohol and medications:** If medications warn that they cause or may cause drowsiness, avoid taking them before driving. If you must take certain prescription medications that cause drowsiness, don't drive immediately after taking them. You should never consume alcohol before driving in the first place, but it is especially important to realize that alcohol interacts with fatigue, increasing sleepiness. If you are already tired, even a small quantity of alcohol may exacerbate your sleepiness and increase your risk of crashing, even if your BAC is well below the legal limit for a DWI conviction.

- **Consult your physician or a local sleep disorders center:** If you suffer frequent daytime sleepiness, experience difficulty sleeping at night, and/or snore loudly on a regular basis, consult your physician or local sleep disorders center for a diagnosis and treatment.

When are drowsy driving crashes most likely to occur?

As intuition dictates and data confirms, most sleep crashes occur in the "middle of the night," during the early morning hours. Less obviously, though, there is also a peak in sleep-related crashes in the mid-afternoon. Our natural circadian rhythms dictate that we will be most sleepy during the middle of our nighttime sleep period, and again about twelve hours later, between 2 p.m. and 4 p.m., and various studies show a peak in crashes believed to be related to sleep somewhere between 2 p.m. and 6 p.m.

What if I'm already driving and I start to feel tired? What should I do?

Take a nap. Naps are beneficial when experiencing drowsiness. Find a safe place (i.e., not the shoulder of the highway) where you can stop, park your car, and sleep for fifteen to twenty minutes. A nap longer than twenty minutes can make you groggy for at least fifteen minutes after awakening.

If you are planning a long trip, or routinely drive for long durations, identify safe places to stop and nap. If you have only a short distance remaining (e.g., an hour or so of driving), the nap might be enough to revive you. If you still have several hours of driving planned and you're already feeling tired, it would probably be best to find a bed for the night, get a full night's sleep, and then resume driving.

What about coffee? Won't that keep me awake?

Not necessarily. The "perk" that comes from drinking a cup of coffee may take a half hour or so to "kick in," is relatively short in duration, and will be less effective for those who regularly consume caffeine (i.e., most people). If you're very sleepy, and rely on caffeine to allow you to continue driving, you are likely to experience "microsleeps," in which you doze off for four or five seconds, which doesn't sound like long, but is still plenty of time to drive off of the road or over the center line and crash.

Should I open the window or turn up the radio to fight fatigue on the road?

No. Some of these tricks may help you to feel more alert for an instant; however, they are not effective ways to maintain an acceptable level of alertness for long enough to drive anywhere. Even with the window rolled all the way down and radio cranked up, if you're sleepy, you're still an unnecessarily great hazard to yourself and to everybody else on the road. If you're sleepy enough that you're seeking special measures to stay awake, you should have stopped driving already. Look for a safe and secure place, park the car, and take a nap.

Are there any devices I can buy that will keep me awake while I'm driving?

There are a few devices on the market, some of which are worn on your body or placed in your car, that are advertised to keep drowsy drivers awake; however, to our knowledge, none of them have been scientifically validated yet. The only driver warning mechanism that has been validated to date is the shoulder rumble strip, which produces noise and mechanical vibration if your vehicle drives on it. If you start driving onto the rumble strip, this is an indication that you are too tired to drive safely. You should not rely on the rumble strip to alert you every time you begin to doze off and drive off course—rumble strips won't prevent you from crashing into other cars.

Part Three

Sleep Disorders

Chapter 15

Breathing Disorders of Sleep

Chapter Contents

Section 15.1

Sleep Apnea

Reprinted from "Sleep Apnea," National Heart Lung and Blood Institute, National Institutes of Health, May 2009.

What Is Sleep Apnea?

Sleep apnea is a common disorder in which you have one or more pauses in breathing or shallow breaths while you sleep.

Breathing pauses can last from a few seconds to minutes. They often occur five to thirty times or more an hour. Typically, normal breathing then starts again, sometimes with a loud snort or choking sound.

Sleep apnea usually is a chronic (ongoing) condition that disrupts your sleep three or more nights each week. You often move out of deep sleep and into light sleep when your breathing pauses or becomes shallow.

This results in poor sleep quality that makes you tired during the day. Sleep apnea is one of the leading causes of excessive daytime sleepiness.

Overview

Sleep apnea often goes undiagnosed. Doctors usually can't detect the condition during routine office visits. Also, there are no blood tests for the condition.

Most people who have sleep apnea don't know they have it because it occurs only during sleep. A family member or bed partner may first notice the signs of sleep apnea.

The most common type of sleep apnea is obstructive sleep apnea. This most often means that the airway has collapsed or is blocked during sleep. The blockage may cause shallow breathing or breathing pauses.

When you try to breathe, any air that squeezes past the blockage can cause loud snoring. Obstructive sleep apnea happens more often in people who are overweight, but it can affect anyone.

Central sleep apnea is a less common type of sleep apnea. It happens when the area of your brain that controls your breathing doesn't send the correct signals to your breathing muscles. You make no effort to breathe for brief periods.

Central sleep apnea often occurs with obstructive sleep apnea, but it can occur alone. Snoring doesn't typically happen with central sleep apnea.

This section mainly focuses on obstructive sleep apnea.

Outlook

Untreated sleep apnea can do the following things:

- Increase the risk for high blood pressure, heart attack, stroke, obesity, and diabetes

- Increase the risk for or worsen heart failure

- Make irregular heartbeats more likely

- Increase the chance of having work-related or driving accidents

Lifestyle changes, mouthpieces, surgery, or breathing devices can successfully treat sleep apnea in many people.

Other Names for Sleep Apnea

- Sleep-disordered breathing

- Cheyne-Stokes breathing

What Causes Sleep Apnea?

When you're awake, throat muscles help keep your airway stiff and open so air can flow into your lungs. When you sleep, these muscles are more relaxed. Normally, the relaxed throat muscles don't stop your airway from staying open to allow air into your lungs.

But if you have obstructive sleep apnea, your airways can be blocked or narrowed during sleep for the following reasons:

- Your throat muscles and tongue relax more than normal.

- Your tongue and tonsils (tissue masses in the back of your mouth) are large compared to the opening into your windpipe.

- You're overweight. The extra soft fat tissue can thicken the wall of the windpipe. This causes the inside opening to narrow and makes it harder to keep open.

143

- The shape of your head and neck (bony structure) may cause a smaller airway size in the mouth and throat area.

- The aging process limits the ability of brain signals to keep your throat muscles stiff during sleep. This makes it more likely that the airway will narrow or collapse.

Not enough air flows into your lungs when your airways are fully or partly blocked during sleep. This can cause loud snoring and a drop in your blood oxygen levels.

When the oxygen drops to dangerous levels, it triggers your brain to disturb your sleep. This helps tighten the upper airway muscles and open your windpipe. Normal breaths then start again, often with a loud snort or choking sound.

The frequent drops in oxygen levels and reduced sleep quality trigger the release of stress hormones. These compounds raise your heart rate and increase your risk for high blood pressure, heart attack, stroke, and irregular heartbeats. The hormones also raise the risk for or worsen heart failure.

Untreated sleep apnea also can lead to changes in how your body uses energy. These changes increase your risk for obesity and diabetes.

Who Is at Risk for Sleep Apnea?

It's estimated that more than twelve million American adults have obstructive sleep apnea. More than half of the people who have this condition are overweight.

Sleep apnea is more common in men. One out of twenty-five middle-aged men and one out of fifty middle-aged women have sleep apnea.

Sleep apnea becomes more common as you get older. At least one out of ten people over the age of sixty has sleep apnea. Women are much more likely to develop sleep apnea after menopause.

African Americans, Hispanics, and Pacific Islanders are more likely to develop sleep apnea than Caucasians.

If someone in your family has sleep apnea, you're more likely to develop it.

People who have small airways in their noses, throats, or mouths also are more likely to have sleep apnea. Smaller airways may be due to the shape of these structures or allergies or other medical conditions that cause congestion in these areas.

Small children often have enlarged tonsil tissues in the throat. This can make them prone to developing sleep apnea.

Other risk factors for sleep apnea include smoking, high blood pressure, and risk factors for stroke or heart failure.

What Are the Signs and Symptoms of Sleep Apnea?

Major Signs and Symptoms

One of the most common signs of obstructive sleep apnea is loud and chronic (ongoing) snoring. Pauses may occur in the snoring. Choking or gasping may follow the pauses.

The snoring usually is loudest when you sleep on your back; it may be less noisy when you turn on your side. Snoring may not happen every night. Over time, the snoring may happen more often and get louder.

You're asleep when the snoring or gasping occurs. You will likely not know that you're having problems breathing or be able to judge how severe the problem is. Your family members or bed partner will often notice these problems before you do.

Not everyone who snores has sleep apnea.

Another common sign of sleep apnea is fighting sleepiness during the day, at work, or while driving. You may find yourself rapidly falling asleep during the quiet moments of the day when you're not active.

Other Signs and Symptoms

Other signs and symptoms of sleep apnea may include the following:

- Morning headaches
- Memory or learning problems and not being able to concentrate
- Feeling irritable, depressed, or having mood swings or personality changes
- Urination at night
- A dry throat when you wake up

In children, sleep apnea can cause hyperactivity, poor school performance, and aggressiveness. Children who have sleep apnea also may have unusual sleeping positions, bedwetting, and may breathe through their mouths instead of their noses during the day.

How Is Sleep Apnea Diagnosed?

Doctors diagnose sleep apnea based on your medical and family histories, a physical exam, and results from sleep studies. Usually, your primary care doctor evaluates your symptoms first. He or she then decides whether you need to see a sleep specialist.

These specialists are doctors who diagnose and treat people with sleep problems. Such doctors include lung; nerve; or ear, nose, and throat specialists. Other types of doctors also can be sleep specialists.

145

Medical and Family Histories

Your doctor will ask you and your family questions about how you sleep and how you function during the day. To help your doctor, consider keeping a sleep diary for one to two weeks. Write down how much you sleep each night, as well as how sleepy you feel at various times during the day.

Your doctor also will want to know how loudly and often you snore or make gasping or choking sounds during sleep. Often you're not aware of such symptoms and must ask a family member or bed partner to report them.

If you're a parent of a child who may have sleep apnea, tell your child's doctor about your child's signs and symptoms.

Let your doctor know if anyone in your family has been diagnosed with sleep apnea or has had symptoms of the disorder.

Many people aren't aware of their symptoms and aren't diagnosed.

Physical Exam

Your doctor will check your mouth, nose, and throat for extra or large tissues. The tonsils often are enlarged in children with sleep apnea. A physical exam and medical history may be all that's needed to diagnose sleep apnea in children.

Adults with the condition may have an enlarged uvula or soft palate. The uvula is the tissue that hangs from the middle of the back of your mouth. The soft palate is the roof of your mouth in the back of your throat.

Sleep Studies

A sleep study is the most accurate test for diagnosing sleep apnea. It captures what happens with your breathing while you sleep.

A sleep study is often done in a sleep center or sleep lab, which may be part of a hospital. You may stay overnight in the sleep center.

Polysomnogram

A polysomnogram (poly-SOM-no-gram), or PSG, is the most common study for diagnosing sleep apnea. This test records the following things:

- Brain activity

- Eye movement and other muscle activity

- Breathing and heart rate

- How much air moves in and out of your lungs while you're sleeping

- The amount of oxygen in your blood

A PSG is painless. You will go to sleep as usual, except you will have sensors on your scalp, face, chest, limbs, and finger. The staff at the sleep center will use the sensors to check on you throughout the night.

A sleep specialist reviews the results of your PSG to see whether you have sleep apnea and how severe it is. He or she will use the results to plan your treatment.

How Is Sleep Apnea Treated?

Goals of Treatment

The goals of treating obstructive sleep apnea are as follows:

- To restore regular breathing during sleep

- To relieve symptoms such as loud snoring and daytime sleepiness

Treatment may help other medical problems linked to sleep apnea, such as high blood pressure. Treatment also can reduce your risk for heart disease, stroke, and diabetes.

Specific Types of Treatment

Lifestyle changes, mouthpieces, breathing devices, or surgery are used to treat sleep apnea. Currently, there are no medicines to treat sleep apnea.

If you have sleep apnea, talk to your doctor or sleep specialist about the treatment options that are most appropriate for your specific condition.

Lifestyle changes or mouthpieces may be enough to relieve mild sleep apnea. People who have moderate or severe sleep apnea may need breathing devices or surgery.

Lifestyle Changes

If you have mild sleep apnea, some changes in daily activities or habits may be all that you need:

- Avoid alcohol and medicines that make you sleepy. They make it harder for your throat to stay open while you sleep.

- Lose weight if you're overweight or obese. Even a little weight loss can improve your symptoms.

- Sleep on your side instead of your back to help keep your throat open. You can sleep with special pillows or shirts that prevent you from sleeping on your back.

- Keep your nasal passages open at night with nose sprays or allergy medicines, if needed. Talk to your doctor about whether these treatments might help you.

- Stop smoking.

Mouthpiece

A mouthpiece, sometimes called an oral appliance, may help some people who have mild sleep apnea. Your doctor also may recommend a mouthpiece if you snore loudly but don't have sleep apnea.

A dentist or orthodontist can make a custom-fit plastic mouthpiece for treating sleep apnea. (An orthodontist specializes in correcting teeth or jaw problems.) The mouthpiece will adjust your lower jaw and your tongue to help keep your airways open while you sleep.

If you use a mouthpiece, it's important that you check with your doctor about discomfort or pain while using the device. You may need periodic office visits so your doctor can adjust your mouthpiece to fit better.

Breathing Devices

Continuous positive airway pressure (CPAP) is the most common treatment for moderate to severe sleep apnea in adults. A CPAP machine uses a mask that fits over your mouth and nose, or just over your nose. The machine gently blows air into your throat.

The air presses on the wall of your airway. The air pressure is adjusted so that it's just enough to stop the airways from becoming narrowed or blocked during sleep.

Treating sleep apnea may help you stop snoring. But stopping snoring doesn't mean that you no longer have sleep apnea or can stop using CPAP. Sleep apnea will return if CPAP is stopped or not used correctly.

Usually, a technician will come to your home to bring the CPAP equipment. The technician will set up the CPAP machine and adjust it based on your doctor's orders. After the initial setup, you may need to have the CPAP adjusted on occasion for the best results.

CPAP treatment may cause side effects in some people. These side effects include a dry or stuffy nose, irritated skin on your face, sore eyes, and headaches. If your CPAP isn't properly adjusted, you may get stomach bloating and discomfort while wearing the mask.

If you're having trouble with CPAP side effects, work with your sleep specialist, his or her nursing staff, and the CPAP technician. Together, you can take steps to reduce these side effects. These steps include adjusting the CPAP settings or the size and fit of the mask, or adding moisture to the air as it flows through the mask. A nasal spray may relieve a dry, stuffy, or runny nose.

There are many different kinds of CPAP machines and masks. Be sure to tell your doctor if you're not happy with the type you're using. He or she may suggest switching to a different kind that may work better for you.

People who have severe sleep apnea symptoms generally feel much better once they begin treatment with CPAP.

Surgery

Some people who have sleep apnea may benefit from surgery. The type of surgery and how well it works depend on the cause of the sleep apnea.

Surgery is done to widen breathing passages. It usually involves removing, shrinking, or stiffening excess tissue in the mouth and throat or resetting the lower jaw.

Surgery to shrink or stiffen excess tissue in the mouth or throat is done in a doctor's office or a hospital. Shrinking tissue may involve small shots or other treatments to the tissue. A series of such treatments may be needed to shrink the excess tissue. To stiffen excess tissue, the doctor makes a small cut in the tissue and inserts a small piece of stiff plastic.

Surgery to remove excess tissue is done only in a hospital. You're given medicine that makes you sleep during the surgery. After surgery, you may have throat pain that lasts for one to two weeks.

Surgery to remove the tonsils, if they're blocking the airway, may be very helpful for some children. Your child's doctor may suggest waiting some time to see whether these tissues shrink on their own. This is common as small children grow.

Living with Sleep Apnea

Obstructive sleep apnea can be very serious. However, following an effective treatment plan can often improve your quality of life quite a bit.

Treatment can improve your sleep and relieve daytime tiredness. It also may make you less likely to develop high blood pressure, heart disease, and other health problems linked to sleep apnea.

Treatment may improve your overall health and happiness as well as your quality of sleep (and possibly your family's quality of sleep).

Ongoing Healthcare Needs

Follow up with your doctor regularly to make sure your treatment is working. Tell him or her if the treatment is causing side effects that you can't handle.

This ongoing care is especially important if you're getting continuous positive airway pressure (CPAP) treatment. It may take a while before you adjust to using CPAP.

If you aren't comfortable with your CPAP device or it doesn't seem to be working, let your doctor know. You may need to switch to a different device or mask. Or, you may need treatment to relieve CPAP side effects.

Try not to gain weight. Weight gain can worsen sleep apnea and require adjustments to your CPAP device. In contrast, weight loss may relieve your sleep apnea.

Until your sleep apnea is properly treated, know the dangers of driving or operating heavy machinery while sleepy.

If you're having any type of surgery that requires medicine to put you to sleep, let your surgeon and doctors know you have sleep apnea. They might have to take extra steps to make sure your airway stays open during the surgery.

How Can Family Members Help?

Often, people with sleep apnea don't know they have it. They're not aware that their breathing stops and starts many times while they're sleeping. Family members or bed partners usually are the first to notice signs of sleep apnea.

Family members can do many things to help a loved one who has sleep apnea:

- Let the person know if he or she snores loudly during sleep or has breathing stops and starts.

- Encourage the person to get medical help.

- Help the person follow the doctor's treatment plan, including CPAP.

- Provide emotional support.

Key Points

- Sleep apnea is a common breathing disorder in which you have one or more pauses in breathing or shallow breaths while you sleep.

- Sleep apnea usually is a chronic (ongoing) condition that disrupts your sleep three or more nights each week.

- Sleep apnea often goes undiagnosed. Doctors usually can't detect the condition during routine office visits. Also, there are no blood tests for the condition. Most people who have sleep apnea don't know they have it because it only occurs during sleep.

- The most common type of sleep apnea is obstructive sleep apnea. This most often means that the airway has collapsed or is blocked during sleep. This may cause shallow breathing or breathing pauses.

- Sleep apnea can cause daytime sleepiness, increase the risk for or worsen some medical conditions, and increase the chance of having a work- or driving-related accident.

- It's estimated that more than twelve million American adults have sleep apnea. More than half of the people who have this condition are overweight.

- The most common signs of sleep apnea are loud snoring and choking or gasping during sleep and being very sleepy during the day.

- Doctors diagnose sleep apnea based on your medical and family histories, a physical exam, and results from sleep studies.

- Treatment is aimed at restoring regular breathing during sleep and relieving symptoms. Treatment also may help other medical problems linked to sleep apnea.

- Lifestyle changes, mouthpieces, breathing devices, or surgery are used to treat sleep apnea. Continuous positive airway pressure (CPAP) is the most common treatment for moderate to severe sleep apnea.

- Sleep apnea can be very serious. However, following an effective treatment plan can often improve your quality of life quite a bit. Follow up with your doctor regularly to make sure your treatment is working. Tell him or her if the treatment causes side effects that you can't handle.

- Family members can help a person who snores loudly or stops breathing during sleep by encouraging him or her to get medical help.

- Treatment may improve your overall health and happiness as well as your quality of sleep (and possibly your family's quality of sleep).

Section 15.2

Snoring

Definition

Snoring is a loud, hoarse, or harsh breathing sound that occurs during sleep.

Considerations

Snoring is common in adults and is not necessarily a sign of an underlying disorder.

Sometimes, however, snoring can be a sign of a sleep disorder called sleep apnea. This means you have periods when you are not breathing for more than ten seconds while you sleep. The episode is followed by a sudden snort or gasp when breathing resumes. Then, snoring starts all over again. If you have sleep apnea, this cycle generally happens several times a night. Sleep apnea is not as common as snoring.

A doctor (or a sleep specialist) can tell if you have sleep apnea by doing a sleep study either at home or in a hospital setting.

Snoring is an important social problem. Persons who share a bed with someone who snores can develop sleep difficulties.

Causes

In most people, the reason for snoring is not known. Some potential causes (other than sleep apnea) include:

- being overweight, which leads to excessive neck tissue that puts pressure on the airways;

- last month of pregnancy;

- nasal congestion from colds or allergies, especially if it lasts a long time;

- swelling of the muscular part of the roof of the mouth (soft palate) or uvula, the piece of tissue that hangs down in the back of the mouth;

- swollen adenoids and tonsils that block the airways;

- use of sleeping pills, antihistamines, or alcohol at bedtime.

Home Care

The following tips can help reduce snoring:

- Avoid alcohol and other sedatives at bedtime.

- Don't sleep flat on your back. Sleep on your side, if possible. Some doctors even suggest sewing a golf or tennis ball into the back of your night clothes. This causes discomfort if you roll over and helps reminds you to stay on your side. Eventually, sleeping on your side becomes a habit and you don't need to be reminded.

- Lose weight, if you are overweight.

- Try over-the-counter, drug-free nasal strips that help widen the nostrils. (These are not intended as treatments for sleep apnea.)

When to Contact a Medical Professional

Talk to your doctor if you have:

- excessive daytime drowsiness, morning headaches, recent weight gain, awakening in the morning not feeling rested, or change in your level of attention, concentration, or memory;

- episodes of no breathing (apnea)—your partner may need to tell you if this is happening.

Children with chronic snoring should also be evaluated for apnea. Sleep apnea in children has been linked to growth problems, attention deficit hyperactivity disorder (ADHD), poor school performance, learning difficulties, bedwetting, and high blood pressure. Most children who snore do *not* have apnea, but a sleep study is the only reliable way to tell for sure.

What to Expect at Your Office Visit

Your doctor will ask questions to evaluate your snoring and perform a physical exam, paying careful attention to your throat, mouth, and neck.

Questions may include the following (some of which your partner might have to answer):

- Is your snoring loud?

- Does it occur no matter what position you are lying in or only in certain positions?

- Does your own snoring ever wake you up?

- How often do you snore? Every night?

- Is your snoring persistent during the night?

- Are there episodes when you are not breathing?

- Do you have other symptoms like daytime drowsiness, morning headaches, insomnia, or memory loss?

Referral to a sleep specialist for sleep studies may be needed. Treatment options include:

- dental appliances to prevent tongue from falling back;

- palatoplasty—stiffening of the palate using surgery or injection;

- use of a continuous positive airway pressure (CPAP) mask (a device you wear on the nose while sleeping to decrease snoring and sleep apnea);

- surgery (for example, correction of a deviated septum);

- weight loss.

References

Friedman M, Schalch P. Surgery of the palate and oropharynx. *Otolaryngol Clin North Am*. 2007 Aug;40 (4):829–43.

Patil SP, Schneider H, Schwartz AR, Smith PL. Adult obstructive sleep apnea: pathophysiology and diagnosis. *Chest*. 2007 Jul; 132 (1): 325–37.

Basner RC. Continuous positive airway pressure for obstructive sleep apnea. *N Engl J Med*. 2007 Apr 26; 356 (17):1751–58.

Chapter 16

Circadian Rhythm Disorders

Chapter Contents

Section 16.1

Advanced Sleep Phase Disorder

Delayed sleep phase syndrome (DSPS) is characterized by the habitual need to go to sleep later than usual with a corresponding late awakening time. This causes shift workers much difficulty with early work starting times as well as when they need to retard their sleep habits during schedule changes. For our purposes, we refer to these people as "owls."

Likewise, advanced sleep phase syndrome (ASPS) causes difficulty with persons who must stay up later than usual. ASPS is usually found in people who would call themselves "morning people" or "larks." Larks generally find it easy to go to sleep early, and love to get up early. Larks are full of energy in the morning, love to talk, (and generally make life miserable for those who need time in the morning to "warm up.")

There is a fundamental difference between the way larks and owls adjust to changing schedules. Whereas the owl (who stays up late) simply sleeps longer in response to a delayed bedtime, the lark will still get up at the same time in the morning regardless of the time they went to bed. This makes it extremely difficult for the lark (or person afflicted with ASPS) to adjust to changing schedules. After a few days of going to sleep later than usual, they accumulate sleep deprivation.

Scientists have found that exposing the subject to artificial light strong enough to resemble daylight can alter circadian rhythms. The reason that light therapy works as well as it does is that light affects the pineal gland. The pineal gland secretes melatonin, which helps us sleep. When light is taken away, the secretion of melatonin increases and we begin to get drowsy.

It is thought that in people who have ASPS, the connection between light, the pineal gland, and melatonin secretion is so strong that almost immediately as the sun goes down, melatonin production starts up and the poor ASPS sufferer immediately begins to think that it's bedtime. This may have worked fine for farmers of the nineteenth century, but in today's society (and especially the twenty-four-hour society) it is a real problem.

ASPS may be corrected through exposure to bright light for two hours during the evening, which may shift the body's circadian timing mechanism and delay the onset of sleep until a typical bedtime. Some may ask why typical house lighting in the evening won't keep them awake until bedtime. That is because normal house lighting is well below the level of daylight. In order for light therapy to be effective, the intensity must be at least five times the level of normal house lighting. That means you need an illumination system that is in the neighborhood of 2,500 lux.

But how do we keep the ASPS sufferer from getting up too soon? Remember, with ASPS, the person is likely to get up when the sun comes up regardless of when they went to sleep. The reverse of evening light therapy may be in order. Blackout shades or sleep masks may be prescribed for those who find themselves fully awake as soon as the bedroom gets light in the morning. Empirical evidence indicated this to be quite effective.

If you are experiencing chronic insomnia that originates from a problem of the circadian timing system or any other of a number of causes, it is important to find the underlying reason. There may be more than one cause of a sleep disorder, and they may be difficult to identify. Drug therapy (such as melatonin) may be helpful for a short time, but behavioral modifications in tandem with helpful drugs can be even more effective. It is important to consult with a medical and/or behavior expert to determine the best course of treatment for you.

A typical course of action is to have the patient keep a sleep diary for two weeks. Depending on the findings, a discussion of sleep hygiene could be the first step. For instance, moderate-intensity exercise may be advised, such as brisk walking or low-impact aerobics. Some experts also advise their patients to eliminate habits that aren't compatible with sleep, such as lying in bed and worrying.

The subject of sleep disorders and their treatment is fascinating, and new information continuously comes to light. For the shift worker who suffers from DSPS, ASPS, or other sleep-related problems it is important to know that there are treatments that can help.

Section 16.2

Delayed Sleep Phase Disorder

"Delayed Sleep Phase Syndrome," excerpted from Mindell, J.A. and Owens J.A., *A Clinical Guide to Pediatric Sleep: Diagnosis and Management of Sleep Problems*, Philadelphia: Lippincott Williams & Wilkins. © 2003 Lippincott Williams and Wilkins. Reprinted with permission. Reviewed by David A. Cooke, MD, FACP, March 2010.

What is delayed sleep phase syndrome?

Delayed sleep phase syndrome (DSPS) is a disorder in which the person's sleep wake cycle (internal clock) is delayed by two or more hours. Basically, it is a shift of the internal clock by two or more hours, in that sleep is postponed. For example, rather than falling asleep at 10 p.m. and waking at 7 a.m., an adolescent or adult with DSPS will not fall asleep until 12 a.m. or later and then has great difficulty awakening at 7 a.m. for school or work. If the individual is allowed to sleep until late in the morning, he will feel rested and can function well. Most with DSPS describe themselves as "night owls" and usually feel and function their best in the evening and nighttime hours. They usually get much less sleep on weekdays than on weekends or holidays. Having DSPS, especially adolescents who attend school, can cause significant problems, as they are unable to get up for school or work, often resulting in multiple absences and tardiness, and may perform poorly.

What causes delayed sleep phase syndrome?

Delayed sleep phase syndrome usually develops during adolescence but can start in childhood. It seldom occurs after the age of thirty. Although the cause of DSPS is not completely known, it likely is an exaggerated reaction to the normal shift in sleep times that occurs during adolescence. All adolescents have a shift in their internal clock after puberty of about two hours. In those with DSPS, the clock shifts even more. In addition, for persons who already had a tendency to go to bed late, this normal two-hour shift results in a significantly shifted internal clock. It is important to realize that this shift in sleep is not caused by deliberate behavior. Unfortunately, many with DSPS get labeled as noncompliant, truants, or poor performers. Approximately 7 percent of adolescents have DSPS; thus, it is a common disorder.

What are the symptoms of delayed sleep phase syndrome?

A person with DSPS often experiences the following symptoms:

- **Daytime sleepiness:** Because of the late sleep-onset times and the usual requirement to get up earlier than desired for school or work, individuals with DSPS often experience daytime sleepiness as the result of not getting enough sleep.

- **Inability to fall asleep at the desired time:** On nights that individuals with DSPS try to go to sleep at a "normal" time, they are unable to do so. However, if they were to go to bed at their usual fall-asleep time, they would have no problem falling asleep.

- **Inability to wake up at the desired time:** As a result of the late sleep-onset time, many with DSPS are unable to wake up in the morning for school, work, or other activities. This can result in many absences or latenesses.

- **No other sleep complaints:** Because the internal clock is simply shifted in people with DSPS, once asleep they sleep well with few or no awakenings. In addition, on days that they are able to sleep as long as they wish, especially on weekends or holidays, sleep is normal, and daytime sleepiness is not experienced.

- **Other daytime symptoms:** Some with DSPS experience problems with depression and other behavior problems as a result of the daytime sleepiness and the effects of missing school, work, and social activities. In addition, there are a percentage of adolescents with DSPS who have school refusal, which complicates both diagnosis and treatment.

How is delayed sleep phase syndrome diagnosed?

There is no definitive test for DSPS, so the diagnosis is made based on a description of the problem. An overnight sleep study may be recommended to ensure that no other sleep disorder is present, such as obstructive sleep apnea or restless legs syndrome/periodic limb movement disorder.

How is delayed sleep phase syndrome treated?

Delayed sleep phase syndrome is a difficult disorder to treat and requires significant effort on the part of the patient. Thus, for treatment to be successful, the person has to be very motivated. The goal of treatment is to retrain the internal clock to a more regular schedule. However, making the initial shift in the sleep-wake cycle is easier than maintaining that change. Treatment can involve the following:

- **Sleep hygiene:** Good sleep habits are especially important for individuals with DSPS. These habits should include a regular sleep schedule that encompasses going to bed and waking up at the same time every day; avoidance of caffeine, smoking, and other drugs; a bedroom environment that is cool, quiet, and comfortable; a bedtime routine that is calm and sleep inducing; and avoidance of all stimulating activities before bed, such as computer games and television.

- **Shifting the internal clock:** Treatment for DSPS involves systematically advancing or delaying bedtime on successive nights.

- **Phase advancement:** Phase advancement involves moving the bedtime earlier by fifteen minutes on successive nights. If the individual usually falls asleep at 12:30, then bedtime is set for 12:15 for one or two nights, 12:00 for one to two nights, and so on.

- **Phase delay (chronotherapy):** Phase delay is chosen if their naturally occurring bedtime is three or more hours later than desired. Bedtime is delayed by two to three hours on successive nights. For example, if one usually falls asleep at 2 a.m., bedtime is delayed until 4 a.m. on night one, 6 a.m. on night two, and so on until the desired bedtime is reached (e.g., 10:30 p.m.). Given that it is much easier for the body to adjust to a later bedtime than an earlier one, it is often recommended to delay bedtime rather than try to advance it.

- **Sticking with it:** Once the desired bedtime is reached, the person must stick with it on a nightly basis. Even one night of late-night studying or socializing can return the internal clock to the delayed state. However, usually after several months the schedule can become a bit more flexible.

- **Bright-light therapy:** Sometimes bright-light therapy is recommended, which involves exposing the patient to bright light in the morning for approximately twenty to thirty minutes, and avoiding bright light in the evening. Bright light in the morning helps to reset the body's internal clock. Special light boxes must be purchased for this treatment.

Section 16.3

Irregular Sleep-Wake Syndrome

Irregular sleep-wake syndrome involves different and disorganized periods of sleeping and wakeful behavior.

Causes

Some people have an irregular sleep-wake pattern because of a problem with brain function, the body's internal clock (circadian pacemaker), or other reasons.

This disorder is very uncommon. It typically occurs in someone with a brain dysfunction who does not have a regular routine during the day. The amount of total sleep time is normal, but the body clock loses its normal circadian cycle.

Similar symptoms may be seen in people who have frequently changing work shifts and in travelers who often change time zones. These people have a different condition, such as shift work sleep disorder or jet lag syndrome.

Exams and Tests

People with irregular sleep-wake syndrome may have either insomnia or excessive sleepiness. Patients usually have at least three abnormal sleep episodes during a twenty-four-hour period, but their total amount of sleep time is considered normal for their age.

When to Contact a Medical Professional

Most people may occasionally have disturbances in their sleep. However, if this type of irregular sleep-wake pattern occurs regularly and without cause, you may consider consulting your health care provider.

Alternative Names

Sleep-wake syndrome—irregular

Section 16.4

Jet Lag

Reprinted from "Jet Lag," *2010 Yellow Book*, Centers for
Disease Control and Prevention, July 27, 2009.

Jet lag is a temporary disorder among air travelers who rapidly travel across three or more time zones. Jet lag results from the slow adjustment of the body clock to the destination time, so that daily rhythms and the internal drive for sleep and wakefulness are out of synchrony with the new environment.

The intrinsic body clock resides in the suprachiasmatic nuclei at the base of the hypothalamus, which contains melatonin receptors. The body clock receives information about light from the eyes and is also thought to receive input via the intergeniculate leaflet that carries information about physical activities and general excitement. Melatonin is manufactured in the pineal gland from tryptophan, and its synthesis and release are stimulated by darkness and suppressed by light; consequently, the secretion of melatonin is responsible for setting our sleep-wake cycle. The body clock is adjusted to the solar day by rhythmic cues in the environment known as zeitgebers (time-givers). The main zeitgebers are the light-dark cycle and this rhythmic secretion of melatonin. Exercise might also exert a weaker effect on the body clock than other zeitgebers. Although incompletely understood, the body clock is partly responsible for the daily rhythms in core temperature and plasma hormone concentrations as well.

Occurrence

- Eastward travel is associated with difficulty in falling asleep at the destination bedtime and difficulty arising in the morning.

- Westward travel is associated with early evening sleepiness and predawn awakening.

- Travelers flying within the same time zone typically experience the fewest problems.

- Crossing more time zones or traveling eastward generally increases the time required for adaptation.

- Jet lag lasts for several days, roughly equal to two-thirds the number of time zones crossed for eastward flights, and about half the number of time zones crossed after westward flights.

Risk for Travelers

Individual responses to crossing time zones and the ability to adapt to new time zones vary. The intensity and duration of jet lag are related to the following:

- Number of time zones crossed

- Direction of travel

- Ability to sleep while traveling

- Availability and intensity of local circadian time cues at the destination

- Individual differences in phase tolerance

Although more data are needed, risk factors cited by the American Academy of Sleep Medicine include the following:

- Older individuals tend to experience fewer jet lag symptoms than those who are younger.

- Exposure to local (natural) light-dark cycle usually accelerates adaptation after jet travel over two to ten time zones.

Clinical Presentation

Signs of jet lag include the following:

- Poor sleep, including delayed sleep onset (after eastward flight), early awakening (after westward flight), and fractionated sleep (after flights in either direction).

- Poor performance in both physical and mental tasks during the new daytime.

- Negative subjective changes, such as increased fatigue, frequency of headaches and irritability, and decreased ability to concentrate.

- Gastrointestinal disturbances (indigestion, frequency of defecation, and the altered consistency of stools) and decreased interest in and enjoyment of meals.

Preventive Measures for Travelers

Prior to Travel

- Stay healthy by continuing to exercise, eating a nutritious diet, and getting plenty of rest.
- Consider timed bright light exposure prior to and during travel (although it requires high motivation and strict compliance with the prescribed light-dark schedules).
- Break up the journey with a stop-over.

Note: The use of the nutritional supplement melatonin is controversial for the prevention of jet lag. Some clinicians advocate the use of 0.5 mg to 5 mg of melatonin during the first few days of travel, and there are data to suggest its efficacy. However, the quality control of its production is not regulated by the U.S. Food and Drug Administration, and contaminants have been found in commercially available products.

Current information does not support the use of special diets to ameliorate jet lag.

During Travel

Travelers should be advised to do the following things:

- Avoid large meals, alcohol, and caffeine.
- Drink plenty of water.
- Move around on the plane to promote mental and physical acuity.
- Wear comfortable shoes and clothing.
- Sleep, if possible, during long flights.

On Arrival at the Destination

Travelers should be advised to do the following things:

- Avoid situations requiring critical decision-making, such as important meetings, on the first day after arrival.
- Adapt to the local schedule as soon as possible. However, if the travel period is two days or less, travelers should remain on home time.

- Optimize exposure to sunlight following arrival in either direction.
- Eat meals appropriate to the local time.

Treatment

The 2008 American Academy of Sleep Medicine (AASD) recommendations include promoting sleep with hypnotic medication, although the effects of hypnotics on daytime symptoms of jet lag have not been well studied.

The prescription of nonaddictive sedative hypnotics (nonbenzodiazepines), such as zolpidem, has been shown in some studies to promote longer periods of high-quality sleep. If a benzodiazepine is preferred, a short-acting one, such as temazepam, is recommended to minimize oversedation the following day.

- Because alcohol intake is often high during international travel, the risk for interaction with hypnotics should be emphasized with patients.

References

1. Waterhouse J, Reilly T, Atkinson G, et al. Jet lag: trends and coping strategies. *Lancet*. 2007;369(9567):1117–29.

2. Dubocovich ML, Markowska M. Functional MT1 and MT2 melatonin receptors in mammals. *Endocrines*. 2005;27(2):101–10.

3. Reid KJ, Chang AM, Zee PC. Circadian rhythm sleep disorders. *Med Clin North Am*. 2004;88(3):631–51.

4. Waterhouse J, Edward B, Nevill A. et al. Do subjective symptoms predict our perception of jet lag? *Ergonomics*. 2000;43(10):1514–27.

5. Sack RL, Auckley D, Auger RR, et al. Circadian rhythm sleep disorders: part 1, basic principles, shift work and jet lag disorders: An American Academy of Sleep Medicine Review. *Sleep*. 2007;30(11):1460–83.

6. Jamieson AO, Zammit GK, Rosenberg RS, et al. Zolpidem reduces the sleep disturbance of jet lag. *Sleep Med*. 2001;2(5): 423–30.

7. Daurat A, Benoit O, Buguet A. Effects of zopiclone on the rest/activity rhythm after a westward flight across five time zones. *Psychopharmacology*. 2000;149(3):241–5.

8. Reilly T, Waterhouse J, Edwards B. Jet lag and air travel: implications for performance. *Clin Sports Med*. 2005;24(2):367–80.

9. Herxheimer A. Jet lag. *Clin Evid*. 2005;13:2178–83.

Section 16.5

Shift Work Disorder

"Shift Work Sleep Disorder," Stephen Duntley, MD, and Patricia L. Young. Washington University School of Medicine, St. Louis, Missouri, © 2010. All rights reserved. Reprinted with permission. For additional information about the Washington University Sleep Medicine Center, visit http://sleep .wustl.edu or call 314-362-4342.

Millions of Americans are considered shift workers, which includes, doctors, nurses, pilots, police officers, and commercial drivers.

A shift worker is characterized as someone who follows a work schedule outside the typical 9 a.m. to 5 p.m. day. When compared to individuals who work a normal work day, shift workers get less sleep on a regular basis.

Shift work intolerance, although listed as a circadian rhythm–related sleep disorder, should not be regarded as an internal biological clock issue or a sleep disorder alone. It can actually be a complex of three factors, which include, circadian, sleep, and domestic/social factors.

Circadian rhythm refers to the twenty-four-hour rhythmic output of the body's internal clock that regulates our biological processes. The circadian rhythm is the body's internal resting/wakefulness schedule over the course of a day. It is considered a disorder because so many people suffer from excessive sleepiness and sleep disturbance in trying to adapt to a shift work schedule.

In the past few decades, the nation has become increasingly dependent upon shift workers to meet the demand of our twenty-four-hour society. As a result, shift work tends to leave limited time for sleep.

Many individuals in today's workforce are obliged to work irregular shifts and may be working more than one shift in a day's time. It is estimated that 20 percent of the work force engages in some sort of shift work.

Sleep centers have seen an increase in the number of patients with the complaint of inadequate sleep and difficulty coping with shift work.

Some of the most serious and persistent problems shift workers face are frequent sleep disturbances and associated excessive sleepiness. As a result, this can lead to poor concentration, accidents, absenteeism, errors, injury, and fatalities.

This is an alarming situation since most shift workers in the United States are involved in dangerous occupations. Such catastrophes as the failure of the Space Shuttle Columbia and the crash of the Exxon *Valdez* have been attributed to human fatigue, in part.

There are solutions for the person who must work late night or early morning shifts and may be as simple as adjusting the bedroom environment to promote a more restful atmosphere, allowing for a better quality of sleep. This would include proper bedroom lighting and eliminating environmental factors such as noise that can disrupt sleep.

Domestic and social factors include individuals keeping a set sleep schedule throughout the week. Problems arise when a person tries to switch back to a normal day schedule.

Many people who work night shifts try to run errands and take care of children during the hours that should be used to get an adequate amount of sleep. Working the night shift and using the daytime hours to get other things accomplished can make a person feel more productive, but will result in sleep problems. When sleep becomes a low priority a person will not feel their best, and may suffer from a list of symptoms that can become debilitating over time.

Symptoms

The most common ailment that afflicts people with shift work sleep disorders is excessive sleepiness, while other symptoms may include:

* insomnia;
* disrupted sleep schedule;
* difficulties with personal relationships;
* irritability or a depressed mood;
* reduced work performance;
* sleepiness at work.

Diagnosis

Although some people cope well with shift work, others may need to see a sleep medicine specialist. Often there are underlying sleep disorders contributing to the lack of sleep that make it more difficult to work an alternate shift.

The sleep specialist will take a complete sleep history and physical to determine whether or not a sleep study is indicated. The sleep center physician may also want the patient to meet with the behavioral therapist to work on strategies to better improve the quality of sleep and to make adjustments to the patient's current work schedule.

Treatment

Treatment will be discussed at the time of the consultation and/or after the sleep study if indicated. Treatments may include behavioral or pharmacological remedies that can help alleviate symptoms.

Some people may never fully adapt to shift work, but there are ways of getting adequate sleep while doing shift work that can be beneficial.

Chapter 17

Excessive Sleeping

Chapter Contents

Section 17.1

Hypersomnia

Idiopathic hypersomnia is excessive sleeping (hypersomnia) without an obvious cause. It is different from narcolepsy in that idiopathic hypersomnia does not involve suddenly falling asleep or losing muscle control associated with strong emotions (cataplexy).

Causes

The usual approach is to consider other potential causes of excessive daytime sleepiness.

Other sleep disorders that may cause daytime sleepiness include:

- isolated sleep paralysis;

- narcolepsy;

- obstructive sleep apnea;

- restless leg syndrome.

Other causes of excessive sleepiness include:

- atypical depression;

- certain medications;

- drug and alcohol use;

- low thyroid function (hypothyroidism);

- previous head injury.

Symptoms

Symptoms often develop slowly during adolescence or young adulthood. They include:

- daytime naps that do not relieve drowsiness;

- difficulty waking from a long sleep—may feel confused or disoriented;

- increased need for sleep during the day—even while at work, or during a meal or conversation;

- increased sleep time—up to fourteen to eighteen hours per day.

Other symptoms may include anxiety, feeling irritated, low energy, restlessness, slow thinking or speech, loss of appetite, and memory difficulty.

Cataplexy—suddenly falling asleep or losing muscle control—which is part of narcolepsy, is *not* a symptom of idiopathic hypersomnia.

Exams and Tests

The health care provider will take a detailed sleep history. Tests may include:

- multiple-sleep latency test;

- sleep study (polysomnography, done to identify other sleep disorders).

A psychiatric evaluation for atypical depression may also be done.

Treatment

Idiopathic hypersomnia is usually treated with stimulant medications such as amphetamine, methylphenidate, and modafinil. These drugs may not work as well for this condition as they do for narcolepsy.

Important lifestyle changes that can help ease symptoms and prevent injury include:

- avoiding alcohol;

- avoiding operating motor vehicles or using dangerous equipment;

- avoiding working at night or social activities that delay bedtime.

Alternative Names

Hypersomnia—idiopathic; Drowsiness—idiopathic; Somnolence—idiopathic

References

Consens FB, Chervin RD. Sleep Disorders. In: Goetz, CG, ed. *Textbook of Clinical Neurology*. 3rd ed. Philadelphia, Pa: Saunders Elsevier; 2007: chap 54.

Section 17.2

Kleine-Levin Syndrome

Reprinted from "Kleine-Levin Syndrome Information Page,"
National Institute of Neurological Disorders and Stroke, National
Institutes of Health, March 12, 2009.

What is Kleine-Levin syndrome?

Kleine-Levin syndrome is a rare disorder that primarily affects adolescent males (approximately 70 percent of those with Kleine-Levin syndrome are male). It is characterized by recurring but reversible periods of excessive sleep (up to twenty hours per day). Symptoms occur as "episodes," typically lasting a few days to a few weeks. Episode onset is often abrupt, and may be associated with flu-like symptoms. Excessive food intake, irritability, childishness, disorientation, hallucinations, and an abnormally uninhibited sex drive may be observed during episodes. Mood can be depressed as a consequence, but not a cause, of the disorder. Affected individuals are completely normal between episodes, although they may not be able to remember afterward everything that happened during the episode. It may be weeks or more before symptoms reappear. Symptoms may be related to malfunction of the hypothalamus and thalamus, parts of the brain that govern appetite and sleep.

Is there any treatment?

There is no definitive treatment for Kleine-Levin syndrome and watchful waiting at home, rather than pharmacotherapy, is most often advised. Stimulant pills, including amphetamines, methylphenidate, and modafinil, are used to treat sleepiness but may increase irritability and will not improve cognitive abnormalities. Because of similarities between Kleine-Levin syndrome and certain mood disorders, lithium and carbamazepine may be prescribed and, in some cases, have been shown to prevent further episodes. This disorder should be differentiated from cyclic reoccurrence of sleepiness during the premenstrual period in teen-aged girls, which may be controlled with birth control pills. It also should be differentiated from encephalopathy, recurrent depression, or psychosis.

What is the prognosis?

Episodes eventually decrease in frequency and intensity over the course of eight to twelve years.

What research is being done?

The National Institute of Neurological Disorders and Stroke (NINDS) supports a broad range of clinical and basic research on diseases causing sleep disorders in an effort to clarify the mechanisms of these conditions and to develop better treatments for them.

Chapter 18

Insomnia

What Is Insomnia?

Insomnia is a common condition in which you have trouble falling or staying asleep. This condition can range from mild to severe, depending on how often it occurs and for how long.

Insomnia can be chronic (ongoing) or acute (short-term). Chronic insomnia means having symptoms at least three nights a week for more than a month. Acute insomnia lasts for less time.

Some people who have insomnia may have trouble falling asleep. Other people may fall asleep easily but wake up too soon. Others may have trouble with both falling asleep and staying asleep.

As a result, insomnia may cause you to get too little sleep or have poor-quality sleep. You may not feel refreshed when you wake up.

Overview

There are two types of insomnia. The most common type is called secondary or comorbid insomnia. This type of insomnia is a symptom or side effect of some other problem.

More than eight out of ten people who have insomnia are believed to have secondary insomnia. Certain medical conditions, medicines, sleep disorders, and substances can cause secondary insomnia.

"Insomnia," National Heart Lung and Blood Institute, National Institutes of Health, March 2009.

In contrast, primary insomnia isn't due to a medical problem, medicines, or other substances. It is its own disorder. A number of life changes can trigger primary insomnia, including long-lasting stress and emotional upset.

Insomnia can cause excessive daytime sleepiness and a lack of energy. It also can make you feel anxious, depressed, or irritable. You may have trouble focusing on tasks, paying attention, learning, and remembering. This can prevent you from doing your best at work or school.

Insomnia also can cause other serious problems. For example, you may feel drowsy while driving, which could lead to an accident.

Outlook

Secondary insomnia often resolves or improves without treatment if you can stop its cause—especially if you can correct the problem soon after it starts. For example, if caffeine is causing your insomnia, stopping or limiting your intake of the substance may cause your insomnia to go away.

Lifestyle changes, including better sleep habits, often help relieve acute insomnia. For chronic insomnia, your doctor may recommend a type of counseling called cognitive-behavioral therapy or medicines.

What Causes Insomnia?

Secondary Insomnia

Secondary insomnia is the symptom or side effect of another problem. This type of insomnia often is a symptom of an emotional, neurological, or other medical or sleep disorder.

Emotional disorders that can cause insomnia include depression, anxiety, and posttraumatic stress disorder. Alzheimer disease and Parkinson disease are examples of common neurological disorders that can cause insomnia.

A number of other conditions also can cause insomnia, such as the following:

- Conditions that cause chronic pain, such as arthritis and headache disorders

- Conditions that make it hard to breathe, such as asthma and heart failure

- An overactive thyroid

- Gastrointestinal disorders, such as heartburn

- Stroke

- Sleep disorders, such as restless legs syndrome and sleep-related breathing problems

- Menopause and hot flashes

Secondary insomnia also may be a side effect of certain medicines. For example, certain asthma medicines, such as theophylline, and some allergy and cold medicines can cause insomnia. Beta blockers also may cause the condition. These medicines are used to treat heart conditions.

Commonly used substances also may cause insomnia. Examples include caffeine and other stimulants, tobacco or other nicotine products, and alcohol or other sedatives.

Primary Insomnia

Primary insomnia isn't a symptom or side effect of another medical condition. This type of insomnia usually occurs for periods of at least one month.

A number of life changes can trigger primary insomnia. It may be due to major or long-lasting stress or emotional upset. Travel or other factors, such as work schedules that disrupt your sleep routine, also may trigger primary insomnia.

Even if these issues are resolved, the insomnia may not go away. Trouble sleeping may persist because of habits formed to deal with the lack of sleep. These habits may include taking naps, worrying about sleep, and going to bed early.

Researchers continue to try to find out whether some people are born with a greater chance of having primary insomnia.

Who Is at Risk for Insomnia?

Insomnia is a common disorder. One in three adults has insomnia sometimes. One in ten adults has chronic insomnia.

Insomnia affects women more often than men. The condition can occur at any age. However, older adults are more likely to have insomnia than younger people.

People who may be at higher risk for insomnia include those who:

- have a lot of stress;

- are depressed or who have other emotional distress, such as divorce or death of a spouse;

- have lower incomes;

- work at night or have frequent major shifts in their work hours;
- travel long distances with time changes;
- have certain medical conditions or sleep disorders that can disrupt sleep;
- have an inactive lifestyle.

Young and middle-aged African Americans also may be at increased risk for insomnia. Research shows that, compared to whites, it takes African Americans longer to fall asleep. They also have lighter sleep, don't sleep as well, and take more naps. Sleep-related breathing problems also are more common among African Americans.

What Are the Signs and Symptoms of Insomnia?

The main symptom of insomnia is trouble falling or staying asleep, which leads to lack of sleep. If you have insomnia, you may do any of the following things:

- Lie awake for a long time before you fall asleep
- Sleep for only short periods
- Be awake for much of the night
- Feel as if you haven't slept at all
- Wake up too early

The lack of sleep also can cause other symptoms. You may wake up feeling tired or not well rested, and you may feel tired during the day. You also may have trouble focusing on tasks. Insomnia can cause you to feel anxious, depressed, or irritable.

Insomnia may affect your daily activities and cause serious problems. For example, you may feel drowsy while driving. Driving while sleepy leads to more than one hundred thousand car crashes each year. In older women, research shows that insomnia raises the risk of falling.

If insomnia is affecting your daily activities, see your doctor. Treatment may help you avoid symptoms and problems related to the condition. Also, poor sleep may be a sign of other health problems. Finding and treating those problems could improve both your health and your sleep.

How Is Insomnia Diagnosed?

Usually, your doctor will diagnose insomnia based on your medical and sleep histories and a physical exam. He or she also may recommend a sleep study. For example, you may have a sleep study if the cause of your insomnia is unclear.

Medical History

To find out what's causing your insomnia, your doctor may ask whether you:

- have any new or ongoing health problems;
- have painful injuries or health conditions, such as arthritis;
- take any medicines, either over-the-counter or prescription;
- have symptoms or a history of depression, anxiety, or psychosis;
- are coping with any very stressful life events, such as divorce or death.

Your doctor also may ask questions about your work and leisure habits. For example, he or she may ask about your work and exercise routines; your use of caffeine, tobacco, and alcohol; and your long-distance travel history. Your answers may give clues about what's causing your insomnia.

Your doctor also may ask whether you have any new or ongoing work or personal problems or other stresses in your life. Also, he or she may ask whether you have other family members who have sleep problems.

Sleep History

To get a better sense of your sleep problem, your doctor will ask you details about your sleep habits. Before your visit, think about how to describe your problems, including the following details:

- How often you have trouble sleeping and how long you've had the problem
- When you go to bed and get up on workdays and days off
- How long it takes you to fall asleep, how often you wake up at night, and how long it takes to fall back asleep
- Whether you snore loudly and often or wake up gasping or feeling out of breath
- How refreshed you feel when you wake up, and how tired you feel during the day

- How often you doze off or have trouble staying awake during routine tasks, especially driving

To find out what's causing or worsening your insomnia, your doctor also may ask you the following things:

- Whether you worry about falling asleep, staying asleep, or getting enough sleep
- What you eat or drink, and whether you take medicines before going to bed
- What routine you follow before going to bed
- What the noise level, lighting, and temperature are like where you sleep
- What distractions, such as a TV or computer, are in your bedroom

To help your doctor, consider keeping a sleep diary for one or two weeks. Write down when you go to sleep, wake up, and take naps. (For example, you might note: Went to bed at 10 a.m.; woke up at 3 a.m. and couldn't fall back asleep; napped after work for two hours.)

Also write down how much you sleep each night, as well as how sleepy you feel at various times during the day.

Physical Exam

Your doctor will do a physical exam to rule out other medical problems that might cause insomnia. You also may need blood tests to check for thyroid problems or other conditions that can cause sleep problems.

Sleep Study

Your doctor may recommend a sleep study called a polysomnogram (PSG) if he or she thinks an underlying sleep disorder is causing your insomnia.

A PSG usually is done while you stay overnight at a sleep center. A PSG records brain electrical activity, eye movements, heart rate, breathing, muscle activity, blood pressure, and blood oxygen levels.

How Is Insomnia Treated?

Lifestyle changes often can help relieve acute (short-term) insomnia. These changes may make it easier to fall asleep and stay asleep.

A type of counseling called cognitive-behavioral therapy (CBT) can help relieve the anxiety linked to chronic (ongoing) insomnia. Anxiety tends to prolong insomnia.

Several medicines also can help relieve insomnia and reestablish a regular sleep schedule. However, if your insomnia is the symptom or side effect of another problem, it's important to treat the underlying cause (if possible). Your doctor also may prescribe medicine to help treat your insomnia.

Lifestyle Changes

If you have insomnia, avoid substances that make it worse, such as the following:

- **Caffeine, tobacco, and other stimulants taken too close to bedtime:** Their effects can last as long as eight hours.

- **Certain over-the-counter and prescription medicines that can disrupt sleep (for example, some cold and allergy medicines):** Talk to your doctor about which medicines won't disrupt your sleep.

- **Alcohol:** An alcoholic drink before bedtime may make it easier for you to fall asleep. However, alcohol triggers sleep that tends to be lighter than normal. This makes it more likely that you will wake up during the night.

Try to adopt good bedtime habits that make it easier to fall asleep and stay asleep. Follow a routine that helps you wind down and relax before bed. For example, read a book, listen to soothing music, or take a hot bath.

Try to schedule your daily exercise at least five to six hours before going to bed. Don't eat heavy meals or drink a lot before bedtime.

Make your bedroom sleep-friendly. Avoid bright lighting while winding down. Try to limit possible distractions, such as a TV, computer, or pet. Make sure the temperature of your bedroom is cool and comfortable. Your bedroom also should be dark and quiet.

Go to sleep around the same time each night and wake up around the same time each morning, even on weekends. If you can, avoid night shifts, alternating schedules, or other things that may disrupt your sleep schedule.

Cognitive-Behavioral Therapy

CBT for insomnia targets the thoughts and actions that can disrupt sleep. This therapy encourages good sleep habits and uses several methods to relieve sleep anxiety.

For example, relaxation training and biofeedback at bedtime are used to reduce anxiety. These strategies help you better control your breathing, heart rate, muscles, and mood.

CBT also works on replacing sleep anxiety with more positive thinking that links being in bed with being asleep. This method also teaches you what to do if you're unable to fall asleep within a reasonable time.

CBT also may involve talking with a therapist one-on-one or in group sessions to help you consider your thoughts and feelings about sleep. This method may encourage you to describe thoughts racing through your mind in terms of how they look, feel, and sound. The goal is for your mind to settle down and stop racing.

CBT also focuses on limiting the time you spend in bed while awake. This method involves setting a sleep schedule. At first, you will limit your total time in bed to the typical short length of time you're usually asleep.

This schedule may make you even more tired because some of the allotted time in bed will be taken up by problems falling asleep. However, the resulting tiredness is intended to help you get to sleep more quickly. Over time, the length of time spent in bed is increased until you get a full night of sleep.

For success with CBT, you may need to see a therapist who is skilled in this approach weekly over two to three months. CBT works as well as prescription medicine for many people who have chronic insomnia. It also may provide better long-term relief than medicine alone.

For people who have insomnia and major depressive disorder, CBT combined with antidepressant medicines has shown promise in relieving both conditions.

Medicines

Prescription medicines: Many prescription medicines are used to treat insomnia. Some are meant for short-term use, while others are meant for longer use.

Talk to your doctor about the benefits and side effects of insomnia medicines. For instance, insomnia medicines can help you fall asleep, but some people may feel groggy in the morning after taking them.

Rare side effects may include sleep eating, sleep walking, or driving while asleep. If you have side effects from an insomnia medicine, or if it doesn't work well, tell your doctor. He or she may prescribe a different medicine.

Some insomnia medicines may be habit forming. Talk to your doctor about the benefits and risks of insomnia medicines.

Over-the-counter products: Some over-the-counter (OTC) products claim to treat insomnia. These products include melatonin, L-tryptophan supplements, and valerian teas or extracts.

The Food and Drug Administration doesn't regulate "natural" products and some food supplements. Thus, the dose and purity of these products can vary. How well these products work and how safe they are isn't well understood.

Some OTC products that contain antihistamines are marketed as sleep aids. Although these products may make you sleepy, talk to your doctor before taking them.

Antihistamines pose risks for some people. Also, these products may not offer the best treatment for your insomnia. Your doctor can advise you whether these products can benefit you.

Key Points

- Insomnia is a common condition in which you have trouble falling or staying asleep. The condition can range from mild to severe, depending on how often it occurs and for how long.

- Insomnia can be chronic (ongoing) or acute (short-term). Chronic insomnia means having symptoms at least three nights a week for more than a month. Insomnia that lasts for less time is acute insomnia.

- Insomnia causes you to get too little sleep or poor-quality sleep that may not leave you feeling refreshed when you wake up.

- There are two types of insomnia. The most common type is secondary insomnia. This type of insomnia is a symptom or side effect of an emotional, neurological, or other medical or sleep disorder. Secondary insomnia also may result from using certain medicines or substances, such as caffeine.

- Primary insomnia isn't a symptom or side effect of another medical condition. It is its own disorder. A number of life changes can trigger primary insomnia, such as long-lasting stress or emotional upset. Even if these issues are resolved, the insomnia might not go away.

- Insomnia is a common disorder. One in three adults has insomnia sometimes. One in ten adults has chronic insomnia.

- The main symptom of insomnia is trouble falling or staying asleep, which leads to a lack of sleep. The lack of sleep can cause other symptoms, such as trouble focusing, anxiety, depression, and irritability.

- Usually, your doctor will diagnose insomnia based on your medical and sleep histories and a physical exam. He or she also may recommend a sleep study.

- Lifestyle changes often can help relieve acute insomnia. These changes may make it easier to fall asleep and stay asleep. Lifestyle changes include avoiding substances that make insomnia worse, adopting good bedtime habits, and going to sleep and waking up around the same time each day.

- A type of counseling called cognitive behavioral therapy (CBT) can help relieve the anxiety linked to chronic insomnia. CBT targets the thoughts and actions that can disrupt sleep and uses several methods to relieve sleep anxiety.

- Medicines also are used to treat insomnia. Some medicines are meant for short-term use, while others are meant for longer use. Side effects can occur, so talk to your doctor about the risks and benefits of using medicines to treat insomnia.

- Also, talk to your doctor before taking over-the-counter (OTC) products to treat insomnia. These products may pose risks for some people. Your doctor can advise you whether OTC products will benefit you.

Chapter 19

Sleep-Related Movement Disorders

Chapter Contents

Section 19.1

Periodic Limb Movement Disorder

"Periodic Limb Movement Disorder," excerpted from Mindell, J.A. and Owens, J.A. *A Clinical Guide to Pediatric Sleep: Diagnosis and Management of Sleep Problems.* Philadelphia: Lippincott Williams & Wilkins. © 2003 Lippincott Williams and Wilkins. Reprinted with permission. Reviewed by David. A. Cooke, MD, FACP, March 2010.

What is periodic limb movement disorder?

Periodic limb movement disorder (PLMD) involves periodic episodes of repetitive movements, usually in the legs, that occur approximately every twenty to forty seconds. The movements may appear as brief muscle twitches, jerking movements, or an upward flexing of the feet. These movements occur in clusters, lasting from a few minutes to a few hours. Most people with PLMD are not aware of the movements. PLMD can result in frequent brief arousals throughout the night, leading to daytime sleepiness. People with PLMD may also have restless legs syndrome, a movement disorder in which an individual experiences uncomfortable sensations in the legs during periods of rest or sitting still. The sensations are usually described as creepy, crawly, tingling, or painful and can make it difficult for a child or adolescent to fall asleep at bedtime.

What causes periodic limb movement disorder?

The cause of PLMD is unknown but it may be related to low iron (anemia). In addition, some with chronic diseases, such as diabetes and kidney disease, are at increased risk for developing PLMD. Pregnancy increases the incidence also.

What are the symptoms of periodic limb movement disorder?

The symptoms of PLMD may include any of the following, although many with the condition do not report any symptoms:

- **Leg movements:** Repetitive leg movements in sleep characterize PLMD, but the parson is probably not aware of these movements.

- **Sleep disruption:** People with PLMD may experience waking throughout the night as a result of the multiple arousals from sleep.

- **Restless sleep:** A person with PLMD may be described as a restless sleeper due to the leg movements and frequent arousals.

- **Daytime sleepiness:** The frequent arousals in sleep can result in significant daytime sleepiness.

- **Behavior and performance problems:** Individuals with PLMD may have daytime behavior and academic problems, such as hyperactivity, impulsivity, and irritability, which is the result of the sleep disruption. Personality changes such as irritability, moodiness, and shortened temper may result. Work performance may decrease.

How is periodic limb movement disorder diagnosed?

PLMD is diagnosed by an overnight sleep study. This requires one to stay overnight in a sleep laboratory. In addition, a medical history and physical examination will be conducted.

How is periodic limb movement disorder treated?

Treatment for PLMD may involve any of the following:

- **Use of medication:** For those with PLMD who have significant sleep disruption, medication may be recommended. There are a number of different medications that can help.

- **Avoidance of caffeine:** Caffeine can make PLMD symptoms worse; so all caffeine should be avoided. Caffeine can be found in many sodas, tea, and coffee, but also in chocolate and medications (e.g., Midol®, Excedrin®).

- **Management of iron deficiency:** Low levels of iron or folic acid can contribute to PLMD symptoms, so an iron or folic acid supplement may be prescribed by the doctor.

Section 19.2

Restless Legs Syndrome

"Restless Legs Syndrome,"
National Heart Lung and Blood Institute,
National Institutes of Health, March 2008.

What Is Restless Legs Syndrome?

Restless legs syndrome (RLS) is a disorder that causes a strong urge to move your legs. This urge to move often occurs with strange and unpleasant feelings in your legs. Moving your legs relieves the urge and the unpleasant feelings.

People who have RLS describe the unpleasant feelings as creeping, crawling, pulling, itching, tingling, burning, aching, or electric shocks. Sometimes, the feelings also occur in the arms.

The urge to move and unpleasant feelings occur when you're resting and inactive. They tend to be worse in the evening and at night and are temporarily relieved in the morning.

Overview

RLS can make it hard to fall asleep and stay asleep. It may make you feel tired and sleepy during the day. This can make it hard to learn, work, and do your normal routine. Not getting enough sleep also can cause depression, mood swings, or other health problems.

RLS can range from mild to severe based on: the following things:

- The strength of your symptoms and how often they occur

- How easily moving around relieves your symptoms

- How much your symptoms disturb your sleep

One type of RLS usually starts early in life (before age forty-five) and tends to run in families. It may even start in childhood. Once this type of RLS starts, it usually lasts for the rest of your life. Over time, symptoms slowly get worse and occur more often. If you have a mild case, you may have long periods with no symptoms.

Another type of RLS usually starts later in life (after age forty-five). It generally doesn't run in families. This type tends to have a more abrupt onset. The symptoms usually don't get worse with age.

Some diseases, conditions, and medicines also may trigger RLS. For example, it has been associated with kidney failure, Parkinson disease, diabetes, rheumatoid arthritis, pregnancy, and iron deficiency. When a disease, condition, or medicine causes RLS, the symptoms usually start suddenly.

Medical conditions or medicines often cause or worsen the type of RLS that starts later in life.

Outlook

RLS symptoms often get worse over time. However, some people's symptoms go away for weeks to months.

If a condition or medicine triggers RLS, it may go away if the trigger is relieved or stopped. For example, RLS that occurs due to pregnancy tends to go away after giving birth. Kidney transplants (but not dialysis) relieve RLS linked to kidney failure.

Treatments for RLS include lifestyle changes and medicines. Some simple lifestyle changes often help relieve mild cases of RLS. Medicines usually can relieve or prevent the symptoms of more severe RLS. Research is ongoing to better understand the causes of RLS and to find better treatments.

What Causes Restless Legs Syndrome?

Faulty Use or Lack of Iron

Research suggests that restless legs syndrome (RLS) is mainly due to the faulty use or lack of iron in the brain. The brain uses iron to make the chemical dopamine and to control other brain activities. Dopamine works in the parts of the brain that control movement.

A number of conditions can affect how much iron is in the brain or how it's used. These conditions include kidney failure, Parkinson disease, diabetes, rheumatoid arthritis, pregnancy, and iron deficiency. All of these conditions increase the risk of having RLS.

People whose family members have RLS also are more likely to develop the disorder. This suggests that genetics may contribute to the faulty use or lack of iron in the brain that triggers RLS.

Nerve Damage

Nerve damage in the legs or feet and sometimes in the arms or hands may cause or worsen RLS. Several conditions can cause such nerve damage, including diabetes.

Medicines and Substances

Certain medicines may trigger RLS. These include some of the following:

- Antinausea medicines (used to treat upset stomach)
.• Antidepressants (used to treat depression)
- Antipsychotics (used to treat certain mental health disorders)
- Cold and allergy medicines that contain antihistamines
- Calcium channel blockers (used to treat heart problems and high blood pressure)

RLS symptoms usually get better or may even go away if the medicine is stopped.

Certain substances, such as alcohol and tobacco, also can trigger or worsen RLS symptoms. Symptoms may get better or go away if the substances are stopped.

Who Is at Risk for Restless Legs Syndrome?

Restless legs syndrome (RLS) may affect as many as twelve million people in the United States. More than half of the people who have RLS have family members with the condition.

RLS can affect people of any race or ethnic group, but the disorder is more common in people of Northern European descent. RLS affects both genders, but women are more likely to have it than men.

The number of cases of RLS rises with age. Many people who have RLS are diagnosed in middle age. However, in about 40 percent of RLS cases, symptoms start before age twenty. People who develop RLS early in life usually have a family history of it.

People who have certain diseases or conditions or who take certain medicines are more likely to develop RLS.

For example, RLS is common in pregnant women. It usually occurs during the last three months of pregnancy. The disorder usually improves or goes away after giving birth. Some women may continue to have symptoms after giving birth. Other women may develop RLS again later in life.

What Are the Signs and Symptoms of Restless Legs Syndrome?

The four key signs of restless legs syndrome (RLS) are as follows:

- A strong urge to move your legs. This urge often, but not always, occurs with unpleasant feelings in your legs. When the disorder is severe, you also may have the urge to move your arms.

- Symptoms that start or get worse when you're inactive. The urge to move increases when you're sitting still or lying down and resting.

- Relief from moving. Movement, especially walking, helps relieve the unpleasant feelings.

- Symptoms that start or get worse in the evening or at night.
You must have all four of these signs to be diagnosed with RLS.

The Urge to Move

RLS gets its name from the urge to move the legs when sitting or lying down. This movement relieves the unpleasant feelings that RLS sometimes causes. Typical movements are as follows:

- Pacing and walking

- Jiggling the legs

- Stretching and flexing

- Tossing and turning

- Rubbing the legs

Unpleasant Feelings

People who have RLS describe the unpleasant feelings in their limbs as creeping, crawling, pulling, itching, tingling, burning, aching, or electric shocks. More severe RLS symptoms may cause painful feelings. However, the pain usually is more of an ache than a sharp, stabbing pain.

Children may describe RLS symptoms differently than adults. Sometimes children with RLS are misdiagnosed as having ADHD.

The unpleasant feelings from RLS often occur in the lower legs (calves). But the feelings can occur at any place in the legs or feet. They also can occur in the arms.

The feelings seem to come from deep within the limbs, rather than from the surface. You usually will have the feelings in both legs. However, the feelings can occur in one leg, move from one leg to the other, or affect one leg more than the other.

People who have mild symptoms may notice them only when they're still or awake for a long time, such as on a long airplane trip or when watching TV. If they fall asleep quickly, they may not have symptoms when lying down at night.

The unpleasant feelings from RLS aren't the same as the leg cramps many people get at night. Leg cramps often are limited to certain muscle groups in the leg, which you can feel tightening. Leg cramps cause more severe pain and require stretching the affected muscle for relief.

Sometimes arthritis or peripheral arterial disease (PAD) can cause pain or discomfort in the legs. Moving the limbs usually worsens the discomfort instead of relieving it.

Periodic Limb Movement in Sleep

Most people who have RLS also have a condition called periodic limb movement in sleep (PLMS). PLMS causes your legs or arms to twitch or jerk about every ten to sixty seconds during sleep. These movements cause you to wake up often and get less sleep.

PLMS usually affects the legs, but it also can affect the arms. Not everyone who has PLMS also has RLS.

Related Sleep Problems

The symptoms of RLS can make it hard to fall or stay asleep. If RLS disturbs your sleep, you may feel very tired during the day.

Lack of sleep may make it hard for you to concentrate at school or work. Not enough sleep also can cause depression, mood swings, or other health problems such as diabetes or high blood pressure.

How Is Restless Legs Syndrome Diagnosed?

Your doctor will diagnose restless legs syndrome (RLS) based on your symptoms, your medical and family histories, and the results from a physical exam and tests.

Your doctor will use this information to rule out other conditions that have symptoms similar to those of RLS.

Specialists Involved

Your primary care doctor usually can diagnose and treat RLS. However, he or she also may suggest that you see a sleep specialist or neurologist.

Symptoms

You must have the four key signs of RLS to be diagnosed with the condition.

Your doctor also will want to know how your symptoms are affecting your sleep and how alert you are during the day.

To help your doctor, you may want to keep a sleep diary. Use the diary to keep a daily record of how easy it is to fall and stay asleep, how much sleep you get at night, and how alert you feel during the day.

Medical and Family Histories

Your doctor may ask whether you have any of the diseases or conditions that can trigger RLS. These include kidney failure, Parkinson disease, diabetes, rheumatoid arthritis, pregnancy, and iron deficiency.

Your doctor also may want to know what medicines you take. Some medicines can trigger or worsen RLS.

Because the most common type of RLS tends to run in families, your doctor may ask whether any of your relatives have the disorder.

Physical Exam

Your doctor will do a physical exam to check for underlying conditions that may trigger RLS. He or she also will check for other conditions that have symptoms similar to those of RLS.

Tests

Currently, no test can diagnose RLS. Still, your doctor will likely order blood tests to measure your iron levels. He or she also may order muscle or nerve tests. These tests can show whether you have a condition that may worsen RLS or that has symptoms similar to those of RLS.

Rarely, sleep studies are used to diagnose RLS. A sleep study measures how much and how well you sleep. Although RLS can cause a lack of sleep, this sign isn't specific enough to diagnose RLS.

Researchers continue to study new tests to diagnose RLS.

Drug Therapy Trial

If your doctor thinks you have RLS, he or she may prescribe certain medicines to relieve your symptoms. These medicines, which are used to treat people who have Parkinson disease, also can relieve RLS symptoms. If the medicines relieve your symptoms, your doctor can confirm that you have RLS.

How Is Restless Legs Syndrome Treated?

Restless legs syndrome (RLS) has no cure. If a condition or medicine triggers RLS, it may go away or get better if the trigger is relieved or stopped.

RLS can be treated. The goals of treatment are to do the following things:

- Prevent or relieve symptoms

- Increase the amount and improve the quality of your sleep

- Treat or correct any underlying condition that may trigger or worsen RLS

Mild cases of RLS often are treated with lifestyle changes and sometimes with periodic use of medicines. More severe RLS usually is treated with daily medicines.

Lifestyle Changes

Lifestyle changes can prevent or relieve the symptoms of RLS. For mild RLS, lifestyle changes may be the only treatment needed.

Preventing Symptoms

Many common substances, such as alcohol and tobacco, can trigger RLS symptoms. Avoiding these substances can limit or prevent symptoms.

Some prescription and over-the-counter medicines can cause or worsen RLS symptoms. Tell your doctor about all of the medicines you're taking. He or she can tell you whether you should stop or change certain medicines.

Adopting good sleep habits can help you fall asleep and stay asleep—a problem for many people who have RLS. Good sleep habits include the following:

- Keeping the area where you sleep cool, quiet, comfortable, and as dark as possible.

- Making your bedroom sleep-friendly. Remove things that can interfere with sleep, such as a TV, computer, or phone.

- Going to bed and waking up at the same time every day. Some people who have RLS find it helpful to go to bed later in the evening and get up later in the morning.

- Avoiding staying in bed awake for any long period in the evening or during the night.

Doing a challenging activity before bedtime, such as solving a crossword puzzle, may ease your RLS symptoms. This distraction may make it easier for you to fall asleep. Focusing on your breathing and using other relaxation techniques also may help you fall asleep.

Regular, moderate physical activity also may help limit or prevent RLS symptoms. Often, people who have RLS find that if they increase their activity during the day, they have fewer symptoms.

Relieving Symptoms

Certain activities can relieve RLS symptoms. These include the following:

- Walking or stretching

- Taking a hot or cold bath

- Massaging the affected limb(s)

- Using heat or ice packs on the affected limb(s)

- Doing mentally challenging tasks

Choose an aisle seat at the movies or on airplanes and trains so you can move around, if necessary.

Medicines

You may need medicines to treat RLS if lifestyle changes can't control symptoms. Many medicines can relieve or prevent RLS symptoms, including many new medicines.

No single medicine works for all people who have RLS. It may take several changes in medicines and dosages to find the best approach. Sometimes, a medicine will work for a while and then stop working.

Some of the effective medicines used to treat RLS also are used to treat Parkinson disease. These medicines make dopamine or act like it in the parts of the brain that control movement. (Dopamine is a chemical that helps you move properly.)

If medicines for Parkinson disease don't prevent or relieve your symptoms, your doctor may prescribe other medicines. You may have to take more than one medicine to treat your RLS.

Always talk with your doctor before taking any medicines. He or she can tell you the side effects of each RLS medicine. Side effects may include nausea, headache, and daytime sleepiness.

In some cases, RLS medicines may worsen problems controlling excessive gambling, shopping, or sexual activity. Sometimes, continued use of RLS medicines may make your RLS symptoms worse.

Contact your doctor if you have any of these problems. He or she can adjust your medicines to prevent these side effects.

Living with Restless Legs Syndrome

Restless legs syndrome (RLS) is often a lifelong condition. Symptoms may come and go often or go away for long periods. Symptoms often get worse over time.

If a condition or medicine triggers RLS, the disorder may go away if the trigger is relieved or stopped. For example, RLS that occurs due to pregnancy tends to go away after giving birth.

Although RLS has no cure, treatments can relieve or prevent RLS symptoms. Mild cases of RLS often are treated with lifestyle changes and sometimes with periodic use of medicines. More severe RLS usually is treated with daily medicines.

Ongoing Medical Care

If you have RLS, see your doctor regularly so he or she can watch for changes in your symptoms. This will show whether your treatment is working and whether it will continue to work over time.

Call your doctor if you notice your treatment is no longer working or if you have new symptoms.

Other Considerations

Try to plan long car trips and other long periods of inactivity at the times of day when your symptoms are least severe. Give yourself time to stretch or take walking breaks.

Choose an aisle seat at the movies or on airplanes and trains so you can move around if needed.

Consider finding a work setting where you can stand or walk around.

Support Groups

Many people who have RLS find it helpful to join a support group, such as those that the RLS Foundation offers.

Key Points

- Restless legs syndrome (RLS) is a disorder that causes a strong urge to move your legs. This urge often occurs with strange and unpleasant feelings in your legs. Moving your legs relieves the urge and the unpleasant feelings.

- People who have RLS describe the unpleasant feelings as creeping, crawling, pulling, itching, tingling, burning, aching, or electric shocks.

- The urge to move and unpleasant feelings occur when you're resting and inactive. They tend to be worse in the evening and at night and are temporarily relieved in the morning.

- RLS can make it hard to fall asleep and stay asleep. It may make you feel tired and sleepy during the day. This can make it hard to learn, work, and do your normal routine. Not getting enough sleep also can cause depression, mood swings, and other health problems.

- One type of RLS usually starts early in life (before age forty-five) and tends to run in families. Once this type of RLS starts, it usually lasts for the rest of your life. Over time, symptoms slowly get worse and occur more often.

- Another type of RLS usually starts later in life (after age forty-five). It generally doesn't run in families. This type tends to have a more abrupt onset. The symptoms usually don't get worse with age.

- Some diseases, conditions, and medicines also may trigger RLS. For example, it has been associated with kidney failure, Parkinson disease, diabetes, rheumatoid arthritis, pregnancy, and iron deficiency. When a disease, condition, or medicine triggers RLS, symptoms usually start suddenly. The disorder may go away if the trigger is relieved or stopped.

- Research suggests that RLS is mainly due to the faulty use or lack of iron in the brain. Nerve damage in the limbs and some medicines and substances also may cause RLS.

- The number of cases of RLS rises with age. Many people who have RLS are diagnosed in middle age. However, in about 40 percent of RLS cases, symptoms start before age twenty. People who develop RLS early in life usually have a family history of it.

- The four key signs of RLS are an urge to move your legs (unpleasant feelings in the legs often occur with this urge), symptoms that start or get worse when you're inactive, relief from moving, and symptoms that get worse in the evening or at night.

- Your doctor will diagnose RLS based on your symptoms, your medical and family histories, and the results from a physical exam and tests. Your primary care doctor usually can diagnose and treat RLS. However, he or she also may suggest that you see a sleep specialist or neurologist.

- Treatments for RLS include lifestyle changes and medicines. Mild cases of RLS often are treated with lifestyle changes and sometimes with periodic use of medicines. More severe RLS usually is treated with daily medicines. Lifestyle changes include avoiding certain substances and adopting good sleep habits.

- If you have RLS, see your doctor regularly so he or she can watch for changes in your symptoms. Call you doctor if you notice your treatment is no longer working or if you have new symptoms.

- Try to plan long car trips and other long periods of inactivity at the times of day when your symptoms are least severe. Give yourself time to stretch or take walking breaks. Choose an aisle seat at the movies or on airplanes and trains so you can move around if needed. You might want to consider finding a work setting where you can stand or walk around.

Chapter 20

Narcolepsy

What Is Narcolepsy?

Narcolepsy is a disorder that causes periods of extreme daytime sleepiness. It also may cause muscle weakness.

Rarely, people who have this disorder fall asleep suddenly, even if they're in the middle of talking, eating, or another activity. Most people who have narcolepsy also have trouble sleeping at night.

Narcolepsy also may cause the following things:

- **Cataplexy:** This condition causes a sudden loss of muscle tone while you're awake. Muscle weakness can occur in certain parts of your body or in your whole body. For example, if cataplexy affects your hand, you may drop what you're holding. Strong emotions often trigger this weakness. It may last seconds or minutes.

- **Hallucinations:** These vivid dreams occur while falling asleep or waking up.

- **Sleep paralysis:** This condition prevents you from moving or speaking while waking up and sometimes while falling asleep. Sleep paralysis usually goes away within a few minutes.

"Narcolepsy," National Heart Lung and Blood Institute, National Institutes of Health, November 2008.

Overview

The two main phases of sleep are nonrapid eye movement (NREM) and rapid eye movement (REM). Most people are in the NREM phase when they first fall asleep. After about ninety minutes of sleep, most people go from NREM to REM sleep.

Dreaming occurs during the REM phase of sleep. During REM, your muscles normally become limp. This prevents you from acting out your dreams.

People who have narcolepsy often fall into REM sleep quickly and wake up directly from it. This is linked to vivid dreams while waking up and falling asleep.

Hypocretin, a chemical in the brain, helps control levels of wakefulness. Most people who have narcolepsy have low levels of this chemical. What causes these low levels isn't well understood.

Researchers think that certain factors may work together to cause a lack of hypocretin. Examples include heredity; brain injuries; contact with toxins, such as pesticides; and autoimmune disorders. (Autoimmune disorders occur when the body's immune system attacks the body's healthy cells.)

Outlook

Narcolepsy affects between 50,000 and 2.4 million people in the United States. Symptoms usually begin during the teen or young adult years. Due to extreme tiredness, people who have narcolepsy may find it hard to function at school, at work, at home, and in social situations.

Narcolepsy has no cure, but medicines, lifestyle changes, and other therapies can improve symptoms. Research on the causes of narcolepsy and new ways to treat it is ongoing.

What Causes Narcolepsy?

Most people who have narcolepsy have low levels of hypocretin. This is a chemical in the brain that helps control levels of wakefulness. What causes these low hypocretin levels isn't well understood.

Researchers think that certain factors may work together to cause a lack of hypocretin. These factors may include the following:

- Heredity. Some people may inherit a gene that affects hypocretin. Up to 10 percent of people who have narcolepsy report having a relative with the same symptoms.

- Infections.

- Brain injuries due to conditions such as brain tumors or strokes.

- Contact with toxins, such as pesticides.

- Autoimmune disorders. These are conditions in which the body's immune system attacks the body's healthy cells. An example of an autoimmune disorder is rheumatoid arthritis.

Heredity alone doesn't cause narcolepsy. You also must have at least one other factor, such as one of those listed above, to develop narcolepsy.

Who Is at Risk for Narcolepsy?

Narcolepsy affects between 50,000 and 2.4 million people in the United States. Symptoms usually begin during the teen or young adult years. The disorder also can develop later in life or in children, but it's rare before age five. Narcolepsy affects both men and women.

Researchers think that certain factors may work together to cause narcolepsy. If these factors affect you, you may be at higher risk for the disorder.

What Are the Signs and Symptoms of Narcolepsy?

The four major signs and symptoms of narcolepsy are extreme daytime sleepiness, cataplexy (muscle weakness) while awake, and hallucinations and sleep paralysis during sleep.

If you have narcolepsy, you may have one or more of these symptoms. They can range from mild to severe.

Extreme Daytime Sleepiness

All people who have narcolepsy have extreme daytime sleepiness. This is often the most obvious symptom of the disorder.

During the day, you may have few or many periods of sleepiness. Each period usually lasts thirty minutes or less. Strong emotions, such as laughter, anger, fear, or excitement, can bring on this sleepiness.

People who have this symptom often complain of the following things:

- Mental cloudiness or "fog"

- Memory problems or problems focusing

- Lack of energy or extreme exhaustion

- Depression

Rarely, people who have narcolepsy have sleep episodes in which they fall asleep suddenly. This is more likely to happen when they're not active—for example, while reading, watching TV, or sitting in a meeting.

However, sleep episodes also may occur in the middle of talking, eating, or another activity. Cataplexy also may occur at the same time.

Cataplexy

This condition causes loss of muscle tone while you're awake. Muscle weakness occurs in certain parts of your body or in your whole body.

Cataplexy may make your head nod or make it hard for you to speak. Muscle weakness also may make your knees weak or cause you to drop things you're holding. Some people lose all muscle control and fall.

Strong emotions, such as laughter or excitement, often trigger this symptom. It usually lasts a few seconds or minutes. During this time, you're usually awake.

Cataplexy may occur weeks to years after you first start to have extreme daytime sleepiness.

Hallucinations

If you have narcolepsy, you may have vivid dreams while falling asleep, waking up, or dozing. These dreams can feel very real. You may feel like you can see, hear, smell, and taste things.

Sleep Paralysis

This condition prevents you from moving or speaking while falling asleep or waking up. However, you're fully conscious (aware) during this time. Sleep paralysis usually lasts just a few seconds or minutes, but it can be scary.

Other Symptoms

Most people who have narcolepsy also don't sleep well at night. They may have trouble falling and staying asleep. Vivid, scary dreams may disturb sleep. Not sleeping well at night worsens daytime sleepiness.

Rarely, people who fall asleep in the middle of an activity, such as eating, may continue that activity for a few seconds or minutes. This is called automatic behavior.

During automatic behavior, you're not aware of your actions, so you don't perform them well. For example, if you're writing before falling asleep, you may scribble rather than form words. If you're driving, you may get lost or have an accident. Most people who have this symptom don't remember what happened while it was going on.

Children who have narcolepsy often have trouble studying, focusing, and remembering things. Also, they may seem hyperactive. Some children who have narcolepsy speed up their activities rather than slow them down.

How Is Narcolepsy Diagnosed?

It can take as long as ten to fifteen years after the first symptoms appear before narcolepsy is recognized and diagnosed. This is because narcolepsy is fairly rare. Also, many of the symptoms of narcolepsy are like symptoms of other illnesses, such as infections, depression, and sleep disorders.

Narcolepsy is sometimes mistaken for learning problems, seizure disorders, or laziness, especially in school-aged children and teens. When narcolepsy symptoms are mild, it's even harder to diagnose.

Your doctor will diagnose narcolepsy based on your signs and symptoms, your medical and family histories, a physical exam, and results from tests.

Signs and Symptoms

Tell your doctor about any signs and symptoms of narcolepsy that you have. This is important because your doctor may not ask about them during a routine checkup.

Your doctor will want to know when you first had signs and symptoms and whether they bother your sleep or daily routine. He or she also will want to know about your sleep habits and how you feel and act during the day.

To help answer these questions, you may want to keep a sleep diary for a few weeks. Keep a daily record of how easy it is to fall and stay asleep, how much sleep you get at night, and how alert you feel during the day.

Medical and Family Histories

To learn about your medical and family histories, your doctor may ask whether any of the following are true:

- You're affected by certain factors that can lead to narcolepsy. These include infection, brain injuries, contact with toxins (such as pesticides), or autoimmune disorders.

- You take medicines and which ones you take. Some medicines can cause daytime sleepiness. Thus, your symptoms may be due to medicine, not narcolepsy.
- You have symptoms of other sleep disorders that cause daytime sleepiness.
- You have relatives who have narcolepsy or who have signs or symptoms of the disorder.

Physical Exam

Your doctor will examine you to see whether another condition is causing your symptoms. For example, infections, certain thyroid diseases, drug and alcohol use, and other medical or sleep disorders may cause symptoms similar to those of narcolepsy.

Diagnostic Tests

Sleep studies: If your doctor thinks you have narcolepsy, he or she will likely suggest that you see a sleep specialist. This specialist may advise you to have special sleep studies to find out more about your condition.

Sleep studies usually are done at a sleep center. The results of two tests—a polysomnogram (PSG) and a multiple sleep latency test (MSLT)—are used to diagnose narcolepsy.

For a polysomnogram, you usually stay overnight at a sleep center. The test records brain activity, eye movements, breathing, heart rate, and blood pressure. This test can help find out whether you fall asleep quickly, go into rapid eye movement (REM) sleep soon after falling asleep, or wake up often during the night.

The multiple sleep latency test is a daytime sleep study that measures how sleepy you are. It's often done the day after a PSG. During the test, you relax in a quiet room for about thirty minutes. A technician checks your brain activity during this time. The test is repeated three or four times throughout the day.

An MSLT finds out how quickly you fall asleep during the day (after a full night's sleep). It also shows whether you go into REM sleep soon after falling asleep.

Other Tests

Hypocretin test: This test measures the levels of hypocretin in the fluid that surrounds your spinal cord. Most people who have narcolepsy have low levels of hypocretin.

To get a sample of spinal cord fluid, a spinal tap (also called a lumbar puncture) is done. For this procedure, your doctor inserts a needle into your lower back area and then withdraws a sample of your spinal fluid.

How Is Narcolepsy Treated?

Narcolepsy has no cure. However, medicines, lifestyle changes, and other therapies can relieve many of its symptoms. Treatment for narcolepsy is based on the type of symptoms you have and how severe they are.

Not all medicines and lifestyle changes work for everyone. It may take weeks to months for you and your doctor to find the best treatment.

Medicines

You may need one or more medicines to treat narcolepsy symptoms. These may include the following:

- Stimulants to ease daytime sleepiness and raise your alertness.

- A medicine that helps make up for the low levels of hypocretin in your brain. (Hypocretin is a chemical that helps control levels of wakefulness.) This medicine helps you stay awake during the day and sleep at night. It doesn't always completely relieve daytime sleepiness, so your doctor may tell you to take it with a stimulant.

- Medicines that help you sleep at night.

- Medicines used to treat depression. These medicines also help prevent cataplexy, hallucinations, and sleep paralysis.

Some prescription and over-the-counter medicines can interfere with your sleep. Ask your doctor about these medicines and how to avoid them, if possible.

If you take regular naps when you feel sleepy, you may need less medicine to stay awake.

Lifestyle Changes

Lifestyle changes also may help relieve some narcolepsy symptoms. You can take steps to make it easier to fall asleep at night and stay asleep:

- Follow a regular sleep schedule. Go to bed and wake up at the same time every day.

- Do something relaxing before bedtime, such as taking a warm bath.

- Keep your bedroom or sleep area quiet, comfortable, dark, and free from distractions, such as a TV or computer.

- Allow yourself about twenty minutes to fall asleep or fall back asleep after waking up. After that, get up and do something relaxing (like reading) until you get sleepy.

Certain activities, foods, and drinks before bedtime can keep you awake. Try to follow these guidelines:

- Exercise regularly, but not within three hours of bedtime.

- Avoid tobacco, alcohol, chocolate, and drinks that contain caffeine for several hours before bedtime.

- Avoid large meals and beverages just before bedtime.

- Avoid bright lights before bedtime.

Other Therapies

Light therapy may help you keep a regular sleep and wake schedule. For this type of therapy, you sit in front of a light box, which has special lights, for ten to thirty minutes. This therapy can help you feel less sleepy in the morning.

Living with Narcolepsy

Living with narcolepsy can be hard. It can affect your ability to drive, work, go to school, and have relationships. Besides taking medicine, you can do many things to live a safe and satisfying life.

Driving

Driving can be dangerous for people who have narcolepsy. Ask your doctor whether you can drive safely. To help make it safer for you to drive, do the following things:

- Take naps before driving. This helps some people who have periods of extreme daytime sleepiness.

- Stop often during long drives. Stretch and walk around during the stops.

- Try to have family, friends, or co-workers in the car to keep you aware and engaged, or get rides from them.

Working

People who have narcolepsy can work in almost all types of jobs, but some jobs may be better than others. For example, a job with a flexible work schedule can make it easier to take naps when needed. A job in which you interact with your co-workers can help keep you awake. Jobs that don't require you to drive or are closer to home also may be better.

Certain laws may apply to workers who have medical conditions, such as narcolepsy. These laws include the following:

- **Americans with Disabilities Act (ADA):** This law requires employers to reasonably accommodate the needs of their workers who have disabilities. This includes people who have narcolepsy. For example, employers may allow workers to take short naps during the workday or adjust work schedules to avoid sleepy periods.

- **Family and Medical Leave Act:** This law requires employers who have fifty or more employees to provide unpaid leave to employees with an illness, such as narcolepsy. It also gives leave to family members who need time to care for a close relative who has a serious illness.

- **Social Security Disability Insurance or Supplemental Security Income programs:** These programs may offer financial help if you can't work because of your narcolepsy.

Getting Emotional Support

Getting support from others—friends, family, and co-workers—may help you cope with your disorder. Learn more about narcolepsy, and tell your family and friends about the disorder. Ask them for help.

Seek professional counseling for yourself and your family. Ask your doctor about narcolepsy or sleep disorder support groups in your area.

Narcolepsy in Special Groups

School-aged children: Children who have narcolepsy may have trouble studying, focusing, and remembering things.

To help your child in school, do the following things:

- Talk to your child's teachers and school administrators about your child's narcolepsy and the best ways to meet his or her needs. For example, your child may need to take naps or walks during the day or tape the teacher's lessons.

- Talk to the school nurse about your child's narcolepsy and medicines. Together you can work out a place to keep the medicines and a schedule for taking them at school.

Pregnant women: If you're pregnant or planning a pregnancy, talk to your doctor about whether you should continue taking your narcolepsy medicines. Certain medicines may interfere with your pregnancy.

Key Points

- Narcolepsy is a disorder that causes periods of extreme daytime sleepiness. Rarely, people who have this disorder fall asleep suddenly during routine activities. Most people who have narcolepsy also have trouble sleeping at night.

- Narcolepsy also may cause cataplexy, hallucinations (vivid dreams) during sleep, and sleep paralysis. Sleep paralysis is a condition that prevents you from moving or speaking while waking up and sometimes while falling asleep. Cataplexy is a condition that causes sudden loss of muscle tone while you're awake.

- People who have narcolepsy have low levels of hypocretin. This is a chemical in the brain that helps control levels of wakefulness. Researchers think that certain factors may work together to cause a lack of hypocretin. Examples of these factors include heredity; brain injuries; contact with toxins, such as pesticides; and autoimmune disorders.

- Narcolepsy affects between 50,000 and 2.4 million people in the United States. Symptoms usually begin during the teen or young adult years. Narcolepsy affects both men and women.

- The four major signs and symptoms of narcolepsy are extreme daytime sleepiness, cataplexy (muscle weakness) while awake, and hallucinations and sleep paralysis during sleep. Most people who have narcolepsy also don't sleep well at night. They may have trouble falling and staying asleep. Vivid, scary dreams may disturb sleep.

- It can take as long as ten to fifteen years after the first symptoms appear before narcolepsy is recognized and diagnosed. This is because narcolepsy is fairly rare. Also, many of the symptoms of narcolepsy are liked symptoms of other illnesses.

- Narcolepsy is diagnosed based on your signs and symptoms, your medical and family histories, a physical exam, and results from tests.

- Narcolepsy has no cure. However, medicines, lifestyle changes, and other therapies can relieve many of its symptoms. Treatment for narcolepsy is based on the type of symptoms you have and how severe they are.

- Living with narcolepsy can be hard. It can affect your ability to drive, work, go to school, and have relationships. Besides taking medicine, you can do many things to live a safe and satisfying life. Talk to your doctor about how to cope with your condition.

Chapter 21

Parasomnias

Chapter Contents

Section 21.1

What Are Parasomnias?

"An Introduction to Parasomnias," © 2000 Talk About Sleep (www.talkaboutsleep.com). All rights reserved. Reprinted with permission. Reviewed by David. A. Cooke, MD, FACP, March 2010.

A sleep disorder is a physical and psychological condition or disturbance of sleep and wakefulness caused by abnormalities that occur during sleep or by abnormalities of specific sleep mechanisms. Although the sleep disorder exists during sleep, recognizable symptoms manifest themselves during the day. Accurate diagnosis requires a polysomnogram, widely known as a "sleep test."

It is estimated that some forty million Americans suffer from chronic, long-term sleep disorders. Another twenty to thirty million Americans suffer from some kind of sleep disorder on an irregular basis. The annual costs in productivity, health care, and safety have been estimated in the billions of dollars.

Parasomnia is a broad term used to describe various uncommon disruptive sleep-related disorders. They are intense, infrequent physical acts that occur during sleep. Some common parasomnias include sleepwalking, sleep talking, sleep terrors, nightmares, and teeth grinding.

Sleepwalking

Sleepwalking, also called somnambulism, is when a person is able to perform complicated actions, including walking, while in deep sleep. Sleepwalking is an "arousal" disorder. These occur when a person is in a mixed state of awareness, i.e., both asleep and awake. Researchers believe sleepwalking stems from a temporary sleep mechanism malfunction that occurs during the deeper stages of sleep. Because sleepwalking does not occur during rapid eye movement (REM) sleep, a sleepwalker is not acting out a dream.

Sleepwalking behavior can range from sitting upright in bed to driving a car a long distance. The sleepwalker is awake just enough to be active, but still asleep enough to be unaware of the activity. Sleepwalkers are usually unable to remember the activity. Most sleepwalkers appear awake, with their eyes wide open and dilated. They will not respond if spoken to. In some cases, sleepwalking is associated with incoherent sleep talking.

Injuries to the sleepwalker during such events are common, and simple precautions, like shutting doors and windows, can enhance safety. Sleepwalkers are not easily awakened. If awoken, the sleepwalker will be disoriented and agitated. The best advice is to direct the person back to bed or to a closer location to lie down. Do not inhibit the motion or movement of a sleepwalker, as they have been known to react violently to being detained.

Sleepwalking is a condition that is more prevalent in children. Boys are more likely to sleepwalk than girls. About 10 to 15 percent of children between the ages of five and twelve years old will have at least one episode of sleepwalking.

Researchers estimate about 18 percent of the population is prone to sleepwalking. It typically occurs around the onset of puberty and subsides a short time after. This parasomnia tends to run in families, and rarely indicates any serious underlying medical problem.

When Should I See a Doctor?

Since many young sleepwalkers discontinue their nighttime wanderings after puberty, there is usually no need for treatment. For younger children, a safe sleeping environment, free of harmful or sharp objects, is advised.

For children and adults, sleepwalking is usually a sign of sleep deprivation, intense emotions, stress, or fever. As these circumstances resolve, sleepwalking incidences disappear.

Because most parasomnias are complex in nature, a sleep specialist should carry out diagnosis and treatment. Medical or psychological evaluation should be investigated if any of the following apply:

- The sleepwalker has excessive daytime sleepiness.

- The sleepwalker is violent.

- The sleepwalker has injuries as a result of sleepwalking.

- The sleepwalker disturbs others in the household.

For violent or troublesome sleepwalkers, medications in the benzodiazepine family have proven successful. This class of drugs is a depressant that slows the central nervous system. Forms of benzodiazepine are often prescribed for anxiety, muscle spasms, insomnia, and epilepsy. In sleepwalkers, it reduces motor activity during sleep. Hypnosis has also been found to be helpful for both children and adults.

Sleep Talking

Occasionally, a person may shout out a word or two of gibberish or even recite an entire speech during their sleep. Sleep talking that occurs during REM sleep is understandable, while talking in stage 2 sleep is usually garbled. Sleep talking, or somniloquy, is harmless and usually temporary. The sleeper usually has no memory of their action and it does not affect sleep.

Sleep Terrors

Sleep terrors, also called pavor nocturnus or night terrors, are the most extreme and dramatic of the parasomnias. This disorder is marked by a sudden arousal and a piercing scream or shouting.

The person who has a sleep terror will have signs of intense fear, such as wide eyes with dilated pupils, racing heart, sweating, and rapid breathing. It is not uncommon for a person experiencing a sleep terror to jump out of bed, run around agitated, or hurt themselves and/or others. Fighting is also common and may result in harm to the sleeper or bed partner.

Episodes usually occur during the first hour of falling asleep, the point at which deep sleep begins, and last about fifteen minutes. After the episode, the person returns to sleep, unable to remember the incident in the morning because he or she was never fully awake. A sleep terror patient does not usually experience vivid dream images, but may recall fragments or images of a scene.

Sleep terrors usually occur during stage 3 or stage 4 sleep, the deepest stages of sleep, and children have more deep sleep than adults. Therefore, like sleepwalking, sleep terrors are more common in children. They are also more prevalent in boys. Only 1 to 6 percent of children between the ages of four and twelve experience sleep terrors. Sleep terrors typically do not continue into adulthood (less than 1 percent of the adult population).

Children experiencing a sleep terror may have a strange expression on their face. They are typically unresponsive to their environment; this also includes any comfort that may be offered. In fact, attempting to reassure or calm the child down often results in increased agitation.

For children and adults, sleep terrors can be the result of stress, psychological disturbance, or sleep deprivation. Sleeping in a different bed may also trigger episodes of sleep terrors.

When Should I See a Doctor?

For children under six years of age, occasional sleep terrors usually do not require treatment. Often, sleep terrors in children older than six may be suggestive of an emotional disturbance or a lack of sleep. It is important that a parent be aware of situations in the child's life that may be the trigger of sleep terrors, such as a new school, divorce, or a death in the family.

For children, medical treatment is not necessary unless the child's disturbed sleep causes violent behavior or excessive daytime sleepiness. Bringing up episodes of sleep terrors by parents or siblings only makes the child feel odd or silly. Family members should avoid teasing the child, as it may contribute to the stress or anxiety the child has already. Treatment includes adequate sleep, frequent exercise, and sometimes medication for occasional circumstances, such as sleepovers or summer camp.

In contrast, sleep terrors in adults are serious and abnormal. It is usually indicative of excessive agitation or sleep deprivation, depression, or anxiety. Sleep terrors have also been associated with post-traumatic stress disorder. It is highly recommended that an adult who has sleep terrors see a sleep specialist. In some cases, sleep terrors may be the result of certain medications or withdrawal from a medication. If this is the case, discussing sleep terrors as a side effect with a physician is advocated.

Nightmares

Sleep specialists term a "bad dream" a nightmare if the sleeper is aroused from REM sleep and can recall the dream, often in great detail. A nightmare is composed of a very vivid and frightening dream. Common themes include another person assaulting, attacking, or chasing the person having the dream.

Nightmares are not associated with bodily reactions such as increased heart rate, faster breathing, or sweating. They occur mainly in REM sleep and consequently, late during the sleep cycle in the last third of the night.

Nightmares are normal in children and adults. They are indicative of an unresolved issue or a psychological problem that still troubles the individual, such as what to do if attacked. When the problem is solved, the nightmare disappears.

For young children, having a parent reassure and comfort him or her after a nightmare is helpful in establishing the dream as "not real." Some children will want to discuss the dream, while others maybe fearful at bedtime because of a prior nightmare.

When Should I See a Doctor?

Treatment for nightmares is rarely needed. Only in cases of severe or frequent nightmares are hypnosis or medication required.

Teeth Grinding

Grinding of teeth, or bruxism, is a common nighttime occurrence. In fact, 80 to 90 percent of children and adults grind or clench their teeth during sleep. It is more common in children. Chronic teeth grinding, however, occurs in less than 5 percent of adults.

Most teeth grinders are unaware of their parasomnia. A bed partner who is awakened to the noise, or a dentist who finds teeth with excessive wear more often reports it. Patients may complain of a sore jaw, headaches, or frequent awakenings. Chronic teeth grinding can lead to dental damage or injury.

There is little evidence to suggest that bruxism is associated with any medical or psychological problems. It may be related to stress and uneven alignment of the teeth and jaw.

When Should I See a Doctor?

A chronic teeth grinder should consult with a physician if he or she suffers from excessive daytime sleepiness, frequent nighttime awakenings, or disturbs others in the household. In most cases, the physician will be able to refer the individual to a dental specialist or orthodontist.

There are a number of methods to minimize teeth grinding. If a patient has dental reasons for teeth grinding, the problem can be corrected orthodontically. Rubber mouth guards or dental splints are devices designed by dentists to prevent grinding. Relaxation techniques have also proved helpful.

Other Parasomnias

- **Sleep eating:** a rare variation of sleepwalking. This disorder is characterized by recurrent episodes of eating during sleep, without conscious awareness. It is most common in young women.

- **Hypnagogic hallucinations:** Episodes of dreaming while awake. Common in narcoleptics, but also seen in sleep-deprived individuals.

- **Nocturnal seizures:** Seizures during sleep that cause the victim to cry, scream, or walk; usually treated with medication.

- **REM behavior disorder:** The paralysis that normally occurs during rapid eye movement sleep is incomplete or absent, allowing the sleeper to "act out" dreams.

- **Rhythmic movement disorder:** Most frequently seen in young children, it results in recurrent head banging and body rocking. Behavioral treatments may be effective in severe cases.

Section 21.2

REM Behavior Disorder

"REM Behavior Disorder," Stephen Duntley, MD, and Patricia L. Young, Washington University School of Medicine, St. Louis, Missouri. © 2010. All rights reserved. Reprinted with permission. For additional information about the Washington University Sleep Medicine Center, visit http://sleep .wustl.edu or call 314-362-4342.

REM behavior disorder (RBD) occurs during a stage of sleep known as rapid eye movement (REM) sleep. The characteristic behaviors of this sleep disorder can sometimes be violent and may cause injury, if left untreated.

During the dreaming state, people are normally paralyzed during their dreams and cannot act out their behaviors. Someone with REM behavior disorder is able to act out his dreams due to the loss of muscle atonia.

This particular disorder can be an inherited trait, but tends to present in males more often than females. Sometimes medications such as antidepressants, can cause REM behavior disorder. In these situations the prescribing physician would need to address the situation.

Symptoms

Individuals who experience REM behavior disorder may call out or talk out loud and yell during sleep. Other symptoms may include:

- acting out violent behaviors, such as hitting or thrashing about in or out of the bed;

- sleepiness during the daytime;

- awakening with injury such as lacerations, bleeding, bumps or bruises; and/or

- vivid dreams.

Diagnosis

Patients will have a history and physical evaluation performed by one of the sleep medicine physicians. Because a clinical history alone is insufficient to make the diagnosis, the sleep center physician may decide to proceed with a sleep study or polysomnography.

A sleep study will monitor a patient's sleep, particularly REM sleep and will help in making an accurate diagnosis. Video monitoring and/or a full montage electroencephalogram (EEG) may be performed along with the sleep study to differentiate the unusual behaviors during sleep.

Treatment

Once the diagnosis has been made, the sleep center physician will counsel the patient regarding a treatment plan. Many times medication can help suppress REM sleep and the behaviors associated with this diagnosis. The sleep specialist will also make recommendations for safety measures to be put in place that will help prevent the patient from getting injured during sleep periods.

Section 21.3

Sleep Paralysis

Alternative Names

Sleep paralysis—isolated

Definition

Isolated sleep paralysis is a type of paralysis associated with a sleep disorder. Sleep paralysis is the inability to perform voluntary muscle movements during sleep.

Causes

Isolated sleep paralysis is more likely to happen during the first two hours of sleep. Not getting enough sleep or sleeping on the back may cause more frequent episodes.

Though this condition may be associated with narcolepsy, many people who do not have narcolepsy have isolated sleep paralysis. It is common in adults and is also seen in children.

Most people with isolated sleep paralysis do not have any mental health problems. However, these episodes seem to occur more often in people with:

- bipolar illness;

- depression;

- anxiety disorders;

- post-traumatic stress disorder.

Rarely, it runs in families.

Symptoms

People with isolated sleep paralysis have episodes that last from a few seconds to one or two minutes in which they are unable to move or speak.

These spells end on their own or when the person is touched or moved.

Rarely, the person may have dreamlike sensations or hallucinations, which may be scary to them.

Exams and Tests

If you do not have other symptoms of narcolepsy, there is usually no need to perform sleep studies.

References

Stores G. Parasomnias of childhood and adolescence. *Sleep Med Clin.* 2007;2:405-417.

Mahowald MW. Disorders of sleep. In: Goldman L, Ausiello D, eds. *Cecil Medicine. 23rd ed.* Philadelphia, Pa: Saunders Elsevier; 2007:chap 429.

Section 21.4

Sleepwalking

Alternative Names

Walking during sleep; somnambulism

Definition

Sleepwalking is a disorder that occurs when a person walks or does another activity while they are still asleep.

Causes

The normal sleep cycle has distinct stages, from light drowsiness to deep sleep. During rapid eye movement (REM) sleep, the eyes move quickly and vivid dreaming is most common.

Each night people go through several cycles of non-REM and REM sleep. Sleepwalking (somnambulism) most often occurs during deep, non-REM sleep (stage 3 or stage 4 sleep) early in the night. If it occurs during REM sleep, it is part of REM behavior disorder and tends to happen near morning.

The cause of sleepwalking in children is usually unknown. Fatigue, lack of sleep, and anxiety are all associated with sleepwalking. In adults, sleepwalking may be associated with:

- mental disorders;

- reactions to drugs and alcohol;

- medical conditions such as partial complex seizures.

In the elderly, sleepwalking may be a symptom of an organic brain syndrome or REM behavior disorders.

Sleepwalking can occur at any age, but it happens most often in children aged four to eight. It appears to run in families.

Symptoms

When people sleepwalk, they may sit up and look as though they are awake when they are actually asleep. They may get up and walk around, or do complex activities such as moving furniture, going to the bathroom, and dressing or undressing. Some people even drive a car while they are asleep.

The episode can be very brief (a few seconds or minutes) or it can last for thirty minutes or longer. If they are not disturbed, sleepwalkers will go back to sleep. However, they may fall asleep in a different or even unusual place.

Symptoms of sleepwalking include:

- eyes open during sleep;

- may have blank look on face;

- may sit up and appear awake during sleep;

- walking during sleep;

- performing other detailed activity of any type during sleep;

- not remembering the sleepwalking episode when they wake up;

- acting confused or disoriented when they wake up;

- rarely, aggressive behavior when they are awakened by someone else;

- sleep talking that does not make sense.

Exams and Tests

Usually, people do not need further examinations and testing. If the sleepwalking occurs often, the doctor may do an exam or tests to rule out other disorders (such as partial complex seizures).

If you have a history of emotional problems, you also may need to have a psychological evaluation to look for causes such as excessive anxiety or stress.

Treatment

Some people mistakenly believe that a sleepwalker should not be awakened. It is not dangerous to awaken a sleepwalker, although it is common for the person to be confused or disoriented for a short time when they wake up.

Another misconception is that a person cannot be injured while sleepwalking. Sleepwalkers are commonly injured when they trip and lose their balance.

Most people don't need any specific treatment for sleepwalking.

Safety measures may be needed to prevent injury. This may include moving objects such as electrical cords or furniture to reduce the chances of tripping and falling. You may need to block off stairways with a gate.

In some cases, short-acting tranquilizers have been helpful in reducing sleepwalking episodes.

Outlook (Prognosis)

Sleepwalking usually decreases as children get older. It usually does not indicate a serious disorder, although it can be a symptom of other disorders.

It is unusual for sleepwalkers to perform activities that are dangerous. However, you may need to take care to prevent injuries such as falling down stairs or climbing out of a window.

Possible Complications

The main complication is getting injured while sleepwalking.

When to Contact a Medical Professional

You probably won't need to visit your healthcare provider if you are sleepwalking. However, discuss the condition with your doctor if:

- you also have other symptoms;

- sleepwalking is frequent or persistent;

- you perform potentially dangerous activities (such as driving) while sleepwalking.

Prevention

- Avoid the use of alcohol or central nervous system depressants if you sleepwalk.

- Avoid getting too tired and try to prevent insomnia, because this can trigger a sleepwalking episode.

- Avoid or minimize stress, anxiety, and conflict, which can worsen the condition.

References

Mahowald MW. Disorders of sleep. In: Goldman L, Ausiello D, eds. *Cecil Medicine. 23rd ed.* Philadelphia, Pa: Saunders Elsevier; 2007:chap 429.

Plante DT, Winkelman JW. Parasomnias. *Psychiatr Clin North Am.* 2006; 29:969–87.

Section 21.5

Sleep Eating

Overview

Sleep eating is a sleep-related disorder, although some specialists consider it to be a combination of a sleep and an eating disorder. It is a relatively rare and little known condition that is gaining recognition in sleep medicine. Other names for sleep eating are sleep-related eating (disorder), nocturnal sleep-related eating disorder (NS-RED), and sleep-eating syndrome.

Sleep eating is characterized by sleepwalking and excessive nocturnal overeating (compulsive hyperphagia). Sleep eaters are comparable to sleepwalkers in many ways: they are at risk for self-injury during an episode; they may (or may not) experience excessive daytime sleepiness; and they are usually emotionally distressed, tired, angry, or anxious. Sleep eaters are also at risk for the same health complications as compulsive overeaters, with the added dangers of sleepwalking. Common concerns include excessive weight gain, daytime sleepiness, choking while eating, sleep disruption, and injury from cooking or preparing food such as from knives, utensils, or hot cooking surfaces. There is also the potential for starting a fire.

As with sleepwalkers, sleep eaters are unaware and unconscious of their behavior. If there is any memory of the episode, it is usually

223

sketchy. A sleep eater will roam the house, particularly the kitchen, and may eat large quantities of food (as well as non-food items). In the morning, sleep eaters have no recollection of the episode. However, in many cases there are clues to their behavior. One woman woke up with a stomachache and chocolate smeared on her face and hands. Candy wrappers littered the kitchen floor. The next morning her husband informed her that she had been eating during the night. She was shocked and distressed because she had no recollection of the event.

As in the case described above, food consumed by sleep eaters tends to be either high sugar or high fat. Odd combinations of foods, such as potato chips dipped in peanut butter or butter smeared on hotdogs, as well as non-food items, have been reported. Oddly, one person was discovered cutting a bar of soap into slices and then eating it as if it were a slice of cheese!

Sleep eating is classified as a parasomnia. It is a rare version of sleepwalking, which is an arousal disorder. In 1968, Roger Broughton published a paper in *Science* (159:1070–78) that outlined the major features of arousal disorders. They are:

- abnormal behavior that occurs during an arousal from slow wave sleep;

- the absence of awareness during the episode;

- automatic and repetitive motor activity;

- slow reaction time and reduced sensitivity to environment;

- difficulty in waking despite vigorous attempts;

- no memory of the episode in the morning (retrograde amnesia); and

- no or little dream recall associated with the event.

How Common Is Sleep Eating?

The actual number of sleep-eating sufferers is unknown; however, it is estimated that 1 to 3 percent of the population is affected by sleep eating. A higher percentage of persons with eating disorders, as many as 10 to 15 percent, are affected. For this reason, sleep eating is more common in younger women. Symptoms typically begin in the late twenties. Episodes may reoccur, in combination with a stressful situation, or an episode may occur only once or twice. Additionally, many parasomnias seem to run in families, which may indicate that sleep eating is genetically linked.

When Should I See a Doctor?

In many cases, sleep eating is the outward sign of an underlying problem. Many sufferers are overweight and dieting. When their control is diminished by sleep, these individuals binge at night to satisfy their hunger. Some sleep eaters have histories of alcoholism, drug abuse, or a primary sleep disorder, such as sleepwalking, restless legs syndrome, or sleep apnea. An article in *Sleep* (October 1991:14(5): 419–31) suggested that sleep eating is directly linked to the onset of another medical problem.

Because sleep eating occurs in people that are usually dieting and emotionally distressed, attempts at weight loss may be unsuccessful and cause even more stress. Compounded with the dangers of sleepwalking, compulsive eating while asleep is a sleep disorder that results in weight gain, disrupted sleep, and daytime sleepiness. As these consequences of sleep eating impact daily living, the necessity of seeing a healthcare professional becomes more important.

Parasomnias are complex and often serious in nature. If you think you suffer from sleep eating, consult with your physician or a healthcare professional who can refer you to a sleep disorders treatment center. It is strongly recommended that a sleep specialist carry out the diagnosis and treatment. Medical or psychological evaluation should also be investigated.

How Is Sleep Eating Treated?

The first step in treating any sleep disorder is to ascertain any underlying causes. As with most parasomnias, sleep eating is usually the result of an underlying problem, which may include another sleep disorder, prescription drug abuse, nicotine withdrawal, chronic autoimmune hepatitis, encephalitis (or hypothalamic injury), or acute stress (*Sleep* 1991 Oct; 14(5):419–31).

It is important to keep in mind that throughout life, people experience varying patterns of sleep and nutrition during positive and negative situations. Problems with eating are defined as overeating or not eating enough. Problems with sleeping can be simplified with two symptoms, too much or not enough sleep. Medical attention is required for abnormal behaviors in either or both areas.

For some people who have been diagnosed with sleep eating, interventions without the use of medications have proven helpful. Courses on stress management, group or one-on-one counseling with a therapist, or self-confidence training may alleviate the stress and anxiety that leads to nighttime bingeing. Although considered an alternative treatment, hypnosis may be an option for some sleep eaters. A change in diet that includes avoiding certain foods and eating at specified times of the day, as well as reducing the intake of caffeine or alcohol, may be therapeutic. Professional advice may also suggest avoiding certain medications.

If the underlying problem is diagnosed as sleepwalking, medications in the benzodiazepine family have had some success. In sleepwalkers, this class of drugs reduces motor activity during sleep. Another class of drug found to be effective for sleep eaters has been the dopaminergic agents such as Sinemet® (carbidopa or levodopa) and Mirapex® (pramipexole dihydrochloride).

Night Eating: Another Disorder of Sleep and Eating

A similar sleep-related eating disorder has also been clinically described. It is different from sleep eating in that the individual is awake during episodes of nocturnal bingeing. This disorder has many names: nocturnal eating (or drinking) syndrome, nighttime hunger, nocturnal eating, night eating or drinking (syndrome), or the "Dagwood" syndrome. Affected individuals are physically unable to sleep without food intake.

The *Merck Manual* lists night eating under the heading obesity. It states that the disorder "consists of morning anorexia, excessive ingestion of food in the evening, and insomnia." Because night eating is associated with increased weight gain as well as insomnia, this may cause the individual stress, anxiety, or depression.

Night eating or drinking may occur once or many times during the night. It is diagnosed when 50 percent or more of an individual's diet is consumed between sleeping hours. Unlike sleep eaters, this person will eat foods that are similar to his or her normal diet.

People who are night eaters typically avoid food until noon or later, eat small portions frequently when they do eat, and binge in the evening. They are usually overweight and in adults, overly stressed or anxious. They will also complain of not being able to maintain sleep or not being able to initiate sleep. For night eaters, the urge to eat is an abnormal need, rather than true hunger, according to an article in *Sleep* by Italian researchers (September 1997; 20(9):734–38).

Night eaters/drinkers are usually children, although the disorder can occur in adults. For children, eating or drinking at night is a conditioned behavior. This is a common occurrence for babies, but most infants can sleep the entire night by the age of six months. Sleep disturbance can persist to an older age if the child is allowed a bottle or drinks throughout the night. An older child may consistently wake up during the night and ask for a drink or something to eat and refuse to return to bed until the snack is consumed. In this case, the caregiver should identify actual need versus repeated requests.

According to the International Classification of Sleep Disorders, night eating is characterized as a dyssomnia (as opposed to sleep eating, which is considered a parasomnia). A dyssomnia is a disorder of sleep or wakefulness in which insomnia or excessive daytime sleepiness is a complaint. Within the heading of dyssomnia, night eating is classified as an extrinsic sleep disorder, which means that it originates, develops, or is caused by an external source. Eating or drinking at night is usually a conditioned, conscious behavior; although it is a disorder, in many cases night eating is not caused by a psychological or medical condition.

Night eating may arise because of an ulcer, by dieting during the day, by undue stress, or by a routine expectation (conditioned behavior). Hypoglycemia, or low blood sugar, has also been proposed as possible cause of nighttime bingeing in some people. This can be determined by a glucose tolerance test.

How Is Night Eating Treated?

For children, treatment of this disorder mainly involves the caregiver. For a young child, weaning from the breast, bottle, or drinks during the night is essential. The adult should evaluate if the request for food or drink is based on real need. If the demand is false, the adult should deny the request. Eventually, waking up with the urge for food or drink will be eliminated.

For an adult, it is important to first recognize that the behavior is not normal. (If the pattern of eating at night has been persistent for a long time, a night eater may only complain of insomnia and weight gain.) Secondly, a night eater should schedule an appointment with a physician. Night eating may be the result of a medical condition or hypoglycemia, both of which can be treated. If not, the habit of eating in the middle of the night can be broken with behavior modification and/or stress reduction. Eating frequent small meals during the day beginning in the morning, reducing carbohydrate intake, and increasing protein intake before bedtime are diet patterns that may help. Protein metabolizes slowly and will stabilize blood sugar levels during sleep. Contrary to protein, sugary snacks raise the blood sugar quickly, then cause it to plunge. So, avoid sweet foods before bedtime.

Night eaters who have conquered their uncontrollable need for nocturnal food or drink often sleep equally as well or better than before they started night eating.

Part Four

Other Health Problems that Often Affect Sleep

Chapter 22

Alzheimer's Disease and Changing Sleep Patterns

Introduction

Many people with Alzheimer's experience changes in their sleep patterns. Scientists do not completely understand why this happens. As with changes in memory and behavior, sleep changes somehow result from the impact of Alzheimer's on the brain.

Many older adults without dementia also notice changes in their sleep, but these disturbances occur more frequently and tend to be more severe in Alzheimer's. There is evidence that sleep changes are more common in later stages of the disease, but some studies have also found them in early stages.

Sleep changes in Alzheimer's may include:

- **Difficulty sleeping:** Many people with Alzheimer's wake up more often and stay awake longer during the night. Brain wave studies show decreases in both dreaming and non-dreaming sleep stages. Those who cannot sleep may wander, be unable to lie still, or yell or call out, disrupting the sleep of their caregivers.

- **Daytime napping and other shifts in the sleep-wake cycle:** Individuals may feel very drowsy during the day and then be unable to sleep at night. They may become restless or agitated in the late afternoon or early evening, an experience often called "sundowning." Experts estimate that in late stages of Alzheimer's, individuals spend about 40 percent of their time in bed at night awake and a significant part of their daytime sleeping. In extreme cases, people may have a complete reversal of the usual daytime wakefulness-nighttime sleep pattern.

Treatment of Sleep Changes

A person experiencing sleep disturbances should have a thorough medical exam to identify any treatable illnesses that may be contributing to the problem. Examples of conditions that can make sleep problems worse include:

- depression;
- restless legs syndrome, a disorder in which unpleasant "crawling" or "tingling" sensations in the legs cause an overwhelming urge to move them;
- sleep apnea, an abnormal breathing pattern in which people briefly stop breathing many times a night, resulting in poor sleep quality.

For sleep changes due primarily to Alzheimer's disease, there are non-drug and drug approaches to treatment. Most experts and the National Institutes of Health (NIH) strongly encourage use of non-drug measures rather than medication.

Studies have found that sleep medications generally do not improve overall sleep quality for older adults. Use of sleep medications is associated with a greater chance of falls and other risks that may outweigh the benefits of treatment.

Non-Drug Treatments for Sleep Changes

Non-drug treatments aim to improve sleep routine and the sleeping environment and reduce daytime napping. To create an inviting sleeping environment and promote rest for a person with Alzheimer's:

- Maintain regular times for meals and for going to bed and getting up.
- Seek morning sunlight exposure.
- Encourage regular daily exercise, but no later than four hours before bedtime.

- Avoid alcohol, caffeine, and nicotine.

- Treat any pain.

- If the person is taking a cholinesterase inhibitor (tacrine, done-pezil, rivastigmine, or galantamine), avoid giving the medicine before bed.

- Make sure the bedroom temperature is comfortable.

- Provide nightlights and security objects.

- If the person awakens, discourage staying in bed while awake; use the bed only for sleep.

- Discourage watching television during periods of wakefulness.

Medications for Sleep Changes

In some cases, non-drug approaches fail to work or the sleep changes are accompanied by disruptive nighttime behaviors. For those individuals who do require medication, experts recommend that treatment "begin low and go slow."

The risks of sleep-inducing medications for older people who are cognitively impaired are considerable. They include increased risk for falls and fractures, confusion, and a decline in the ability to care for oneself. If sleep medications are used, an attempt should be made to discontinue them after a regular sleep pattern has been established.

The type of medication prescribed by a doctor is often influenced by behaviors that may accompany the sleep changes. Examples of medications used to treat sleep changes include:

- tricyclic antidepressants, such as nortriptyline and trazodone;

- benzodiazepines, such as lorazepam, oxazepam, and temazepam;

- "sleeping pills" such as zolpidem, zaleplon, and chloral hydrate;

- "atypical" antipsychotics such as risperidone, olanzapine, and quetiapine;

- older "classical" antipsychotics such as haloperidol.

Chapter 23

Cancer Patients and Sleep Disorders

Overview

Sleep disorders occur in some people with cancer and may be caused by physical illness, pain, treatment drugs, being in the hospital, and emotional stress. Sleep has two phases: rapid eye movement (REM) and non-REM (NREM). REM sleep, also known as "dream sleep," is the phase of sleep in which the brain is active. NREM is the quiet or restful phase of sleep. The stages of sleep occur in a repeated pattern of NREM followed by REM. Each sleep cycle lasts about ninety minutes and is repeated four to six times during a seven- to eight-hour sleep period. The four major categories of sleep disorders that interfere with normal sleep patterns include the following:

- The inability to fall asleep and stay asleep (insomnia)

- Disorders of the sleep-wake cycle

- Disorders associated with sleep stages, or partial waking (parasomnia)

- Excessive sleepiness

PDQ® Cancer Information Summary. National Cancer Institute; Bethesda, MD. Sleep Disorders (PDQ®): Patient Version. Updated January 2010. Available at http://cancer.gov. Accessed August 2, 2010.

Risk Factors

The sleep disorders most likely to affect patients with cancer are insomnias and disorders of the sleep-wake cycle. Effects of tumor growth and cancer treatment that may cause sleep disturbances include the following:

- Anxiety or depression
- Pain or itching
- Fever, cough, or trouble breathing
- Fatigue
- Seizures
- Headaches
- Night sweats or hot flashes
- Diarrhea, constipation, nausea, or incontinence

Long-term use of certain drugs commonly used during cancer treatment may cause insomnia. Stopping or decreasing the use of certain drugs may also cause insomnia.

Some drugs that help patients sleep (such as hypnotics and sedatives) should not be stopped suddenly without the advice of a doctor. Suddenly stopping these medicines may cause nervousness, seizures, and a change in REM sleep that increases dreaming, including nightmares. This change in REM sleep may be dangerous for patients with peptic ulcers or heart conditions.

Patients may have sleep interruptions due to treatment schedules, hospital routines, and roommates. Other factors affecting sleep during a hospital stay include noise, temperature, pain, anxiety, and the patient's age. Chronic sleep disturbances can cause irritability, inability to concentrate, depression, and anxiety. While in the hospital, sleep disorders may make it hard for the patient to continue with cancer therapy.

Diagnosis

To diagnose sleep disorders in cancer patients, the doctor will get the patient's complete medical history and give a physical examination. The doctor may get information about the patient's sleep history and patterns of sleep from the patient, from observations, and from the patient's family and friends. A polysomnogram, an instrument that measures brain waves, eye movements, muscle tone, heart rate, and breathing during sleep, may also be used to diagnose sleep disorders in patients with cancer.

Treatment

Sleep disorders that are related to cancer may be treated by eliminating the cancer and side effects of cancer treatment. To promote rest and treat sleep disorders the following may be considered:

- Create an environment that decreases sleep interruptions by:
  - Lowering noise
  - Dimming or turning off lights
  - Adjusting room temperature
  - Keeping bedding, chairs, and pillows clean, dry, and wrinkle-free
  - Using bedcovers for warmth
  - Placing pillows in a supportive position
  - Encouraging the patient to dress in loose, soft clothing
- Encourage regular bowel and bladder habits to minimize sleep interruptions, such as:
  - No drinking before bedtime
  - Emptying the bowel and bladder before going to bed
  - Increasing consumption of fluids and fiber during the day
  - Taking medication for incontinence before bedtime

Rest in patients with cancer may also be promoted by:

- Eating a high-protein snack two hours before bedtime
- Avoiding heavy, spicy, or sugary foods four to six hours before bedtime
- Avoiding drinking alcohol or smoking four to six hours before bedtime
- Avoiding drinks with caffeine
- Exercising (which should be completed at least two hours before bedtime)
- Keeping regular sleeping hours

It is important for the patient to talk about sleep problems with family and the healthcare team so education and support can be offered. Some treatments help the patient change thoughts and behaviors to decrease anxiety and relax mentally, so sleep can happen more easily:

- Relaxation exercises
- Self- hypnosis at bedtime
- Cognitive-behavior therapy, in which the patient learns to change the goal from "I need to sleep" to "just relax." This may help the patient relax enough to fall asleep.

Drugs may also be used to help patients with cancer manage their sleep disorders.

Chapter 24

Gastroesophageal Reflux Disorder and Sleep

Gastroesophageal reflux is a very common condition, and most of us experience at least a mild degree of it at some point or another. While it is little more than an annoyance to most, gastroesophageal reflux sometimes becomes a serious issue, and can impact upon on many activities, including sleep.

To understand gastroesophageal reflux, it is helpful to first understand how the esophagus and stomach normally function. The esophagus is a long, muscular tube that connects to the throat and carries food down into the stomach. When a lump of food is swallowed, it is pushed downward by esophageal muscles, much like squeezing a tube of toothpaste. Upon reaching the bottom of the esophagus, a circular muscle known as the lower esophageal sphincter (LES) relaxes and allows food to pass into the stomach. The LES promptly closes, and food in the stomach is washed with gastric fluids to create a soupy mixture.

The stomach produces powerful acids and digestive enzymes, which mix with food to kill harmful bacteria and break the food down into small enough pieces to be absorbed. Because of the resulting harsh acidic environment, the stomach has a special lining that resists the corrosive fluids. When the stomach has completed its work, the semi-digested mixture moves into the small intestine, where the acid is neutralized and the next phase of digestion begins.

"Gastroesophageal Reflux and Sleep" by David A. Cooke, MD, FACP, © 2010 Omnigraphics.

239

Unfortunately, the stomach and esophagus do not always function according to design. A variety of problems can arise in the transport of food from the mouth to the esophagus to the stomach and beyond. The most common issue is gastroesophageal reflux.

When the stomach contracts to churn its contents, the food-acid mixture may wash back up into the esophagus (reflux) if the LES is not tightly closed. The LES normally loosens and tightens at intervals as part of its normal function. Some individuals have unusually frequent episodes of LES loosening. This can be problematic, because the esophagus does not share the stomach's protective lining. The acids and digestive enzymes from the stomach cause chemical burns in the esophagus.

The esophageal damage is most often experienced as heartburn; a painful, burning sensation behind the breastbone, which often seems to ascend toward the throat. This may range from mild and occasional to severe and constant. Reflux can also be sensed in other ways, such as burping, chest pain resembling a heart attack, a need to cough, wheezing, or a sensation that something is stuck in the throat. Sometimes, stomach contents will wash all the way up to the mouth, causing an unpleasant sour taste (acid brash). If reflux is frequent and severe, it can lead to deep ulcerations, difficulty swallowing, and scarring of the esophagus. Infrequently, individuals may have few or no symptoms, despite quite severe reflux and esophageal damage.

Reflux will occur at least occasionally in almost everyone. It is termed gastroesophageal reflux disease (GERD) when it causes frequent symptoms or complications.

It is not known why GERD occurs, although a number of factors are known to contribute to it. An anatomic variation known as a hiatal hernia is very frequent in the general population, and is almost universally present in GERD suffers. Hiatal hernia reduces the effectiveness of the LES, and predisposes to GERD. Obesity is a major risk factor for GERD; excess fat in the abdomen puts pressure on the stomach, encouraging reflux. Many common foods affect the function of the LES. Caffeine, alcohol, fats, and mint all relax the LES muscle, making it easier for reflux to occur. Nicotine from tobacco products has a similar effect on the LES, as do many prescription and nonprescription medications. For example, many antihistamines, medications for high blood pressure, and some antidepressants tend to aggravate GERD. Finally, while it is relatively uncommon, the LES is found to be almost completely nonfunctional in some cases of severe GERD.

GERD symptoms may occur at any time, but they are often more severe and bothersome during sleep. The reasons for this are relatively simple. When a person stands upright, the force of gravity tends to limit upward reflux of the stomach contents. However, most people sleep lying down. In this position, gravity does not oppose liquid movement into the esophagus, and the gastric contents may flow more freely.

Many individuals develop painful heartburn when they lay down in bed for sleep, or they may be awakened by heartburn once they have fallen asleep. Some people who do not experience heartburn nonetheless have evidence of sleep disruption–related episodes of reflux if they are carefully monitored during sleep studies. More severe GERD may lead to complaints of awakening with a mouthful of acid, or even regurgitating during sleep.

It has also been noted that GERD coexists with sleep apnea more frequently than would be expected by chance alone. Evidence to date has suggested that the two do not directly affect one another, but rather share similar risk factors. However, treatment of sleep apnea with continuous positive airway pressure (CPAP) frequently has a beneficial effect on GERD.

Fortunately, there are a number of ways that GERD can be effectively treated. Solving this problem can greatly improve sleep quality for many affected individuals.

Relatively simple dietary and lifestyle adjustments are frequently effective for GERD. Modest weight loss will often significantly improve GERD. Avoiding caffeine, chocolate, alcohol, mint, fatty foods, and tobacco, particularly in the evening hours, will often substantially improve reflux. Scheduling evening meals to be several hours before bedtime is also helpful, as this gives the stomach an opportunity to empty before lying down to sleep. Limiting the size of evening meals is also helpful, as a very full stomach puts pressure on the LES and promotes reflux.

Elevating the head during sleep is a commonly used treatment. Some nighttime reflux sufferers find that sleeping in a chair will give good relief. However, most people with GERD need not take measures this drastic. Elevating the head end of the bed by a few inches relative to the foot will allow you to sleep on a slight upward angle. This is usually not enough to cause discomfort, but is enough to utilize gravity's downward pull to keep food in the stomach. Supports under the head posts of the bed or soft wedges under the mattress are widely available for this use.

These measures are effective for many GERD sufferers, but not everyone sees adequate relief. Further medical intervention is sometimes necessary.

The ideal therapy for GERD would be one that prevents relaxation of the LES so that reflux cannot occur. Unfortunately, there has been little progress in developing medications that accomplish this. Baclofen (Lioresal®) has been reported to be effective, but it has significant side effects that prevent routine use.

Surgical procedures can tighten the LES, and are performed in resistant cases of GERD. However, they are invasive and carry significant risks. If the procedure is too effective, a person may not be able to swallow at all. Therefore, while addressing LES function is the most obvious solution for GERD, it is not usually the preferred approach.

Medications that promote prompt emptying of the stomach may help by removing most of the gastric contents. However, their effectiveness tends to be relatively limited. In addition, most of the drugs used for this purpose have potentially serious side effects. Metoclopramide (Reglan®) can cause neurologic problems known as tardive dyskinesia, which are sometimes permanent. Cisapride (Propulsid®) is available only under very tight restrictions, as it has been linked to fatal heart rhythm disturbances. Domperidone (Motilium®) has not been approved for use in the United States due to similar concerns about effects on the heart, and can be used legally only under exceptional circumstances.

The primary approach to treatment of GERD is reducing the acidity of the stomach contents. This does not prevent the backwash of fluids into the esophagus, but it limits the damage that may occur.

Antacids react directly with stomach acid and neutralize it. Calcium carbonate is the most commonly used antacid, found in Tums® and many other preparations, but others are available. They typically give prompt but short-term relief, and are often the most practical approach for occasional GERD. Some people find that taking a dose of antacids before bed greatly improves sleep quality.

When antacids are inadequate, medications that suppress the production of stomach acid may be used. Histamine type 2 receptor antagonists (H2RAs) have been in wide use for several decades. H2RAs block the hormonal signals that stimulate acid production in the stomach. Commonly used H2RAs include cimetidine (Tagamet®), ranitidine (Zantac®), famotidine (Pepcid®), and nizatidine (Axid®), and are available in both over-the-counter and prescription forms. They are generally effective and usually have few side effects. However, it is worth recognizing that cimetidine (Tagamet®) may cause more side effects than other H2RAs and can have serious interactions with a number of common drugs.

For the most severe cases of GERD, proton pump inhibitors (PPIs) are the drugs of choice. PPIs sabotage the cellular machinery that produces stomach acid, resulting in a dramatic decrease in stomach acidity.

A number of PPIs are available, including omeprazole (Prilosec®, Zegerid®), lansoprazole (Prevacid®), pantoprazole (Protonix®), rabeprazole (AcipHex®), esomeprazole (Nexium®), and dexlansoprazole (Dexilant®, Kapidex®). Some of these medications are also available over the counter, although others are still prescription-only.

PPIs are generally the most effective medications for GERD. However, they can cause stomach upset, diarrhea, and headache in some individuals. Concerns have also been raised about increased risk of gastrointestinal infections and pneumonia in patients taking PPIs, probably due to reduced killing of bacteria in the stomach. There is also limited evidence that long-term use of PPIs may increase the risk of certain vitamin deficiencies and osteoporosis by altering absorption. However, these risks appear to be small, and should not prevent their use for most individuals.

If you believe that GERD may be impacting on your sleep, discuss these concerns with your physician. Nighttime heartburn is an obvious sign, but keep in mind that poor quality sleep is sometimes the only sign of GERD, and the diagnosis needs to be considered if other causes of sleep disruption have been excluded.

As stated above, lifestyle and dietary approaches are sufficient to provide relief for many GERD sufferers. Your physician may also identify medications you are taking that aggravate GERD, and determine whether they can be substituted or stopped.

In addition, your physician may be able to identify more serious conditions that could be mistaken for GERD. Generally speaking, GERD symptoms associated with difficulty swallowing, unintentional weight loss, or vomiting are considered "warning signs" and require more in-depth investigation and testing.

If non-medication approaches fail, your physician can determine which medications are most appropriate for treating your symptoms. Many individuals who take PPIs for GERD don't need them long term, and may be able to transition to an H2RA. Therefore, it's worthwhile discussing your GERD with your doctor from time to time, even if you are already on therapy. For the most severe and persistent cases, surgical options do exist, and your physician can help determine whether and when these are appropriate.

Chapter 25

Mental Health and Sleep

Chapter Contents

Section 25.1

Anxiety and Sleep Disorders

A good night's sleep is important to good health. Many of us toss and turn or watch the clock when we can't sleep for a night or two. But for some, a restless night is routine. More than forty million Americans suffer from chronic, long-term sleep disorders, and an additional twenty million report sleeping problems occasionally, according to the National Institutes of Health. Stress and anxiety may cause sleeping problems or make existing problems worse. And having an anxiety disorder can only exacerbate the problem.

What is an anxiety disorder?

Anxiety disorders are a unique group of illnesses that fill people's lives with persistent, excessive, and unreasonable anxiety, worry, and fear. They include generalized anxiety disorder (GAD), obsessive-compulsive disorder (OCD), panic disorder, posttraumatic stress disorder (PTSD), social anxiety disorder (SAD), and specific phobias. Anxiety disorders are real, serious medical conditions, but they can be treated.

What is a sleep disorder?

Sleep disorders are conditions characterized by abnormal sleep patterns that interfere with physical, mental, and emotional functioning. Stress or anxiety can cause a serious night without sleep, as do a variety of other problems. Insomnia is the clinical term for people who have trouble falling asleep, difficulty staying asleep, waking too early in the morning, or waking up feeling unrefreshed. Other common sleep disorders include sleep apnea (loud snoring caused by an obstructed airway), sleepwalking, and narcolepsy (falling asleep spontaneously). Restless leg syndrome and bruxism (grinding of the teeth while sleeping) are conditions that also may contribute to sleep disorders.

Does an anxiety disorder lead to a sleep disorder, or does a sleep disorder cause an anxiety disorder?

Either is possible. Anxiety does cause sleeping problems, and new research suggests sleep deprivation can cause an anxiety disorder. That's because a lack of sleep stimulates the part of the brain most closely associated with depression, anxiety, and other psychiatric disorders. Research also shows that some form of sleep disruption is present in nearly all psychiatric disorders.

For those living with anxiety disorders, insomnia is part of a vicious cycle. Many symptoms of anxiety disorders, including excessive stress, persistent worry, obsessive thoughts, gastrointestinal problems, and nightmares are likely to rob precious sleep. And some antidepressants commonly prescribed for anxiety disorders may cause sleep difficulties. The results of a study published in the July 2007 issue of *Sleep* suggest that people with chronic insomnia are at high risk of developing an anxiety disorder.

Other research suggests that sleep deprivation results in people focusing on negative emotions, according to Mark H. Pollack, MD, director of the Center for Anxiety and Traumatic Stress Disorders at Massachusetts General Hospital. Pollack says this can decrease the effectiveness of exposure-based cognitive-behavioral therapy.

If I have a sleep disorder, does that put me at risk for other health issues?

The risks of inadequate sleep extend way beyond tiredness. Sleeplessness can lead to poor performance at work or school, increased risk of injury, and health problems.

"Ninety percent of the time people who have insomnia also have another health condition," says Thomas Roth, PhD, director of the Sleep Disorders and Research Center at Henry Ford Hospital. "Most frequently those include anxiety and mood disorders, and treating each condition impacts the course of the other." Those with sleep disorders may also be at risk for heart disease, heart failure, irregular heartbeat, heart attack, high blood pressure, stroke, and diabetes. And some researchers say that adults who sleep less than six hours a night are 50 percent more likely to become obese than those who sleep seven to eight hours a night.

What are my treatment options?

It's important to obtain an accurate diagnosis for any medical conditions that may contribute to a sleep disorder or anxiety disorder, as well as to determine which is the primary condition. This information will help you and your doctor determine the most appropriate treatment plan.

If you suspect you have a sleep disorder, see a primary care physician or mental health professional, or visit a clinic that specializes in sleep disorders. Treatment options include sleep medicine and cognitive-behavior therapy, which teaches how to identify and modify behaviors that perpetuate sleeping problems.

Treatment options for an anxiety disorder include cognitive-behavior therapy, relaxation techniques, and medication. Your doctor or therapist may recommend one or a combination of these treatments.

What else can I do to reduce anxiety and sleep more soundly?

To reduce anxiety and stress:

- **Meditate:** Focus on your breath—breathe in and out slowly and deeply—and visualize a serene environment such as a deserted beach or grassy hill.

- **Exercise:** Regular exercise is good for your physical and mental health. It provides an outlet for frustrations and releases mood-enhancing endorphins. Yoga can be particularly effective at reducing anxiety and stress.

- **Prioritize your to-do list:** Spend your time and energy on the tasks that are truly important, and break up large projects into smaller, more easily managed tasks. Delegate when you can.

- **Play music:** Soft, calming music can lower your blood pressure and relax your mind and body.

- **Get an adequate amount of sleep:** Sleeping recharges your brain and improves your focus, concentration, and mood.

- **Direct stress and anxiety elsewhere:** Lend a hand to a relative or neighbor, or volunteer in your community. Helping others will take your mind off of your own anxiety and fears.

- **Talk to someone:** Let friends and family know how they can help, and consider seeing a doctor or therapist.

To sleep more soundly:

- **Make getting a good night's sleep a priority:** Block out seven to nine hours for a full night of uninterrupted sleep, and try to wake up at the same time every day, including weekends.

- **Establish a regular, relaxing bedtime routine:** Avoid stimulants like coffee, chocolate, and nicotine before going to sleep, and never watch TV, use the computer, or pay bills before going to bed. Read a book, listen to soft music, or meditate instead.

- **Make sure your bedroom is cool, dark, and quiet:** Consider using a fan to drown out excess noise, and make sure your mattress and pillows are comfortable.

- **Use your bedroom as a bedroom—not for watching TV or doing work—and get into bed only when you are tired:** If you don't fall asleep within fifteen minutes, go to another room and do something relaxing.

- **Exercise:** Regular exercise will help you sleep better, but limit your workouts to mornings and afternoons.

- **Avoid looking at the clock:** This can make you anxious in the middle of the night. Turn the clock away from you.

Talk to your doctor if you still have problems falling asleep You may need a prescription or herbal sleep remedy.

Section 25.2

Sleep and Depression

"Sleep and Depression," by David A. Cooke, MD, FACP,
© 2010 Omnigraphics.

Sleep and depression are deeply interrelated issues. The term "losing sleep" has made its way into our language, and reflects an intuitive understanding of this relationship.

Sleep disturbances are considered once of the hallmarks of depression. Studies indicate that greater than 80 percent of depressed patients have symptoms of sleep disturbance, and sleep disturbances are one of the diagnostic criteria for depression in the *Diagnostic and Statistical Manual IV-TR*, the gold standard for psychiatric diagnosis. Depression-related sleep changes most often consist of insomnia, including difficulty initiating or maintaining sleep, as well as early morning awakenings. However, some depressed individuals instead complain of excessive sleep.

Interestingly, there is evidence that not only does depression lead to sleep disturbance, but sleep disturbance can also lead to depression. Sleep deprivation can produce many of the symptoms of depression, and may be the inciting cause of a major depressive episode in predisposed individuals.

Biological explanations for these interrelationships between sleep and depression have been identified. The normal sleep-wake cycle is controlled by regions of the brain that act as tiny clocks. These timers are able to keep time independently of outside stimuli, although they normally reset according to exposures to light and dark conditions. The clock regions control production of hormonal systems that regulate body functions including temperature, digestion, and the onset of sleep.

The neurochemical disturbances that lead to depression affect many of the same brain regions that regulate sleep. This may disrupt the normal rhythms of sleep, and sleep disturbances are often among the first symptoms to appear with depression.

Inability to sleep can also considerably aggravate depressive symptoms, and severe insomnia is a marker of increased suicide risk. Anxiety and worry often intrude upon sleep, and may prevent falling asleep, or cause recurrent awakenings.

When insomnia is due to depression, treatment of depression is usually the most helpful course of action. Psychological therapies for depression such as cognitive behavior therapy and interpersonal therapy often produce improvements in sleep.

Nearly all antidepressant medications improve sleep quality in people with depression. While the exact manner in which these drugs improve depression is not fully understood, it is noteworthy that changes in sleep patterns occur even when they are given to individuals who are not depressed.

While nearly all antidepressants improve sleep, they may not all be equal in this respect. Nefazodone, mirtazapine, and trazodone all tend to increase sleep, and may be ideal for depression with severe insomnia. The tricyclic class of antidepressants, which includes imipramine, amitriptyline, desipramine, nortriptyline, and doxepin, is also sedating, and may be useful in this setting. The selective serotonin reuptake inhibitor (SSRI) class of antidepressants, which includes fluoxetine, paroxetine, fluvoxamine, sertraline, citalopram, and escitalopram, typically improves sleep, although these medications are not sedating in and of themselves. The same is true for the serotonin-norepinephrine reuptake inhibitor (SNRI) class, which includes venlafaxine, desvenlafaxine, and duloxetine. Bupropion is one of the few antidepressant drugs that does not improve sleep, and must be used with caution when insomnia is an issue, as it can aggravate the problem.

Improvement in sleep on antidepressant therapy typically correlates with resolution of other depressive symptoms. Conversely, lack of improvement in sleep problems during treatment often indicates incomplete recovery from depression, and a higher risk for relapse of depression.

Some patients complain of persistent sleep problems, despite resolution of other symptoms of depression. Often, adding a sedating antidepressant such as trazodone or one of the tricyclic drugs before bed will improve sleep quality.

Sleep medications without antidepressant properties may also be helpful for depression-associated sleep disorders. They are generally considered less desirable because they can lead to dependence, but can still have an important place in therapy. Benzodiazepines such as temazepam, triazolam, alprazolam, diazepam, lorazepam, and clonazepam can often improve sleep. A newer class of non-benzodiazepine agents including zolpidem, zaleplon, and eszopiclone can be used in a similar manner.

If you have problems with depression, you should definitely discuss your sleep problems with your doctor or therapist. Treating them may be important to improving your mood and your quality of life. Conversely, if you have persistent and unexplained sleep problems, a careful assessment for depression is definitely in order.

Section 25.3

Posttraumatic Stress Disorder and Its Impact on Sleep

"Sleep and Posttraumatic Stress Disorder (PTSD)," National Center for Post-traumatic Stress Disorder, U.S. Department of Veterans Affairs, June 1, 2007.

Many people have trouble sleeping sometimes. This is even more likely if you have posttraumatic stress disorder (PTSD). Having trouble sleeping and nightmares are two symptoms of PTSD.

Why do people with PTSD have sleep problems?

There are many reasons why people with PTSD may have trouble sleeping:

- **Changes in your brain:** PTSD can cause changes in the brain, making it difficult to sleep. Many people with PTSD may feel they need to be on guard or "on the lookout," to protect themselves from danger. It is difficult to have restful sleep when you feel the need to be always alert.

- **Medical problems:** There are medical problems that are commonly found in people with PTSD such as chronic pain, stomach problems, and pelvic-area problems in women. These physical problems can make going to sleep difficult.

- **Your thoughts:** Your thoughts can make it difficult to fall asleep. People with PTSD often worry about general problems or worry that they are in danger. If you have not been able to sleep for several nights (or even weeks), you may start to worry that you won't be able to fall asleep. These thoughts can keep you awake.

- **Drugs or alcohol:** Some people with PTSD use drugs or alcohol to help them cope with their symptoms. Drinking and using drugs can make it more difficult to fall asleep.

- **Upsetting dreams or nightmares:** Nightmares are common for people with PTSD. Nightmares can wake you up in the middle of the night, making your sleep less restful. Or, you may find it difficult to fall asleep because you are afraid you might have a nightmare.

- **Hearing a noise:** Many people with PTSD wake up easily if they hear a noise. You may feel that you need to get up and check your room to make sure you are safe.

What can you do if you have problems?

Whatever the cause, there are things you can do.

Your sleeping area: Your sleeping area and what you do during the day can affect how well you sleep. Too much noise, light, or activity in your bedroom can make sleeping harder. Creating a quiet, comfortable sleeping area can help.

Here are some things you can do to sleep better:

- Use your bedroom only for sleeping and sex.

- Move the TV and radio out of your bedroom.

- Keep your bedroom quiet, dark, and cool. Use curtains or blinds to block out light. Consider using soothing music or a "white noise" machine to block out noise.

Your evening and bedtime routine: Having an evening routine and a set bedtime will help your body get used to a sleeping schedule. You may want to ask others in your household to help you with your routine.

Here are some guidelines that may help:

- Don't do stressful or energizing things in the evening.

- Create a relaxing bedtime routine. You might want to take a warm shower or bath, listen to soothing music, or drink a cup of noncaffeinated tea.

- Go to bed at the same time every night and get up at the same time every morning, even if you feel tired.

- Use a sleep mask and earplugs if light and noise bother you.

If you can't sleep, try the following things:

- Imagine yourself in a peaceful, pleasant scene. Focus on the details and feelings of being in a place that is relaxing.

- Get up and do a quiet or boring activity until you feel sleepy.

- Don't drink any liquids after 6 p.m. if you wake up often because you have to go to the bathroom.

Your activities during the day: Your habits and activities can affect how well you sleep.

Here are some tips:

- Exercise during the day. Don't exercise after 5 p.m. because it may be harder to fall asleep.

- Get outside during daylight hours. Spending time in sunlight helps to reset your body's sleep and wake cycles.

- Don't drink or eat anything that has caffeine in it, such as coffee, tea, cola, and chocolate.

- Don't drink alcohol before bedtime. Alcohol can cause you to wake up more often during the night.

- Don't smoke or use tobacco, especially in the evening. Nicotine can keep you awake.

- Don't take naps during the day, especially close to bedtime.

- Don't take medicine that may keep you awake, or make you feel hyper or energized, right before bed. Your doctor can tell you if your medicine may do this and if you can take it earlier in the day.

Talk to your doctor: If you can't sleep because you are in great pain or have an injury, you often feel anxious at night, or you often have bad dreams or nightmares, talk to your doctor.

There are a number of medications that are helpful for sleep problems in PTSD. Depending on your sleep symptoms and other factors, your doctor may prescribe some medication for you. There are also other skills you can learn to help improve your sleep.

Chapter 26

Multiple Sclerosis and Sleep Disorders

Diane Hart, age forty-three, struggled to fall asleep every night for almost half a year. On her "good" nights, she awoke as frequently as every hour; on the worst ones she lay awake until breakfast. She moved through her days in a fog. Nighttime was a battleground, and she lost all zest for life. Not until a magnetic resonance imaging (MRI) was done did she learn that multiple sclerosis (MS) was behind her almost continual headaches, stiff neck, and the nighttime body jerks that made falling and staying asleep so difficult. Now, Ms. Hart reports, she sleeps "like a baby."

She found relief when her primary care physician referred her to the Providence Sleep Center in Seattle, where she underwent tests and learned to change some habits. The changes included restricting caffeine to early morning; exercising early enough in the evening to insure she is sufficiently tired for sleep, but not so close to bedtime that the endorphin release (the surge of well-being that exercise brings) will interfere with falling asleep. She now does a deep-breathing relaxation exercise just before bedtime and has a regular time for retiring and rising. In addition, Ms. Hart received a prescription for an antidepressant that releases the sleep-inducing chemical serotonin.

Her natural upbeat attitude has returned. "I'm finally getting the deep sleep I craved," she said. Her MS is also more controlled since her neurologist prescribed a disease-modifying drug.

"Sleep Disorders and MS: The Basic Facts," © 2003 National Multiple Sclerosis Society (www.nationalmssociety.org). Reprinted with permission. Reviewed by David A. Cooke, MD, FACP, April 2010.

Things that Go Bump in the Night

Ms. Hart's problems are eased, but every night people with MS lie awake, gripped by anxiety and plagued by physical symptoms. These include painful muscle spasms from spasticity, the need to make frequent trips to the bathroom (called "nocturia"), or involuntary twitching and kicking called "periodic limb movements in sleep," or PL MS.

Smaller numbers of people with MS have difficulty swallowing during sleep or suffer from sleep apnea—temporary pauses in breathing, often accompanied by gasping, choking, or violent snoring.

MS symptoms and the sleep problems that tangle up with them are many and diverse. Some are directly related to symptoms; some may be caused by the location of MS lesions (areas of damage) within the brain. Others may stem from stress. Sleep specialists—psychiatrists, psychologists, neurologists, and neuropsychologists who specialize in sleep disorders—have a smorgasbord of pharmaceutical and behavioral treatments to offer.

ZZZs with Ease

"Behavioral techniques for sleep disorders empower people with a feeling that they can do something to take control of their sleep problems," said Campbell M. Clark, professor of psychiatry at the University of British Columbia in Vancouver, Canada. The techniques he teaches include:

- Repetitive mental exercises such as counting sheep or repeating a mantra. (Some people fall asleep just from the tedium!)

- Visualization (seeing yourself being lulled to sleep in a tranquil environment, perhaps a spot with a rippling mountain brook or palm trees swaying in a cool breeze).

- Progressive relaxation (mentally "putting to sleep" each part of the body through tensing and then relaxing muscles). People with spasticity should be careful with this one, he suggests, as tensing could trigger muscle spasms.

Sound Sleeping Is a Habit

Lauren Caruso, Ph.D., a neuro-psychologist at the MS Research and Treatment Center at St. Luke's-Roosevelt Hospital Center, in New York City, helps people create consistent bedtime routines that set the stage for falling and staying asleep.

"Establish habits that announce, 'now I can relax,'" Dr. Caruso advises. "Try listening to music or meditating. People who aren't bothered by nocturia might try a cup of chamomile tea or warm milk as part of their bedtime ritual. Then adjust the pillows, nightclothes, the room temperature, turn out the light, and position yourself comfortably."

If slumber is still elusive after about ten minutes, don't lie there watching the clock, she advises. Get up! Find something quiet to do—a puzzle, a game, reading, or writing. (If you are angry or worried, this may be the time to write letters you will never send.) Rather than doing something passive, such as watching TV or listening to music, do something mildly active so that natural tiredness can build up.

Sleeping Pills? Naps?

Dr. Caruso cautions against over-reliance on sleep medications, though some physicians do prescribe them for short-term use. "They have potential sleep-altering properties and may interact with other prescription medications. Just because a remedy is available over the counter doesn't mean it's harmless. Melatonin, which has been shown to be useful for jet lag, has been associated with adverse side effects when used for more than a few days," she commented. It's important to avoid alcohol, tobacco, or caffeine near bedtime. (Caffeine is found in many teas, cocoa, chocolate, cola drinks, and some over-the-counter pain relievers. Check labels.) Long daytime naps may also interfere with nighttime sleep.

"For a quick pick-me-up, a short rest period, whether you sleep or not, can be very helpful," Dr. Caruso said. "Simply sit comfortably, or lie down, close your eyes, clear your mind, and do absolutely nothing for about fifteen minutes. Listen to music if you like, but don't read, watch TV, or talk on the phone."

Treat Symptoms, Not Sleeplessness

The best habits and behavioral remedies won't alleviate sleep problems caused by PLMS ("periodic limb movements in sleep"), spasticity, or nocturia. But there are effective treatments available for all of them.

"PLMS, such as bending at the hips or knees, can awaken people with a start," said Dr. Art Walters, clinical professor of neurology at the Robert Wood Johnson Medical School, University of Medicine and Dentistry of New Jersey, in New Brunswick, New Jersey. "But sometimes PLMS are not so obvious. They can occur as flexions of a toe that are so slight the person doesn't remember the sleep disruption."

257

People who consistently begin the day feeling weary and unrested might ask the person who shares their bedroom if any PLMS were noticed. Mates are often aware of nighttime disturbances, which can mess with rest on both sides of the bed.

If MS symptoms are under control, and self-help hasn't worked, ask your physician for a referral to a sleep specialist. Sleeplessness doesn't have to be a permanent problem.

Chapter 27

Nocturia: When the Need to Urinate Interrupts Sleep

Nocturia is defined as being awakened at night one or more times in order to pass urine. This can occur at any age, although it is less frequent in the age range below sixty years, and becomes more common as a person ages. A common pattern seen among people with this condition is an increased number of times to wake to pass urine per decade of life (i.e., once in your sixties, twice in your seventies, etc.). Though this is not a consistent pattern among all individuals with nocturia, it is seen among most.

Nocturnal polyuria is an important cause of nocturia in which there is an overproduction of urine at night.

Global polyuria is an important cause of nocturia in which there is an overproduction of urine at night. According to the International Continence Society, it is defined to be nighttime urine volume that is greater than 20 to 30 percent of the total twenty-four-hour urine volume and is an age-dependent observation.

Studies and research have been few, causing nocturia to be misunderstood. Yet, it has recently been recognized as a clinical entity in its own right; in other words it is not just seen by doctors as a symptom, but rather a condition.

How Urination Occurs

Urine is produced by the kidneys and travels through the ureters to the bladder to be stored. The bladder is a muscular sac that holds urine until it is ready to be released into the urethra, the tube that connects the bladder to the outside of the body. The bladder is emptied when the detrusor muscle, the muscle within the bladder wall, contracts thereby squeezing urine out of the body. At the same time the bladder contracts, the urinary sphincter relaxes. The relaxed sphincter acts like an open door, which allows the urine to pass and exit the body.

Causes of Nocturia

As stated previously, nocturia occurs more commonly among older people. It also occurs in women and men differently since the anatomy is different. Women generally experience nocturia as a result of the consequences from childbirth, menopause, and pelvic organ prolapse. Nocturia in men can be linked to benign prostatic hyperplasia (BPH), or enlarged prostate. For men and women multiple factors could cause nocturia including:

• behavioral patterns;

• diuretic medications;

• caffeine;

• alcohol;

• excessive fluids before bedtime;

• diminished nocturnal bladder capacity—urine production exceeds the bladder capacity, causing an individual to be awakened in order to void;

• fluid redistribution—when a person lies down to sleep, fluid is reabsorbed into the blood stream.

During the day, gravity causes fluid to accumulate in the body's lower extremities. When this happens, the kidneys clean the increased fluid in the blood by producing more urine, which leads to excess fluid in legs, ankles, and fingers causing them to swell.

Possible Underlying Conditions

Sometimes nocturia is a symptom of a greater problem. Certain conditions can alter the way in which your body functions causing urine to be passed in the evening and during sleep. Such conditions include:

• diabetes mellitus;

• diabetes insipidus;

- high blood pressure;
- heart disease;
- congestive heart failure;
- vascular disease;
- restless leg syndrome;
- sleep disorders;
- insomnia.

What to Do If You Have Nocturia

Seek information about symptoms and general habits to discuss circumstances to your healthcare provider so they can diagnosis the condition. A two-day diary must be maintained to help a healthcare provider determine the cause of the problem and the appropriate treatment. When organizing a diary be sure to note some of these points:

- When you void during the day and night
- The number of times you wake in order to void
- Amount of urine voided
- Drinking patterns (Do you drink a lot of fluids in the later afternoon/evening?)
- What you drink (sugary, caffeinated, artificially sweetened, carbonated, alcoholic drinks, etc.)
- Medications (Do you take diuretics? Do you take them in the evening?)
- Any recurrent urinary tract infections
- Note any other symptoms that accompany nocturia

At the time of the appointment, be prepared to supply such details related to personal and family medical history as well as medication usage. In addition to helping you find options to help cure nocturia, it is also important to see a healthcare provider to rule out any other serious problems that may cause nocturia as a side effect. At the appointment you can expect a physical examination and urinalysis and urine culture, which are tests that determine the contents of the urine.

Further tests include post-void residual urine measurements, which require an ultrasound and are non-invasive procedures that determine the volume of urine left in the bladder after voiding.

If other problems are suspected, you can expect further tests for diagnosis.

Types of Professional to Visit

If you believe that you are experiencing nocturia and/or nocturnal polyuria, you should first see a primary care professional such as a family care physician, nurse practitioner, physician's assistant, or general practitioner. Once your provider has determined if, in fact, you have this condition, you should be referred to a specialist:

- Urologist (urinary tract)
- Urogynecologist (female reproductive system and urinary tract)
- Gynecologist (female reproductive system)
- Neurologist (brain)
- Sleep expert
- Endocrinologist (glands)

Treatment Options

Behavioral Therapy

- Restriction of fluid intake (limiting the intake of fluids in the evening results in a decreased amount of urine produced in the late evening into the night)
- Afternoon naps
- Elevation of legs
- Compression stockings

The combination of the last three behavioral treatments may reduce fluid buildup and help alleviate nocturia, but in some individuals one of these three options is sufficient in reduction and alleviation.

Pharmacological Therapy

Different medicinal options exist to alleviate and even treat nocturia. These may be used alone or combined with some of the behavioral treatments listed above, which generally have been proven to be more effective. While pharmacological treatment may be initially effective in lowering the number of times awakened to void, the medicine is generally effective only as long as it is taken.

Anticholinergic medications: These prescription medications are effective for treating nocturia due to detrusor overactivity. The main side effects with anticholinergic medications are dry mouth, dizziness, and blurred vision:

- Darifenacin

- Oxybutynin

- Tolterodine

- Trospium chloride

- Solifenacin

Desmopressin: Desmopressin is also known as DDAVP. This medication mimics the hormone ADH or vasopressin, which causes the kidneys to produce less urine. This has been proven to reduce and/or eliminate nocturia in patients experiencing diabetes insipidus, autonomic dysfunction, and Parkinson disease.

Imipramine: Although the mechanism of this tricyclic antidepressant is not known, it has been shown to decrease the production of urine in order to eliminate being awakened to void.

Furosemide: This loop diuretic is used in order to regulate urine production in the daytime hours in order to decrease urine production during sleep. Furosemide functions to block ion flow in the kidneys allowing urine production to be more controlled.

Bumetanide: This loop diuretic is often used when high doses of furosemide are ineffective. It assists an individual in regulation of urine production prior to sleep so waking during the nighttime does not occur.

Conclusion

Nocturia can be a debilitating problem for many people who experience it because of the negative effects of chronic sleep impairment. However, with proper management, motivation, and dedication this condition can be overcome to better the quality of life.

For Further Information

Get into the habit of visiting a healthcare provider to discuss symptoms and receive proper treatment. Always consult a physician, and seek a second opinion from a different provider if you feel that your needs are not being met as best as possible.

Chapter 28

Pain Disorders that Impact Sleep

Chapter Contents

Section 28.1

Pain and Sleep: An Overview

"How Pain Affects Sleep," © 2000 Scottsdale Sleep Center. Reprinted
with permission. For additional information, visit www.scottsdalesleep
center.com. Reviewed by David A. Cooke, MD, FACP, April 2010.

Pain is a leading cause of insomnia. Difficulty falling asleep, staying
asleep, and waking earlier than desired are all symptoms of insomnia.
When pain makes it hard to sleep, falling asleep is often a major problem. However, 65 percent of those with pain and sleep problems in a
2005 National Sleep Foundation (NSF) Gallup survey indicated that
they were awakened during the night by pain. And 62 percent woke up
too early because of pain. Many people who experience pain wake up
feeling unrefreshed, and also find it difficult to function at their best.
Insomnia may be a short-term problem experienced for only a night or
two now and then, or it may be chronic, lasting for a month or more.

Understanding Your Pain: Common Causes

The major causes of sleep loss due to pain are back pain, headaches,
and facial pain caused by temporomandibular joint (TMJ) syndrome,
which is characterized by pain in and around the ears and soreness of
the jaw muscles. Also, musculoskeletal pain, which includes arthritis
and fibromyalgia, can lead to poor sleep. Pain from cancer, the disease
itself and treatment, is also a major offender in causing poor sleep.

If your sleep difficulty is chronic, you should consult your doctor or a
sleep specialist. If you don't get enough sleep, or your sleep is troubled,
you, and those around you, may suffer. You could be more susceptible
to accidents or at risk for falling asleep at the wheel.

There are a variety of treatments available to ease the sleep problems
of chronic pain sufferers, including medication and physical therapy.
Doctors may also recommend seeing a psychiatrist or psychologist.

What You Can Do to Get Good Sleep

Some sleep tips for people with chronic pain are:

- Stop or limit caffeine and alcohol consumption.

- Avoid vigorous exercise. However, a gentle, preferably supervised, fitness program (e.g., walking, swimming, light weight-bearing exercise) carried out on a regular basis is very helpful for improving the quality of sleep and controlling muscle and joint pain.

- Avoid regular naps. If you need to take a nap, do so by mid-afternoon and make it no more than fifteen to twenty-five minutes.

- Practice relaxation techniques, such as deep abdominal breathing and/or guided imagery.

- Use of pain medication and/or sleeping pills is effective, but they should be used under the supervision of a physician.

Section 28.2

Fibromyalgia and Sleep Problems

"Fibromyalgia and Sleep" by David A. Cooke, MD, FACP,
© 2010 Omnigraphics.

Sleep problems are a very common complaint among people with fibromyalgia. Improving quality of sleep can make a major difference in quality of life for fibromyalgia sufferers.

Fibromyalgia is a commonly diagnosed but poorly understood disorder that causes widespread pain. People with fibromyalgia typically complain of muscular pain not attributable to other causes, and frequently have multiple specific tender points. Fibromyalgia sufferers also commonly complain of generalized fatigue, headaches, sleep disturbances, difficulty concentrating, and bowel symptoms.

There has been intense debate over the years regarding what fibromyalgia represents, and how to diagnose it. There are no lab tests that determine the presence or absence of fibromyalgia. It is diagnosed when a minimum number of symptoms from a list are present, without alternate explanations. More than one definition is in use, so experts can disagree about whether a given patient has fibromyalgia.

Originally, it was believed that fibromyalgia was a disease of muscle. However, evidence suggests it is a problem with pain processing in the brain. People with fibromyalgia experience pain differently and more intensely than others. Even normal body functions may be painful in fibromyalgia, and this explains their widespread pain.

With increasing evidence that fibromyalgia is a brain disorder, it's not surprising that sleep is also disturbed in fibromyalgia. Most people with fibromyalgia complain that they do not feel refreshed when they wake up, and may also have difficulty falling asleep. Studies of fibromyalgia patients have shown brain wave abnormalities during sleep in many cases. Additionally, it appears that a high percentage of people with fibromyalgia have restless leg syndrome, which can also disrupt sleep. Pain may interfere with achieving deep sleep.

What can be done for sleep disturbances associated with fibromyalgia? There is no single answer for this, but there are a few steps that can be taken:

- Determine whether a specific sleep disorder is present by performing a sleep study. Restless leg syndrome can often be treated by correcting iron deficiency, or with any of a number of medications if iron levels are normal. It's not clear whether sleep apnea is more common in people with fibromyalgia than those without, but this also should be identified and treated if it is present.

- Identify depression, if it is present. Mood disorders are strongly associated with fibromyalgia, and they can also affect sleep. Treating depression can often greatly improve sleep.

- Regular aerobic exercise is helpful for many sleep disorders, and also helps with many of the symptoms of fibromyalgia. Keeping to a regular program of physical activity may improve sleep.

- Follow good sleep hygiene. The recommendations that apply to other types of sleep disorders, such as keeping a consistent bedtime, avoiding reading or watching TV in bed, are at least as important for fibromyalgia sufferers as other people.

- Recognize that the sleep problem is a real issue. Because the signs of fibromyalgia are not easily apparent to others, sleep complaints may be dismissed. Validating these symptoms may help reduce the level of emotional distress they would otherwise cause.

Section 28.3

Headaches and Sleep

Headaches and sleep relate to each other in many ways. Headaches can disrupt sleep. Headache treatments can lead to insomnia or sleepiness. Some sleep disorders can lead to headaches, while healthy sleep may relieve them.

Healthy sleep for most adults consists of about eight hours a night, at about the same time each night. Children need more. The same amount of sleep broken up into shorter segments is not as refreshing. Sleep disruption may also make headaches more likely. So, for people with chronic headaches, getting a full night's sleep may be a helpful strategy for headache prevention.

Sleep Disorders

Sleep disorders can cause insomnia (difficulty getting to sleep or staying asleep), excessive daytime sleepiness, or unwanted behavior in sleep. Sleep apnea is a syndrome of repeated episodes of stopping breathing in sleep. While morning headaches are a complaint of many patients with sleep apnea, many different sleep disorders have been linked to morning headache. In people with frequent headaches upon waking, sleep apnea should be considered, but so should other causes of sleep disruption.

Obstructive sleep apnea, due to collapse of the upper airway, is the most common type of apnea and the most commonly diagnosed sleep disorder. It is typically associated with snoring and often causes excessive daytime sleepiness. An episode of apnea often causes reduced blood oxygen level, increased blood pressure, and brief awakening.

Treatment of sleep apnea may help prevent headaches that awaken one from sleep or occur first thing in the morning. Most apnea is easily treated. CPAP (continuous positive airway pressure) provides pressurized air through a mask worn over the nose during sleep, and almost always controls apnea. Weight loss can also help and sometimes cure apnea. Others may benefit from surgery to remove the uvula and some of the soft palate at the back of the throat, but this is only effective in fewer than half of patients. An oral appliance can be worn during sleep to reposition the jaw forward. This treats some people with mild to moderate sleep apnea, but is not generally effective in severe cases.

Since low oxygen (such as at high altitude) can trigger cluster headaches, and sleep apnea can cause low oxygen levels, some have speculated that sleep apnea may trigger cluster headaches in some people. A relationship between cluster headache and sleep has long been known, but it is still not well understood. Cluster headache is a brief but severe one-sided head pain with associated symptoms such as tearing or redness of the eye, facial swelling, nasal congestion or runny nose on the side with the pain. The headaches often occur in REM (rapid eye movement) sleep. Sleep apnea is also worse in REM sleep. There is now some evidence to show that treatment of sleep apnea can reduce the cluster headaches that occur during sleep.

Improving Poor Sleep

The relationship between headache and insomnia is complex, varying greatly among individuals. Some patients with chronic headaches may awaken from sleep aware of the pain that led to the awakening. Others may have sleep disruption from increased arousal without fully awakening, causing sleep to be less refreshing. Insomnia for other reasons may make headaches more frequent at other times, but this relationship is not clear. Insomnia is a symptom, not a diagnosis, and the underlying causes should be identified and treated. Sleeping pills may help temporarily, but eliminating the actual cause is more helpful in the long run.

Our sleep habits (sleep hygiene) have great impact on how well we sleep each night. Keeping a regular schedule and avoiding behavior that promotes sleep disruption can help minimize insomnia, allow an adequate amount of sleep, and may reduce sleep-related headaches in some. The following are guidelines for healthy sleep hygiene:

- Go to bed when you are sleepy, not earlier. Going to bed before you are sleepy will promote lying awake in bed, which can condition (teach) the brain to be awake in bed. Limiting your time in bed helps consolidate and deepen your sleep. Excessively long times in bed lead to fragmented and shallow sleep. When you wake up refreshed, get up. Don't linger in bed for long.

- Get up at the same time every day, seven days a week. A regular wake time will help you fall asleep more easily at night, and helps set your "internal clock."

- Sleep only in bed. Sleeping in other locations at home may make it more difficult to sleep in bed.

- Use the bedroom only for sleeping and sexual activity. Avoid reading, watching TV, eating, or talking on the phone in bed. Also avoid lying awake thinking in bed. If you need to problem-solve, make plans, or sort things out in your mind, do it else-where. Get up and sit in another room to "process" your thoughts. Do not take your problems to bed. It is often helpful to spend time earlier in the evening to work on your problems or plan the next day's activities. Some people find it helpful to desig-nate "worry time" before bed to work through difficult issues that might otherwise keep them awake. All this should be done in a room other than the bedroom.

- Cover the clock or put it where you cannot see it. Looking at the clock when you either can't fall asleep or have awakened and can't get back to sleep only perpetuates the problem.

- Regular daily exercise may help deepen sleep. Exercise too close to bedtime may disturb sleep. Finish exercising at least three hours before bedtime.

- Insulate your bedroom against sounds. Carpeting, wearing ear-plugs, and closing the door may help. Noise may disturb your sleep even if you are not fully aware of it. This is especially prob-lematic for third-shift workers who need to sleep during the day when most people are awake.

- Keep the room temperature moderate. Excessively warm rooms may disturb sleep, even more than you might be aware of.

- Don't go to bed hungry, as it may keep you from falling asleep. A light snack at bedtime may help sleep, but avoid having a big meal. Stomach and intestinal activity slow down and food is not well digested during sleep.

- Avoid excessive fluid intake in the evening to minimize the need for nighttime trips to the bathroom. While it is generally healthy to drink plenty of water during the day, limiting this for the last two to three hours before bedtime can help you sleep through the night.

- Avoid caffeine, especially in the afternoon or evening. A single cup of coffee in the morning can affect sleep at night, even if you are not aware of it. This doesn't mean caffeine should be avoided

271

by everyone, but it does mean that anyone with trouble sleeping should stop it completely, at least until the insomnia is in control. Many people say "caffeine doesn't affect me," or "I stopped caffeine once and it didn't do any good." If a person has insomnia and uses any caffeine, there could be a relationship. And, stopping caffeine without following all the points of good sleep hygiene may not have been enough on its own. Use of caffeine to treat headaches may actually disrupt sleep. If sleep disruption is an issue for an individual, other treatments should be considered.

- Avoid alcohol, especially in the evening. Although alcohol may help some people fall asleep at the start of the night, the sleep through the night becomes fragmented. Occasional social use of alcohol in modest amounts is fine for most people, but regular use or drinking large quantities may be a significant problem for sleep.

- Avoid using tobacco in any form, especially at bedtime or if you awaken at night. Tobacco use disturbs sleep.

- If you cannot fall asleep, do not "try harder" to fall asleep. This often makes the problem worse. Instead, get out of bed, go to another room, and do something quietly (such as reading a book) until you become sleepy again. Avoid television, computer use, snacks, or tobacco use, as these can make you more alert. Return to bed only when you become sleepy again. Get up at your regular time in the morning, no matter how much you slept.

- Avoid naps. If you have an irresistible urge to sleep during the day, a single nap of thirty minutes or less may be taken in bed. Longer or more numerous naps can disturb sleep the following night.

The relationship between headaches and sleep is complex, but important for many people with chronic headaches. Pain control with medication may be essential for some to be able to sleep through the night. Maintaining healthy sleep hygiene and treating specific sleep disorders may in turn be necessary for relief of chronic headaches.

Chapter 29

Parkinson Disease and Sleep

Sleep disorders in Parkinson disease (PD) have long been recognized, however their causes remain ill-defined and treatment strategies not well established. These deficiencies derive from the heterogeneity of PD and coincident factors such as medication, again, and cognitive and mood disturbances, each of which are independently known to affect sleep. The sleep of PD patients is profoundly disturbed, even relative to other neurodegenerative conditions. One survey has estimated the prevalence of sleep disturbance in PD at 98 percent.

For discussion purposes it is convenient to consider sleep complaints in three broad categories: sleep onset insomnia, sleep maintenance problems, and daytime sleepiness. It should be stressed that these complaints are not mutually exclusive; i.e., many patients suffer from two or more of these symptoms.

Sleep Onset Insomnia

Difficulties with sleep onset, surprisingly, seem no greater a problem in the PD patient than in the general population. In most instances, sleep onset problems can be related to anxiety or to agitated depression, which, if identified, should then be the focus of treatment. On occasion, I have seen anxiety related to anticipation of an "off" period

"Sleep Disorders and Parkinson's Disease," David B. Rye, M.D., Ph.D., © 2000 American Parkinson Disease Association (www.apdaparkinson.org). Reprinted with permission. Reviewed by David A. Cooke, MD, FACP, April 2010.

severely interferes with sleep onset, and in such an instance more attention must be paid to optimizing anti-parkinsonian medications. Additional contributors to sleep onset insomnia in small subpopulations of PD patients include restless legs syndrome (which, incidentally, appears no more common in PD than in the general population) and akathisia (i.e., inner restlessness) and dyskinesias usually reflective of overmedication with anti-parkinsonian drugs. When treatment with L-dopa is instituted, some patients may experience sleep onset insomnia that typically resolves with time. In such an instance it is best to administer medication earlier and to wait patiently.

When insomnia is severe enough to produce a significant and persistent delay of sleep onset (viz., delayed sleep phase syndrome), the use of fairly rapidly absorbed and/or short acting benzodiazepines such as Restoril®, Xanax®, ProSom®, or Halcion® seems warranted. We have been most satisfied with Halcion® with the comment that it should be used with caution in elderly and cognitively affected patients. Our own attempts to treat advanced patients with Ambien®, a very rapidly absorbed and commonly prescribed medication, have met with limited success even at therapeutic doses. Many patients are prescribed sedating, antidepressant medications to enhance sleep onset and in many cases these seem effective. We have been less inclined to employ these medications due to: 1) fear of morning "hangover" effects; and 2) the potential to enhance nocturnal movement and thereby further fragment sleep (see below).

Sleep Maintenance Insomnia

Sleep maintenance insomnia, i.e., sleep fragmentation, is the most common nocturnal complaint in PD patients. In many instances it can precede the waking manifestations of the disease (e.g., in the form of dream sleep behavior disorder) or more commonly be apparent at initial presentation/diagnosis. The complaint of sleep fragmentation, as correlated with objective findings during recording of sleep in the laboratory, represents a continuum from unexplained awakenings to awakenings associated with quite specific nighttime motor disturbances. Early in the course of treatment of PD, daytime administration of L-dopa improves motor symptoms and may not disrupt sleep. Frequent awakenings, for the most part unassociated with nighttime movements, are treated with sedating antidepressants. Some caution is warranted in anti-depressant use, as they are known to precipitate confusion/hallucinations, exacerbate arousing movements at night, and even worsen daytime PD in some patients. As PD progresses, patients may experience "off" periods during the night. Immobility with subsequent inability to rise to use the bathroom is therefore a common complaint. In this instance, L-dopa dosing may need to be moved closer to bedtime, particularly in the sustained release form, because this is felt to diminish sleep fragmentation. It may also be prudent to consider use of a dopamine agonist, e.g., Permax®, Mirapex®, or Requip®, in such instances, as they tend to be sedating. Unfortunately, these agents, like some antidepressants, may precipitate hallucinations, although they are preferred in that they diminish nocturnal movement.

It is increasingly recognized that many—an estimated 15 percent of PD patients—experience exaggerated nocturnal movements and dream-enactment (viz. dream-sleep behavior disorder) behaviors. Treatment is usually in the form of Klonopin® and precautions should be taken in insuring that injury is not incurred by the patient or bed partner (e.g., bed rails, and removal of breakable objects from nearby the bed). Finally, it is important to respect proper sleep hygiene so as to not worsen the quality of sleep. Measures should include abstinence from caffeinated beverages or foods (e.g., chocolates) within four to five hours of bedtime. Alcohol, while promoting sleep onset, is well known to fragment sleep once achieved, and thereby should be avoided.

Daytime Sleepiness

Daytime sleepiness, and even near instances of sudden onset sleep, are increasingly recognized in the PD patient population. Unfortunately, because of its insidious nature, many patients and caregivers do not endorse sleepiness as a significant complaint and most physicians fail to inquire about this symptom. Sleepiness should be taken very seriously, as it can contribute to significant morbidity and even mortality (e.g., automobile accidents). Most importantly, quality of life can be significantly improved if it is identified and properly treated.

Sleepiness in PD has many potential causes. First, dopamine deficiency itself or other brain pathologies in PD render some patients sleepy. Some may even approach the level of excessive sleepiness seen in narcolepsy. Such a diagnosis requires careful assessment and exclusion of other contributors to sleepiness by a trained sleep specialist. Treatments include activating antidepressants such as Wellbutrin®, the new wake-promoting agent Provigil®, or even classic amphetamine-like stimulants (e.g., Ritalin®, Dexedrine®). Second, the dopamine agonists such as Permax®, Mirapex®, or Requip® are themselves sedating and recently have been reported to precipitate excessive somnolence and sudden onset of sleep in some PD patients. If sleepiness coincides with dosing of any of these medications, the dose should be lowered or discontinued. Third, insufficient quantity or quality of prior nights' sleep can contribute to daytime sleepiness. In this instance, any disorder delaying sleep onset or interfering with sleep maintenance needs to be identified and properly treated (see above). In so saying, it has been surprising in our practice that this third instance is actually quite rare. We have made the somewhat counterintuitive observation that PD patients that sleep less and have more fragmented sleep actually tend to be the most alert group of patients in the day.

In closing, there is much yet we need to learn about the effect of PD and anti-parkinsonian medications upon sleep/daytime alertness. The above is meant to provide just a brief guide to some of the more common sleep complaints of PD patients and treatments. It should be emphasized, however, that each patient is unique. When straightforward solutions, such as those preferred, fail to significantly improve the quality of sleep or daytime alertness, examination by a sleep specialist trained in managing patients with brain disorders is recommended.

Chapter 30

Respiratory Disorders and Sleep Disruption

Chapter Contents

277

Section 30.1

Allergic Rhinitis and Sleep

Overview

Allergic rhinitis, sometimes called hay fever, literally means allergic nose inflammation. It can affect a person during certain seasons, such as spring or fall. People can also suffer from allergic rhinitis all year round. It is a common condition. Allergic rhinitis is a reaction of the nose to something in the air which the person is allergic to. This could be pollen, dust, animal dander, or mold.

Symptoms

Symptoms of allergic rhinitis include: nasal congestion, sore throat, coughing, sneezing, running nose, and headache.

How Does Allergic Rhinitis Affect Sleep?

Sleep problems are common in people with allergic rhinitis.[1] This is especially true when the condition is severe. The sleep problems include: difficulty falling asleep, as well as disturbed sleep. People with allergic rhinitis are more likely to snore. The problems with sleep lead to daytime sleepiness along with a decrease in memory and quality of life. Allergic rhinitis can also interfere with continuous positive airway pressure (CPAP) therapy.

Treatment

- The first step is to avoid, if possible, the cause of the reaction. Allergy shots are sometimes used for severe cases of allergic rhinitis.

- Antihistamines can relieve mild to moderate symptoms.

278

- Nasal corticosteroid sprays and longer acting antihistamines are available by prescription.

References

1. Leger D. Annesi-Maesano I, et al, Allergic Rhinitis and Its Consequences on Quality of Sleep *Archives of Internal Medicine*, Vol.166 No 16, Sept 18, 2006.

Tips for Coping with Allergic Rhinitis

- Stay indoors on days with high pollen count.
- Keep windows closed and air-conditioning on to avoid pollen.
- Use a dehumidifier to prevent mold spore from growing.
- Wash pets regularly, and do not sleep in the same room as them.
- Vacuum often.
- Change air filters monthly.

Section 30.2

Asthma and Sleep

Pruitt, B. "Sleeping—or Not—with Asthma." *RT: For Decision Makers in Respiratory Care*. 2008; 21(2): 22–26. Copyright 2008 Allied Media LLC. Reprinted with permission.

Mark had not had a good night's sleep in two weeks. Every night he woke up coughing and wheezing, so he finally went to his doctor. After a thorough examination and a series of questions about his symptoms, his doctor finally concluded, "Mark, I think you have asthma. You complain of wheezing and frequent cough, and say that every year you have trouble with pollen. In addition, you are allergic to cat hair and dust mites, plus you suffer from heartburn."

Upon confirmation of the asthma diagnosis, Mark's doctor prescribed bronchodilators and steroids, added an antacid medication, a leukotriene modifier, and recommended that Mark elevate the head of his bed to help relieve the nighttime gastric reflux. "I feel much better now," Mark told his doctor. "I'm sleeping through the night without wheezing and coughing, as long as I take my medicine as you ordered."

As we have seen with this case, asthma can play havoc with a good night's sleep, but with the right management, it can be minimized and good sleep restored. Asthma is described as an obstructive airway disease that involves inflammation and airway hyperresponsiveness (sometimes referred to as twitchy airways). Asthma is partially or fully reversible, either with treatment or spontaneously.[1] The main underlying problem with asthma is tied to the inflammatory process, with acute attacks involving bronchospasm of the airways.

Asthma is often referred to as allergic, where the problem is linked to an allergen such as pollen or pet dander, and nonallergic, where the problem is linked to exposure to an irritant such as smoke, fresh paint, or air pollution.[2] When an asthma attack occurs, a flood of cellular mediators is released that causes the inflammatory response (vascular congestion and leakage, release of histamine and leukotrienes, airway swelling, and an influx of mast cells, eosinophils, and lymphocytes) and bronchospasm or sudden contraction of the smooth muscles that surround the airways. Airflow obstruction is a result of the inflammation and bronchospasm. In an acute attack, the patient may exhibit wheezing, shortness of breath, coughing, and chest tightness. Serious asthma attacks require hospitalization and may be critical situations involving intubation and mechanical ventilation. According to the Centers for Disease Control and Prevention (CDC), in 2002 there were an estimated 30.8 million people in the United States who had diagnoses of asthma during their lifetime. About 20 million people in 2002 were diagnosed with asthma, and 11.9 million had experienced an asthma episode/attack in the previous year (2001). Asthma accounted for 13.9 million outpatient visits, 1.9 million emergency department visits, and 484,000 hospitalizations. In 2001, asthma accounted for 4,269 deaths.[3] Asthma is categorized by frequency of symptoms and by forced expiratory volume (FEV1) and/or peak expiratory flow measurements. Daytime and nighttime symptoms are examined separately when classifying severity due to the fact that asthmatics have increased symptoms at night. A study involving 3,129 asthmatic patients revealed that 94 percent of nighttime complaints of dyspnea occurred between 10 p.m. and 7 a.m. with the peak in symptoms occurring at 4 a.m.[4]

Asthma and Sleep

Many physiologic changes occurring during sleep affect patients with asthma. There is a reduced response to chemical, mechanical, and cortical input during sleep that is magnified in REM sleep. The response to high CO_2 and low O_2 levels is blunted during sleep and is even more of a problem during REM sleep. There is reduced responsiveness in muscles of respiration to respiratory center output with a resultant decrease in minute ventilation due to reduced tidal volume. Airway resistance is higher and peak expiratory flow rates are lower in asthmatics compared to normal subjects. There is increased parasympathetic tone and increased bronchoconstriction during sleep.

In studies of asthma and sleep that looked at hormonal changes, researchers found that hormones follow a circadian cycle. Cortisol is a naturally occurring glucocorticoid—a steroid that inhibits inflammation in the body. Cortisol levels were at the lowest level at midnight in both normal and asthma patients. Histamine, one of the naturally occurring mediators involved in inflammation and bronchoconstriction, was found to be at its highest level at 4 a.m. Airway hyperresponsiveness (as measured by bronchial challenge) was also increased in the nighttime hours versus daytime.[5] Likewise, response to the bronchodilator albuterol was decreased at 4 a.m. as compared to 4 p.m. Nocturnal asthma is also associated with gastroesophageal reflux disease

(GERD). However, achieving improvement in symptoms of GERD is not clearly tied to improvements in nocturnal asthma control.[6]

Nocturnal asthma has a detrimental effect on quality of life. In a study of some four hundred asthmatic children, 40 percent had night-time sleep interruptions due to asthma symptoms during the previous four weeks. In addition, these sleep disturbances were linked to an increased number of missed school days, more severe asthma symptoms, and increased reliance on rescue medications. Moreover, the parents of these children had an increase in the number of absences from work.[6] (A child who is home from school sick with asthma will generally translate into a parent who is at home from work to care for the child.) Research has also shown that nocturnal asthma has a detrimental effect on testing for intelligence, aptitude, and personality. Some forty asthmatic students were tested for performance in intelligence, aptitude, and personality before and after a randomized, controlled treatment regime of either fluticasone (an inhaled steroid that reduces inflammation), salmeterol (a long-acting inhaled broncho-dilator that relieves bronchospasm), or a combination of the two. The asthmatic students showed abnormalities in baseline testing compared to the control group, but each treatment group showed improvement in the concluding psychometric testing (as well as in pulmonary function test results), regardless of the treatment protocol used.[6]

Possible Mechanisms for Nocturnal Asthma

Besides the presence of GERD and increased parasympathetic tone, nocturnal asthma may be linked to several other factors. These include airway cooling due to lower ambient temperatures, and increased allergen exposure due to the use of fans at night and the fact that mattresses and pillows tend to harbor dust mites. Mucociliary transport tends to decrease during the night and coughing is suppressed, with the end result of increased airway secretions and subsequent irritation, decreased airflow, and increased work of breathing.[5,6]

Treatment Options for Asthma during Sleep

Controlling asthma symptoms is a key focus in the national asthma guidelines found in the National Asthma Education and Prevention Program (NAEPP).[7] There are several strategies for controlling nocturnal asthma symptoms. The sleeping environment should be well ventilated with clean, dust-free, cool air with optimal humidity to minimize allergen exposure. Use of high-efficiency filtration systems can also reduce allergen exposure. Mattresses and pillows should be covered in dust mite–proof covers. Carpets should be removed, and use of fans at night should be minimized. Pets should not be allowed to sleep on the bed in order to reduce exposure to pet dander. Stuffed animals and plush toys should be removed or washed in hot water (greater than 130 degrees Fahrenheit) to reduce dust mites.[6,7] Cockroaches should be controlled and mold eliminated to remove these allergens from the environment. Appropriate use of long-acting bronchodilators, inhaled steroids, sustained-release theophylline, leukotriene modifiers, and anticholinergic medications can help relieve allergic response, inflammation, and bronchospasm. The NAEPP guidelines recommend treating GERD with appropriate medications and suggest elevating the head of the bed on six- to eight-inch blocks to help relieve reflux and aspiration. The full range of asthma strategies are found in the NAEPP guidelines on the National Heart, Lung, and Blood Institute web site.[7]

There are also asthmatic patients who suffer from obstructive sleep apnea (OSA). If this is diagnosed, the addition of CPAP is needed to provide appropriate care. Moreover, the addition of continuous positive airway pressure (CPAP) often aids in relief of nocturnal asthma due to the relief of some of the work of breathing, reduction in GERD, and the elimination of snoring with the associated irritation/inflammation of the laryngopharyngeal tissues.[8]

Improving Quality of Life

It is well known that during sleep changes in the body take place. Normally, these changes do not impact health, but they can result in serious concerns for asthma patients. Fortunately, there are treatment options available for asthmatics and strategies that can help provide quality sleep. For the asthmatic, control of symptoms and adequate self-management are the top priority. Due to the added burden asthma places on the body, sleep professionals need to know and understand the impact of asthma on sleep. By studying treatment options and available research, sleep professionals will be more capable of addressing the needs of patients impacted by asthma.

References

1. Centers for Disease Control and Prevention. Facts about COPD. www.cdc.gov/nceh/airpollution/copd/copdfaq.htm. Accessed May 22, 2007.

2. GlaxoSmithKlineAsthma.com. Available at: www.asthma.com/types_of_asthma.html. Accessed May 21, 2007.

3. Centers for Disease Control and Prevention. National Asthma Control Program. Available at: www.cdc.gov/asthma/program.htm. Accessed May 22, 2007.

4. Sutherland ER. Nocturnal asthma. *J Allergy Clin Immunol.* 2005116:1179–86, quiz 1187.

5. D'Ambrosio CM, Mohsenin V. Sleep in asthma. *Clin Chest Med.* 1998;19:127–37.

6. Calhoun WJ. Nocturnal asthma. *Chest.* 2003;123(3 suppl):399–405.

7. National Heart, Lung, and Blood Institute. National Asthma Education and Prevention Program Expert Panel Report 2: Guidelines for the Diagnosis and Management of Asthma. Available at: www.nhlbi.nih.gov/guidelines/asthma/asthgdln.htm. Accessed May 23, 2007.

8. Kasasbeh A, Kasasbeh E, Krishnaswamy G. Potential mechanisms connecting asthma, esophageal reflux, and obesity/sleep apnea complex—a hypothetical review. *Sleep Med Rev.* 2007;11:47–58.

Section 30.3

Chronic Obstructive Pulmonary Disease and Sleep

This section begins with "Facts about COPD," excerpted from "What Is COPD?" National Heart Lung and Blood Institute, National Institutes of Health, 2007. Additional information from Dove Medical Press, the American College of Chest Physicians, and the National Institutes of Health is cited separately within the text.

Facts about COPD

What Is COPD?

Chronic obstructive pulmonary disease (COPD) is a serious lung disease that, over time, makes it hard to breathe. You may also have heard COPD called other names, like emphysema or chronic bronchitis. In people who have COPD, the airways—tubes that carry air in and out of your lungs—are partially blocked, which makes it hard to get air in and out.

When COPD is severe, shortness of breath and other symptoms of COPD can get in the way of even the most basic tasks, such as doing light housework, taking a walk, even washing and dressing.

How Does COPD Affect Breathing?

The "airways" are the tubes that carry air in and out of the lungs through the nose and mouth. Healthy airways and air sacs in the lungs are elastic—they try to bounce back to their original shape after being stretched or filled with air, just the way a new rubber band or balloon does. This elastic quality helps retain the normal structure of the lung and helps to move the air quickly in and out.

In people with COPD, the air sacs no longer bounce back to their original shape. The airways can also become swollen or thicker than normal, and mucus production might increase. The floppy airways are blocked, or obstructed, making it even harder to get air out of the lungs.

Symptoms

Many people with COPD avoid activities that they used to enjoy because they become short of breath more easily.

Symptoms of COPD include the following:

- Constant coughing, sometimes called "smoker's cough"
- Shortness of breath while doing activities you used to be able to do
- Excess sputum production
- Feeling like you can't breathe
- Not being able to take a deep breath
- Wheezing

COPD develops slowly, and can worsen over time, so be sure to report any symptoms you might have to your doctor as soon as possible, no matter how mild they may seem.

Getting Tested

Everyone at risk for COPD who has cough, sputum production, or shortness of breath, should be tested for the disease. The test for COPD is called spirometry.

Spirometry can detect COPD before symptoms become severe. It is a simple, non-invasive breathing test that measures the amount of air a person can blow out of the lungs (volume) and how fast he or she can blow it out (flow). Based on this test, your doctor can tell if you have COPD, and if so, how severe it is. The spirometry reading can help your doctor determine the best course of treatment.

Treatment Options

Once you have been diagnosed with COPD, there are many ways that you and your doctor can work together to manage the symptoms of the disease and improve your quality of life. Your doctor may suggest one or more of the following options.

Medications (such as bronchodilators and inhaled steroids): Bronchodilators are medicines that usually come in the form of an inhaler. They work to relax the muscles around your airways, to help open them and make it easier to breathe. Inhaled steroids help prevent the airways from getting inflamed. Each patient is different—your doctor may suggest other types of medications that might work better for you.

Pulmonary rehabilitation: Your doctor may recommend that you participate in pulmonary rehabilitation, or "rehab." This is a program that helps you learn to exercise and manage your disease with physical activity and counseling. It can help you stay active and carry out your day-to-day tasks.

Physical activity training: Your doctor or a pulmonary therapist recommended by your doctor might teach you some activities to help your arms and legs get stronger or breathing exercises that strengthen the muscles needed for breathing.

Lifestyle changes: Lifestyle changes such as quitting smoking can help you manage the effects of COPD.

Oxygen treatment: If your COPD is severe, your doctor might suggest oxygen therapy to help with shortness of breath. You might need oxygen all of the time or just some of the time—your doctor will work with you to learn which treatment will be most helpful.

Surgery: COPD patients with very severe symptoms may have a hard time breathing all the time. In some of these cases, doctors may suggest lung surgery to improve breathing and help lessen some of the most severe symptoms.

Recent Research Regarding Sleep and COPD

Respiratory Disturbance during Sleep in COPD Patients without Daytime Hypoxemia

Krieger, A., et al., "Respiratory Disturbances during Sleep in COPD Patients without Daytime Hypoxemia," International Journal of Chronic Obstructive Pulmonary Disease, December 2007. © 2007 Dove Medical Press. All rights reserved. Reprinted with permission.

Chronic obstructive pulmonary disease (COPD) is associated with significant morbidity and mortality. Its possible association with obstructive sleep apnea is a major cause of concern for clinicians. As the prevalence of both COPD and sleep apnea continues to rise, further investigation of this interaction is needed. In addition, COPD patients are at risk for hypoventilation during sleep due to the underlying respiratory dysfunction. In this study, thirteen COPD subjects and thirteen non-COPD control subjects were compared for the presence and severity of obstructive sleep apnea and nocturnal hypoventilation. All twenty-six subjects had presented to a sleep clinic and showed no signs of daytime hypoxemia. After matching for body mass index (BMI) and age, COPD subjects had a similar prevalence of sleep apnea with a lower degree of severity compared to the control subjects. However, less severe events, such as respiratory effort related arousal (RERA), occurred at similar rates between the two groups. There was no significant difference between groups in the magnitude of oxyhemoglobin desaturation during sleep. Interestingly, severity and presence of nocturnal hypoxemia correlated with that of sleep apnea in the control group, but not in the COPD subjects. In conclusion, COPD without daytime hypoxemia was not a risk factor for sleep apnea or nocturnal hypoventilation in this study.

Impact of Sleep in COPD

Excerpted from "Impact of Sleep in COPD," by Walter McNichols, MD, FCCP, CHEST, February 1, 2000. Copyright 2000 American College of Chest Physicians. Reproduced with permission of the American College of Chest Physicians via Copyright Clearance Center. Reviewed by David A. Cooke, MD, FACP, April 2010.

Sleep has well-recognized effects on breathing, including changes in central respiratory control, airways resistance, and muscular contractility, which do not have an adverse effect in healthy individuals but may cause problems in patients with COPD. Sleep-related hypoxemia and hypercapnia are well recognized in COPD and are most pronounced in rapid eye movement sleep. However, sleep studies are usually only indicated in patients with COPD when there is a possibility of sleep apnea or when cor pulmonale and/or polycythemia are not explained by the awake PaO_2 level. Management options for patients with sleep-related respiratory failure include general measures such as optimizing therapy of the underlying condition; physiotherapy and prompt treatment of infective exacerbations; supplemental oxygen; pharmacologic treatments such as bronchodilators, particularly ipratropium bromide, theophylline, and almitrine; and noninvasive positive pressure ventilation.

The Impact of Salmeterol-Fluticasone on Sleep in Patients With COPD (AQuOS-COPD)

Excerpted from "The Impact of Salmeterol-Fluticasone on Sleep in Patients with COPD (AQuOS-COPD)," ClinicalTrials.gov, National Institutes of Health, September 17, 2009.

Chronic obstructive pulmonary disease (COPD) is a common and clinically important disease characterized by chronic, irreversible airflow obstruction. Poor sleep quality and insomnia are well-described phenomena in patients with COPD. Several studies suggest sleep disturbance adversely affects quality of life and may worsen daytime pulmonary function in COPD patients. Improving sleep quality in patients with COPD, therefore, may not only improve health quality, but also attenuate the decline in daytime pulmonary function.

Previous studies investigating the effects of inhaled bronchodilators on sleep quality in COPD have shown conflicting results. These conflicting data prompted us to perform a retrospective study on patients with COPD and co-existing sleep apnea (OSA) investigating the effects of mechanical lung function impairment and lung hyperinflation on sleep. Our study found a significant correlation between increased lung hyperinflation and reduced sleep efficiency (a measure of sleep quality), and this relationship was preserved in a multivariable regression model.

We hypothesize that Advair Diskus® improves sleep quality by reducing lung hyperinflation in COPD. To test this hypothesis, we propose a double-blinded, placebo controlled crossover study of Advair Diskus® in patients with COPD and lung hyperinflation.

It was mutually decided by the sponsor and principal investigator to terminate the study early due to study subject enrollment difficulties.

Part Five

Preventing, Diagnosing, and Treating Sleep Disorders

Chapter 31

Sleep Hygiene: Tips for Better Sleep

Do you have trouble falling asleep, or toss and turn in the middle of the night? Awaken too early, or find yourself not feeling refreshed in the morning? You are not alone: millions of people struggle with falling and staying asleep.

Unless you're suffering from a serious sleep disorder, simply improving your daytime habits and creating a better sleep environment can set the stage for good sleep. By developing a good bedtime routine and designing a plan that works with your individual needs, you can avoid common pitfalls and make simple changes that bring you consistently better sleep.

Better Sleep Tips I: Improving Your Daytime Habits

How can what you do during the day affect your sleep at night? Better sleep starts with good daytime habits, from when (and how often) you exercise to what you eat and drink.

"Tips for Getting Better Sleep: How to Sleep Well Every Night," by Joanna Saisan, MSW, Robert Segal, M.A., and Suzanne Barston. © 2008 Helpguide.org. All rights reserved. Reprinted with permission. Helpguide provides a detailed list of references and resources for this article, including links to related Helpguide topics and information from other websites. For a complete list of these resources, including information about sleep disorders and habits that promote healthy sleep, go to http://www.helpguide.org/life/sleep_tips.htm.

Regular Day Exercise Can Help Sleep

Regular exercise, aside from many other wonderful health benefits, usually makes it easier to fall asleep and sleep better. You don't have to be a star athlete to reap the benefits—as little as twenty to thirty minutes of activity helps. And you don't need to do all thirty minutes in one session: break it up into five minutes here, ten minutes there. A brisk walk, a bicycle ride, or a run is time well spent. However, be sure to schedule your exercise in the morning or early afternoon. Exercising too late in the day actually stimulates the body, raising its temperature. That's the opposite of what you want near bedtime, because a cooler body temperature is associated with sleep. Don't feel glued to the couch in the evening, though. Exercise such as relaxation yoga or simple stretching shouldn't hurt.

Get Some Light to Set Your Body Clock

We all have an internal body clock that helps regulate sleep. This clock is sensitive to light and dark. Light tells your body clock to move to the active daytime phase. When you get up, open the shades or go outside to get some sunlight. If that's not possible, turn on the lights to make your environment bright.

Napping Can Interfere with Sleep

Perhaps the English had the right idea in having teatime in the late afternoon when you naturally get sleepy. Some people can take a short afternoon nap and still sleep well at night. However, if you are having trouble sleeping at night, try to eliminate napping. If you must nap, do it in the early afternoon, and sleep no longer than about thirty minutes.

Alcohol, Caffeine, Smoking

Alcohol reduces overall quality of sleep: Many people think that a nightcap before bed will help them sleep. While it may make you fall asleep faster, alcohol reduces your sleep quality, waking you up later in the night. To avoid this effect, stay away from alcohol in the last few hours before bed.

Caffeine: You might be surprised to know that caffeine can cause sleep problems up to ten to twelve hours after drinking it! If you rely on coffee, tea, or caffeinated soda to keep you going during the day, consider eliminating caffeine after lunch or cutting back your overall intake.

Smoking: Smoking causes sleep troubles in numerous ways. Nicotine is a stimulant, which disrupts sleep. Additionally, smokers actually experience nicotine withdrawal as the night progresses, making it hard to sleep.

Better Sleep Tips II: Creating a Better Sleep Environment

The key to better sleep might be as simple as making some minor changes to your bedroom. Take a careful look around your sleep environment to see what might be disrupting your sleep.

Your Bed

Is your bed large enough? Do you have enough room to stretch and turn comfortably in bed, or are you cramped? Having a bedmate makes this even more important—both of you should have plenty of room to stretch out. Consider getting a larger bed if you don't have enough space.

Your mattress, pillows, and bedding: Waking up with a cramp in your back or a sore neck? You may want to experiment with different levels of mattress firmness and pillows that provide more support. If your mattress is too hard, you can add a foam topper for additional softness. Experiment with different types of pillows—feather, synthetic, and special pillows for side, back, or stomach sleepers. Consider your bedding—scratchy sheets might be making you uncomfortable in the middle of the night, or your comforter might not be keeping you warm enough. Consider soft, breathable cotton sheets. Flannel sheets may be cozy for the winter months.

Your Room

Ideally, to maximize sleep, your room should be quiet, dark, and at a comfortable temperature and ventilation.

Keep the noise level down: Too much noise—loud outside conversations, televisions blaring, traffic noise—can make it difficult to sleep well. When the source of outside noise can't be eliminated, sometimes it can be masked. A fan or white noise machine can help block outside noise. Some people enjoy recordings of soothing sounds such as waves, waterfalls, or rain. Earplugs may also help, although you want to make sure they don't block out important noises like an alarm clock if you use one.

Keep your room dark during sleep hours: Early morning light can send your body clock the wrong signal that it is time to wake up. Or perhaps there is a street lamp shining right in your window at night. Heavy shades can help block light from windows, or you can try an eye mask to cover your eyes.

Room temperature and ventilation: Who can sleep in a hot, stuffy room? Or, for that matter, a cold, drafty one? If you can, experiment with the room temperature. Most people sleep best in a slightly cooler room. Make sure that you have adequate ventilation as well—a fan can help keep the air moving. You also might want to check your windows and doors to make sure that drafts are not interfering with sleep.

Reserve your bed for sleeping: Do you sometimes balance your checkbook propped up on your pillows? Or jot down some notes for tomorrow's meeting? It might feel relaxing to do tasks like these on a comfortable bed. However, if you associate your bed with events like work or errands, it will only make it harder to wind down at night. Use your bed only for sleep and sex.

Better Sleep Tips III: Preparing for Sleep

Keep a Regular Bedtime Schedule, Including Weekends

Time of day serves as a powerful cue to your body clock that it is time to sleep and awaken. Go to bed and wake up at the same time each day, and it will be easier and easier to fall asleep. However tempting it may be, try not to break this routine on weekends when you may want to stay up much later or sleep in. Your overall sleep will be better if you don't.

In setting your bedtime, pay attention to the cues your body is giving you. When do you feel sleepy? Set your bedtime for when you normally feel tired, within reason—you may not want to make your bedtime 2 a.m. if you have to work at 8 a.m.! If you regularly go to bed when you don't feel sleepy, not only is it harder to fall asleep, but you may start worrying about not sleeping, which can end up keeping you up longer! If you want to change your bedtime, try doing it in small daily increments, such as fifteen minutes earlier or later each day.

Foods that Help You Sleep

Maybe a rich, hearty dinner, topped off with a big slice of chocolate cake might seem like the perfect way to end the day, but it's wise not to eat a large meal within two hours of bed. Try to make dinnertime earlier in the evening, and avoid heavy, rich foods as bedtime snacks.

However, a light snack before bed, especially one which contains the amino acid tryptophan, can help promote sleep. When you pair tryptophan-containing foods with carbohydrates, it helps calm the brain and allow you to sleep better. For even better sleep, add some calcium to your dinner or nighttime snack. Calcium helps the brain use and process tryptophan. On the other hand, you might want to avoid eating too much protein before bedtime—protein-rich foods contain tyrosine, an amino acid that stimulates brain activity. Experiment with your food habits to determine your optimum evening meals and snacks.

Some bedtime snacks to help you sleep:

- A glass of warm milk and half a turkey or peanut butter sandwich

- Whole-grain, low-sugar cereal or granola with low-fat milk or yogurt

- A banana and a cup of hot chamomile tea

Foods that Can Interfere with Sleep

Some food and drinks that can interfere with your sleep, including the following:

- **Too much food, especially fatty, rich food**: These take a lot of work for your stomach to digest and may keep you up. Spicy or acidic foods in the evening can cause stomach trouble and heartburn, which worsens as you are laying down.

- **Too much liquid:** Drinking lots of fluid may result in frequent bathroom trips throughout the night.

- **Alcohol:** Although it may initially make you feel sleepy, alcohol can interfere with sleep and cause frequent awakenings. Also some people are also sensitive to tyrosine, found in certain red wines.

- **Caffeine:** Avoid food and drinks that contain caffeine, and that doesn't just mean coffee. Hidden sources of caffeine include chocolate, caffeinated sodas, and teas.

If you suspect a food or drink is keeping you up, try eliminating it for a few days to see if sleep improves.

Develop a Relaxing Bedtime Routine

A consistent, relaxing routine before bed sends a signal to your brain that it is time to wind down, making it easier to fall asleep.

Start by keeping a consistent bedtime as much as possible. Then, think about what relaxes you. It might be a warm bath, soft music, or some quiet reading. Relaxation techniques, such as yoga, visualization, or muscle relaxation not only tell your body it is time for sleep but also help relieve anxiety.

Avoid bright light or activities which cause stress and anxiety. Here are some ideas to help prepare for sleep:

- Reading a light, entertaining book or magazine

- Visualization/meditation

- Listening to soft music or a radio broadcast

- A light bedtime snack or a glass of warm milk

- Hobbies such as knitting or jigsaw puzzles

- Listening to books on tape

Worry, Anxiety, and Sleep

With busy schedules and family lives, it's hard to leave the worries of daily life behind when it is time to sleep. Worrying and anxiety trigger the "fight or flight" mechanism in the body, releasing chemicals that prepare us to be alert and ready for action. That not only makes it difficult to fall asleep, but can wake you up frequently in the night as well. Stop stress and worry from disrupting your rest by doing the following things:

- **Making the time before sleep a time of peace and quiet:** As much as possible, avoid things that may trigger worry or anxiety before bed, like upsetting news or gory television shows.

- **Quieting your mind:** There are many things you can do to help your brain wind down and prepare for sleep. Relaxation techniques set the stage for quieting the mind. Make some simple preparations for the next day, like a to-do list or laying out the next day's clothes and shoes. Some people find jotting down a list of worries makes them more manageable.

Better Sleep Tips IV: Getting Back to Sleep, Television, and Sleep Medications

Getting Back to Sleep

It's normal to wake briefly during the night—a good sleeper won't even remember it. However, there are times when you may wake during the night and not be able to fall back asleep. You may get more and more frustrated about not being able to sleep, which raises your anxiety level, ironically making it even harder to achieve the sleep you crave!

Stay relaxed: The key to getting back to bed is continuing to cue your body for sleep. Some relaxation techniques, such as visualization and meditation, can be done without even getting out of bed. The time honored technique of "counting sheep" works by engaging the brain in a repetitive, nonstimulating activity, helping you wind down.

Do a quiet, nonstimulating activity if you can't sleep: If you've been awake for more than fifteen minutes, try getting out of bed and doing a quiet activity. Keep the lights dim so as not to cue your body clock that it's time to wake up. A light snack or herbal tea might help relax you, but be careful not to eat so much that your body begins to expect a meal at that time of the day.

Television

Many people use the television to fall asleep or relax at the end of the day. You may even have a television in your bedroom. However, it's best to get rid of the television, or related activities like video games, for several reasons.

First, television programming is frequently stimulating rather than calming. Late-night news or prime time shows frequently have disturbing, violent material. Even nonviolent programming can have commercials, which are jarring and louder than the actual program. Remember, commercials want to get your attention! Processing this type of material is a stimulating activity, the opposite of what you want to help you sleep.

In addition, the light coming from the TV (or a computer screen) can interfere with the body's clock, which is sensitive to any light. Television is also noisy, which can disturb sleep if the set is accidentally left on.

Take the television out of the bedroom: The optimum setup for better sleep is to have your bedroom reserved for sleeping. So if you watch TV in bed, even if you don't fall asleep watching it, you are unconsciously associating another activity with the area you use to sleep. It's best to remove the TV from the bedroom entirely, saving your viewing for the living room or den.

Trouble falling asleep without the TV: You may be so used to falling asleep with the TV that you have trouble without it. Be patient. It takes time to develop new habits. If you miss the noise, try turning on soft music or a fan. If your favorite show is on late at night, record it for viewing earlier in the day. Although the first few days might be difficult, better sleep pays off in the long run.

Medications and Sleep

If only sleeplessness could be completely cured by a simple pill! There are certainly plenty of over-the-counter sleep aids. However, these medications are not meant for long-term use. They can cause side effects and even rebound insomnia, where your sleep ends up worse than before. Prescription medications are no magic pill, either. If you must take sleep prescription medications, work carefully with your healthcare professional.

Learning about medical treatment options can help you make an informed choice about treating your sleep problems. Behavioral modifications often make the largest difference in good sleep.

Have you started a new medication lately? Some medications have sleeplessness as a side effect. If you suspect this may be the case, be sure to communicate with your healthcare professional.

Quality sleep is important to your health. Make a commitment to yourself—don't "rest" until you find the solution to your sleep problems!

Chapter 32

Identifying Common Sleep Disrupters

Chapter Contents

Section 32.1

Common Causes of Disturbed Sleep

Excerpted from "A Good Night's Sleep," © 2005 Department of Health, Government of Western Australia. Reproduced with permission from the Prevention Branch, Drug and Alcohol Office, Western Australia. Reviewed by David A. Cooke, MD, FACP, April 2010.

Many of us have experienced some sort of sleep problems at some time in our lives. Some of the things that may affect a good night's sleep are described here.

Personal Factors

Medical Conditions

Asthma, coronary heart disease, depression, chronic fatigue syndrome, chronic pain and tinnitus may affect sleep.

Sleep Disorders

Restless legs syndrome, narcolepsy, snoring, and sleep apnea can affect sleep. Snoring is a common condition caused by vibration of the throat with the muscle relaxation that accompanies sleep. Factors that increase the likelihood of snoring include:

- being overweight;
- having large tonsils;
- having a small receding chin;
- suffering from nasal obstruction and/or congestion;
- taking sleeping tablets;
- sleeping on your back;
- consuming alcohol before bed;
- smoking and chronic exposure to other inhaled irritants;
- suffering from chronic exposure to allergens.

Often snoring has no serious consequences, but it can be a symptom of a condition called sleep apnea.

Sleep apnea occurs when someone stops breathing for a few seconds while asleep. This may result in broken sleep. Sleep apnea has been linked with poor work performance, relationship problems, and other health concerns.

A simple test, like the one below, can help decide if you may have sleep apnea:

- Are you a loud habitual snorer?
- Do you feel tired and groggy on awakening?
- Do you experience sleepiness and fatigue during the day?
- Are you overweight?
- Have you been observed to choke, or hold your breath during sleep?
- Do you often wake up in the morning with a headache?

If you answer yes to at least three of these questions it is worthwhile visiting your doctor for further tests. You may be referred to a sleep disorders center for full assessment and treatment.

Parasomnias

Some specific conditions can interfere and disrupt the sleep process. Examples include sleep talking and walking, night terrors, nightmares, bedwetting (sleep enuresis), and grinding of teeth (bruxism).

Grief

Grief can be experienced from losses such as breaking up with a partner, the death of a close friend or family member and can cause intense emotional and psychological distress.

Grieving may lead to a range of sleep disturbances. Talking to someone about the loss may help make the feelings more bearable. Someone experiencing prolonged or very strong grief reactions may require specialized assistance.

Stress

Stress is the body's response to anything that is threatening. Experts suggest that 60 to 80 percent of sleep problems may be due to stress and worry.

Anxieties and worries about family, money, friends or work, relationship problems, nervousness, or overexcitement about an event can often cause stress.

Stress is a normal part of being alive and we respond and react to it in many different ways.

While a certain level of stress drives people to achieve goals, too much stress can cause problems. Getting the right balance of stress is important to living a satisfying and healthy life.

Lifestyle Factors

Circadian Rhythm Sleep Disorders

Going to sleep late at night, going to sleep too early at night, having an irregular sleep-wake cycle, jet lag, and shift work may interfere with sleep.

Physical Activity

Physical activity reduces the time taken to fall asleep and increases the length and amount of deep sleep, leading to a more refreshing sleep.

Physical activity during the afternoon will improve sleep, but it can make getting to sleep difficult if too close to bedtime.

Nutrition

Eating late at night or going to bed hungry tends to keep you awake. Maintaining a well-balanced healthy diet is one way of improving your sleep.

Alcohol and Other Drugs

Drugs such as the caffeine in tea, coffee, cola drinks, cocoa, and chocolate, nicotine in cigarettes, alcohol, and the side-effects of medications, may interfere with sleep.

Alcohol may help people to fall asleep but may not lead to deep refreshing sleep. Drug use may cause decreased quality of sleep, insomnia, daytime sleepiness, and more frequent waking.

Shift Work

It can be difficult to sleep well when working shifts because people are working when they would normally be sleeping.

The internal body clock of shift workers is often affected and may result in a lack of sleep. This can cause sleepiness and difficulty in keeping awake, affecting the ability to function and causing safety issues at work, irritability, depression, and family problems. Long-term shift workers can suffer from chronic sleep disturbances.

Some strategies that may help shift workers improve their sleep include:

- having a sleep environment which is dark, quiet, and not too warm;

- eating a carbohydrate-rich meal before sleeping;

- carrying out physical activity during the night shift (this may help the circadian rhythm of night shift workers adapt more quickly to sleeping during the day);

- eating food containing protein during work time (this may help keep the shift worker more alert).

Jet Lag

Traveling across time zones can make it difficult to fall asleep at the appropriate time in a new location. The symptoms that result are called jet lag. These symptoms include:

- daytime sleepiness;
- insomnia;
- poor concentration;
- disorientation;
- slower reaction time;
- gastrointestinal problems;
- irritability;
- depression;
- alterations to the menstrual cycle;
- a tendency to catch colds.

It can take about one day per hour of time difference to recover from the sleep-related symptoms of jet lag.

Strategies to overcome jet lag include:

- drinking water and avoiding alcohol during the flight;

- going to sleep at the normal time for the country you are in, rather than sleeping during the day;

- doing less activity for the first two days after changing time zones.

Environmental Factors

Noise, excess light, a lumpy pillow or mattress, or a stuffy atmosphere can contribute to sleep problems.

Section 32.2

Alcohol and Its Effects on Sleep

Reprinted from "Alcohol and Sleep," National Institute on Alcohol Abuse and Alcoholism, National Institutes of Health, October 2000. Reviewed by David A. Cooke, MD, FACP, April 2010.

The average adult sleeps 7.5 to 8 hours every night. Although the function of sleep is unknown, abundant evidence demonstrates that lack of sleep can have serious consequences, including increased risk of depressive disorders, impaired breathing, and heart disease. In addition, excessive daytime sleepiness resulting from sleep disturbance is associated with memory deficits, impaired social and occupational function, and car crashes.[1,2] Alcohol consumption can induce sleep disorders by disrupting the sequence and duration of sleep states and by altering total sleep time as well as the time required to fall asleep (i.e., sleep latency). This section explores the effects of alcohol consumption on sleep patterns, the potential health consequences of alcohol consumption combined with disturbed sleep, and the risk for relapse in those with alcoholism who fail to recover normal sleep patterns.

Sleep Structure, Onset, and Arousal

Before discussing alcohol's effects on sleep, it is helpful to summarize some basic features of normal sleep. A person goes through two alternating states of sleep, characterized in part by different types of brain electrical activity (i.e., brain waves). These states are called slow wave sleep (SWS), because in this type of sleep the brain waves are very slow, and rapid eye movement (REM) sleep, in which the eyes undergo rapid movements although the person remains asleep.

Most sleep is the deep, restful SWS. REM sleep occurs periodically, occupying about 25 percent of sleep time in the young adult. Episodes of REM normally recur about every ninety minutes and last five to thirty minutes. REM sleep is less restful than SWS and is usually associated with dreaming. Although its function is unknown, REM appears to be essential to health. In rats, deprivation of REM sleep can lead to death within a few weeks.[3] In addition, a transitional stage of light sleep occurs at intervals throughout the sleep period.[4]

Sleep was formerly attributed to decreased activity of brain systems that maintain wakefulness. More recent data indicate that sleep, like consciousness, is an active process. Sleep is controlled largely by nerve centers in the lower brain stem, where the base of the brain joins the spinal cord. Some of these nerve cells produce serotonin, a chemical messenger associated with sleep onset[5] and with the regulation of SWS. Certain other nerve cells produce norepinephrine, which helps regulate REM sleep and facilitates arousal.[6] The exact roles and interactions of these and other chemical messengers in orchestrating sleep patterns are not known.[6] Significantly, however, alcohol consumption affects the function of these and other chemical messengers that appear to influence sleep.

Alcohol and Sleep in Those Without Alcoholism

Alcohol consumed at bedtime, after an initial stimulating effect, may decrease the time required to fall asleep. Because of alcohol's sedating effect, many people with insomnia consume alcohol to promote sleep. However, alcohol consumed within an hour of bedtime appears to disrupt the second half of the sleep period.[7] The subject may sleep fitfully during the second half of sleep, awakening from dreams and returning to sleep with difficulty. With continued consumption just before bedtime, alcohol's sleep-inducing effect may decrease, while its disruptive effects continue or increase.[8] This sleep disruption may lead to daytime fatigue and sleepiness. The elderly are at particular risk, because they achieve higher levels of alcohol in the blood and brain than do younger persons after consuming an equivalent dose. Bedtime alcohol consumption among older persons may lead to unsteadiness if walking is attempted during the night, with increased risk of falls and injuries.[3]

Alcoholic beverages are often consumed in the late afternoon (e.g., at "happy hour" or with dinner) without further consumption before bedtime. Studies show that a moderate dose of alcohol (a standard drink is generally considered to be 12 ounces of beer, 5 ounces of wine, or 1.5 ounces of distilled spirits, each drink containing approximately 0.5 ounces of alcohol) consumed as much as six hours before bedtime can increase wakefulness during the second half of sleep. By the time this effect occurs, the dose of alcohol consumed earlier has already been eliminated from the body, suggesting a relatively long-lasting change in the body's mechanisms of sleep regulation.[7,8]

The adverse effects of sleep deprivation are increased following alcohol consumption. Subjects administered low doses of alcohol following a night of reduced sleep perform poorly in a driving simulator, even with no alcohol left in the body.[9,10] Reduced alertness may potentially increase alcohol's sedating effect in situations such as rotating sleep-wake schedules (e.g., shift work) and rapid travel across multiple time zones (i.e., jet lag).[9] A person may not recognize the extent of sleep disturbance that occurs under these circumstances, increasing the danger that sleepiness and alcohol consumption will co-occur.

Alcohol and Breathing Disorders

Approximately 2 to 4 percent of Americans suffer from obstructive sleep apnea (OSA), a disorder in which the upper air passage (i.e., the pharynx, located at the back of the mouth) narrows or closes during sleep.[11] The resulting episode of interrupted breathing (i.e., apnea) wakens the person, who then resumes breathing and returns to sleep. Recurring episodes of apnea followed by arousal can occur hundreds of times each night, significantly reducing sleep time and resulting in daytime sleepiness. Those with alcoholism appear to be at increased risk for sleep apnea, especially if they snore.[12] In addition, moderate to high doses of alcohol consumed in the evening can lead to narrowing of the air passage,[13,14] causing episodes of apnea even in persons who do not otherwise exhibit symptoms of OSA. Alcohol's general depressant effects can increase the duration of periods of apnea, worsening any preexisting OSA.[14]

OSA is associated with impaired performance on a driving simulator as well as with an increased rate of motor vehicle crashes in the absence of alcohol consumption.[9,10] Among patients with severe OSA, alcohol consumption at a rate of two or more drinks per day is associated with a fivefold increased risk for fatigue-related traffic crashes compared with OSA patients who consume little or no alcohol.[15] In addition, the combination of alcohol, OSA, and snoring increases a person's risk for heart attack, arrhythmia, stroke, and sudden death.[16]

Age-Related Effects and the Impact of Drinking

Little research has been conducted on the specific effects of alcohol on sleep states among different age groups. Scher[17] investigated the effects of prenatal alcohol exposure on sleep patterns in infants. Measurements of brain electrical activity demonstrated that infants of mothers who consumed at least one drink per day during the first trimester of pregnancy exhibited sleep disruptions and increased arousal compared with infants of nondrinking women. Additional studies revealed that infants exposed to alcohol in mothers' milk fell asleep sooner but slept less overall than those who were not exposed to alcohol.[18] The exact significance of these findings is unclear.

Normal aging is accompanied by a gradual decrease in SWS and an increase in nighttime wakefulness. People over sixty-five often awaken twenty times or more during the night, leading to sleep that is less restful and restorative.[3] Age-related sleep deficiencies may encourage the use of alcohol to promote sleep, while increasing an older person's susceptibility to alcohol-related sleep disturbances.[3,19] Potential sources of inconsistency among study results include different doses of alcohol employed and failure to screen out subjects with preexisting sleep disorders.[3]

Effects of Alcohol on Sleep in Those With Alcoholism

Active Drinking and Withdrawal. Sleep disturbances associated with alcoholism include increased time required to fall asleep, frequent awakenings, and a decrease in subjective sleep quality associated with daytime fatigue.[3] Abrupt reduction of heavy drinking can trigger alcohol withdrawal syndrome, accompanied by pronounced insomnia with marked sleep fragmentation. Decreased SWS during withdrawal may reduce the amount of restful sleep. It has been suggested that increased REM may be related to the hallucinations that sometimes occur during withdrawal. In patients with severe withdrawal, sleep may consist almost entirely of brief periods of REM interrupted by numerous awakenings.[3,20]

Recovery and relapse: Despite some improvement after withdrawal subsides, sleep patterns may never return to normal in those with alcoholism, even after years of abstinence.[3,21] Abstinent alcoholics tend to sleep poorly, with decreased amounts of SWS and increased nighttime wakefulness that could make sleep less restorative and contribute to daytime fatigue.[22] Resumption of heavy drinking leads to increased SWS and decreased wakefulness. This apparent improvement in sleep continuity may promote relapse by contributing to the mistaken impression that alcohol consumption improves sleep.[23–25] Nevertheless, as drinking continues, sleep patterns again become disrupted.[3]

309

Researchers have attempted to predict relapse potential using measures of sleep disruption. Gillin and colleagues[26] measured REM sleep in patients admitted to a one-month alcoholism treatment program. Higher levels of REM predicted those who relapsed within three months after hospital discharge in 80 percent of the patients. A review of additional research[3] concluded that those who eventually relapsed exhibited a higher proportion of REM and a lower proportion of SWS at the beginning of treatment, compared with those who remained abstinent. Although additional research is needed, these findings may facilitate early identification of patients at risk for relapse and allow clinicians to tailor their treatment programs accordingly.

Alcohol and Sleep—A Commentary by National Institute of Alcohol Abuse and Alcoholism Director Enoch Gordis, M.D.

According to recent news reports, Americans are at risk for a variety of sleep-related health problems. Alcohol use affects sleep in a number of ways and can exacerbate these problems. Because alcohol use is widespread, it is important to understand how this use affects sleep to increase risk for illness. For example, it is popularly believed that a drink before bedtime can aid falling asleep. However, it also can disrupt normal sleep patterns, resulting in increased fatigue and physical stress to the body. Alcohol use can aggravate sleeping disorders, such as sleep apnea; those with such disorders should be cautious about alcohol use. Many nursing mothers are still regularly advised by their physicians to have a drink to promote lactation (so-called let-down reflex). Babies who receive alcohol in breast milk are known to have disrupted sleeping patterns. Because researchers do not yet know what effect this disruption has on nursing infants, physicians should reconsider this advice.

Alcoholism treatment also can be complicated by sleep problems during withdrawal and during subsequent behavioral treatment, where sleeping problems experienced by many recovering alcoholics may increase their risk for relapse. Because it is likely that alcohol may act on the same neurotransmitters involved in sleep, increased knowledge of alcohol's effects on the brain will help to promote new therapeutic techniques for alcohol-related sleep disorders and, perhaps, improve the chance for long-term sobriety.

References

1. Roehrs, T., and Roth, T. Alcohol-induced sleepiness and memory function. *Alcohol Health Res World* 19(2):130–35, 1995.

2. Kupfer, D.J., and Reynolds, C.F. Management of insomnia. *N Engl J Med* 336(5):341–46, 1997.

3. Aldrich, M.S. Effects of alcohol on sleep. In: Lisansky Gomberg, E.S., et al., eds. *Alcohol Problems and Aging.* NIAAA Research Monograph No. 33. NIH Pub. No. 98-4163. Bethesda, MD: NIAAA, 1998.

4. Guyton, A.C. *Human Physiology and Mechanisms of Disease.* 5th ed. Philadelphia: W.B. Saunders, 1992.

5. Zajicek, K., et al. Rhesus macaques with high CSF 5-HIAA concentrations exhibit early sleep onset. *Neuropsychopharmacology*, in 1997.

6. Shepherd, G.M. *Neurobiology.* 3d ed. New York: Oxford University Press, 1994.

7. Landolt, H.-P., et al. Late-afternoon ethanol intake affects nocturnal sleep and the sleep EEG in middle-aged men. *J Clin Psychopharmacol* 16(6):428–36, 1996.

8. Vitiello, M.V. Sleep, alcohol and alcohol abuse. *Addict Biol* (2):151–58, 1997.

9. Roehrs, T., et al. Sleepiness and ethanol effects on simulated driving. *Alcohol Clin Exp Res* 18(1):154–58, 1994.

10. Krull, K.R., et al. Simple reaction time event-related potentials: Effects of alcohol and sleep deprivation. *Alcohol Clin Exp Res* 17(4):771–77, 1993.

11. Strollo, P.J., and Rogers, R.M. Obstructive sleep apnea. *N Engl J Med* 334(2):99–104, 1996.

12. Aldrich, M.S., et al. Sleep-disordered breathing in alcoholics: Association with age. *Alcohol Clin Exp Res* 17(6):1179–83, 1993.

13. Mitler, M.M., et al. Bedtime ethanol increases resistance of upper airways and produces sleep apneas in asymptomatic snorers. *Alcohol Clin Exp Res* 12(6):801–5, 1988.

14. Dawson, A., et al. Effect of bedtime ethanol on total inspiratory resistance and respiratory drive in normal nonsnoring men. *Alcohol Clin Exp Res* 17(2):256–62, 1993.

15. Aldrich, M.S., and Chervin, R.D. Alcohol use, obstructive sleep apnea, and sleep-related motor vehicle accidents. *Sleep Res,* 1998.

16. Bassetti, C., and Aldrich, M.S. Alcohol consumption and sleep apnea in patients with TIA and ischemic stroke. *Sleep Res* 25:400, 1996.

17. Scher, M., et al. The effects of prenatal alcohol and marijuana exposure: Disturbances in neonatal sleep cycling and arousal. *Pediatr Res* 24(1):101–5, 1988.

18. Mennella, J.A., and Gerrish, C.J. Effects of exposure to alcohol in mothers' milk on the infants' sleep and activity levels. *Pediatrics*, 1998.

19. Block, A.J., et al. Effect of alcohol ingestion on breathing and oxygenation during sleep. *Am J Med* 80(4):595–600, 1986.

20. Allen, R.P., et al. Electroencephalographic (EEG) sleep recovery following prolonged alcohol intoxication in alcoholics. *J Ner and Ment Dis* 153(6):424–33, 1971.

21. Williams, H.L., and Rundell, Jr., O.H. Altered sleep physiology in chronic alcoholics: Reversal with abstinence. *Alcohol Clin Exp Res* 5(2):318–25, 1981.

22. Gillin, J.C., et al. EEG sleep studies in "pure" primary alcoholism during subacute withdrawal: Relationships to normal controls, age, and other clinical variables. *Bio Psychiatry* 27:477–88, 1990.

23. Lester, B.K., et al. Chronic alcoholism, alcohol and sleep. In: Gross, M.M., ed. *Advances in Experimental Medicine and Biology: Volume 35. Alcohol Intoxication and Withdrawal: Experimental Studies*. New York: Plenum Press, 1973. pp. 261–79.

24. Skoloda, T.E., et al. Sleep quality reported by drinking and non-drinking alcoholics. In: Gottheil, E.L., et al., eds. *Addiction Research and Treatments: Converging Trends*. New York: Pergamon Press, 1979, pp. 102–12.

25. Zarcone, V., et al. Alcohol, sleep and cerebrospinal fluid changes in alcoholics: Cyclic AMP and biogenic amine metabolites in CSF. In: Gross, M.M., ed. *Advances in Experimental Medicine and Biology: Volume 85A. Alcohol Intoxication and Withdrawal--IIIa: Biological Aspects of Ethanol*. New York: Plenum Press, 1977. pp. 593–99.

26. Gillin, J.C., et al. Increased pressure for rapid eye movement sleep at time of hospital admission predicts relapse in nondepressed patients with primary alcoholism at 3-month follow-up. *Arch Gen Psychiatry* 51:189–97, 1994.

Section 32.3

Caffeine: Is It Keeping You Awake at Night?

Excerpted from "Information about Caffeine Dependence," adapted from Griffiths, R. R., Juliano, L. M., & Chausmer, A. L. (2003). Caffeine pharmacology and clinical effects. In: Graham A. W., Schultz T. K., Mayo-Smith M. F., Ries R. K. & Wilford, B. B. (eds.) *Principles of Addiction Medicine, Third Edition,* 193–224. Chevy Chase, MD: American Society of Addiction. Reprinted with permission from Johns Hopkins Bayview Medical Center. Reviewed by David A. Cooke, MD, FACP, April 2010.

Use and Common Sources of Caffeine

Caffeine is the most commonly used mood-altering drug in the world. Caffeine is found in numerous plants, the most widely consumed being coffee, tea, cola nut, cocoa pod, guarana, and maté. It is estimated that in North America between 80 and 90 percent of adults and children habitually consume caffeine. About 15 percent of the general population report having stopped caffeine use completely, citing concern about health and unpleasant side effects.

In the United States the average per capita daily intake among adult caffeine consumers is 280 milligrams (the equivalent of 17 ounces of brewed coffee or 84 ounces of soft drink). Studies show that 30 milligrams (mg) or less of caffeine can alter self-reports of mood and affect behavior and 100 mg per day can lead to physical dependence and withdrawal symptoms upon abstinence.

Coffee is the leading dietary source of caffeine among adults in the United States, while soft drinks represent the largest source of caffeine for children. Caffeine consumption from soft drinks has dramatically increased over the last few decades and 70 percent of all soft drinks contain caffeine.

Table 32.1 shows the range of caffeine contents from common foods and medications as well as estimated "typical" caffeine contents. Of the three major dietary sources of caffeine, servings of tea and soft drinks usually contain about one-half to one-third the amount of caffeine in a serving of coffee.

Although most people are aware that coffee, tea, and most cola beverages contain caffeine, there are several sources of caffeine about which

313

there is less awareness. In the United States, about 70 percent of all soft drinks consumed contain caffeine. A number of non-cola drinks such as root beer, orange soda, cream soda, and lemon-lime drinks contain caffeine in amounts similar to those in the cola drinks. Some, but not all, coffee ice creams and yogurts deliver a significant dose of caffeine. Although chocolate milk, cocoa, and milk chocolate candy also contain caffeine, the dose delivered in a usual serving is generally below the threshold for readily detectable mood and behavioral effects (<10 mg). The one exception is that a serving of dark chocolate candy may contain about 30 mg of caffeine.

Medicinal products also often contain significant amounts of caffeine. Over-the counter stimulant medications such as NoDoz® and Vivarin® contain between 100 and 200 milligrams per tablet, while caffeine-containing analgesics such as Anacin®, Excedrin®, and Midol® deliver 64 to 130 milligrams per two-tablet dose.

As shown in Table 32.1, it can be difficult for a person to accurately estimate his or her caffeine consumption because of the wide differences in the amount of caffeine delivered in common foods as well as large differences in common serving sizes. For instance, the amount of caffeine in a serving of coffee can vary over a ten-fold range, from as little as 20 mg for a small five-ounce cup of instant coffee to 300 mg for a large twelve-ounce cup of strong drip coffee. A similar ten-fold variation can occur with soft drinks, with a small glass of one of the weaker cola drinks containing as little as 12 mg of caffeine in contrast to about 120 mg from a twenty-ounce bottle one of the stronger colas.

Caffeine and Health

Caffeine use can be associated with several distinct psychiatric syndromes: caffeine intoxication, caffeine withdrawal, caffeine dependence, caffeine-induced sleep disorder, and caffeine-induced anxiety disorder. Studies have not proven that caffeine produces significant life-threatening health risks such as cancer, heart disease, and human reproduction abnormalities. Nevertheless, individuals with various conditions such as generalized anxiety disorder, panic disorder, primary insomnia, gastroesophageal reflux, pregnancy, and urinary incontinence are often advised to reduce or eliminate regular caffeine use. With regard to cardiovascular health, caffeine produces modest increases in blood pressure and studies have established that unfiltered caffeinated and decaffeinated coffee (including espresso and French press) contain lipids that raise serum cholesterol. In addition, concerns have been raised about a role of caffeine in cardiovascular disease. Finally, studies suggest that there may be an association between high daily caffeine consumption and delayed conception and lower birth weight.

Table 32.1. Typical Caffeine Content of Common Foods and Medications

Substance	Serving Size (volume or weight)	Caffeine Content (range)	Caffeine Content (typical)
Coffee			
Brewed/Drip	6 oz	77–150 mg	100 mg
Instant	6 oz	20–130 mg	70 mg
Espresso	1 oz	30–50 mg	40 mg
Decaffeinated	6 oz	2–9 mg	4 mg
Tea			
Brewed	6 oz	30–90 mg	40 mg
Instant	6 oz	10–35 mg	30 mg
Canned or Bottled	12 oz	8–32 mg	20 mg
Caffeinated Soft Drinks	12 oz	22–71 mg	40 mg
Caffeinated Water	16.9 oz	50–125 mg	100 mg
Cocoa/Hot Chocolate	6 oz	2–10 mg	7 mg
Chocolate Milk	6 oz	2–7 mg	4 mg
Coffee Ice Cream or Yogurt	1 cup (8 oz)	8–85 mg	50 mg
Chocolate Bar			
Milk Chocolate	1.5 oz	2–10 mg	10 mg
Dark Chocolate	1.5 oz	5–35 mg	30 mg
Caffeinated Gum	1 stick	50 mg	50 mg
Caffeine-Containing Over-the-Counter Products			
Analgesics	2 tablets	64–130 mg	64 or 130 mg
Stimulants	1 tablet	75–350 mg	100 or 200 mg
Weight-Loss Products	2–3 tablets	80–200 mg	80–200 mg
Sports Nutrition	2 tablets	200 mg	200 mg

Mood-Altering and Reinforcing Effects of Caffeine

Mood-altering effects: The mood-altering effects of caffeine depend on the amount of caffeine consumed and whether the individual is physically dependent on or tolerant to caffeine. In caffeine non-users or intermittent users, low dietary doses of caffeine (20–200 mg) generally produce positive mood effects such as increased well-being, happiness, energetic arousal, alertness, and sociability. Among daily caffeine consumers, much of the positive mood effect experienced with consumption of caffeine in the morning after overnight abstinence is due to suppression of a low-grade withdrawal symptoms such as sleepiness and lethargy. Large caffeine doses (200 mg or greater) may produce negative mood effects. Although generally mild and brief, these effects include increased anxiety, nervousness, jitteriness, and upset stomach. However, individual differences in sensitivity and tolerance affect the severity and likelihood of experiencing negative effects.

Reinforcing effects: Drug reinforcement refers to the ability of a drug to sustain regular self-administration (i.e., drug-taking). As the most widely consumed mood-altering drug in the world, it is clear that caffeine is a reinforcer. Furthermore, historical efforts to restrict or eliminate use of caffeine-containing foods in various cultures have invariably met with failure. Contemporary research has shown that caffeine functions as a reinforcer when it is delivered in coffee, soft drinks, tea, or capsules. For regular caffeine users, the avoidance of low-grade withdrawal symptoms, such as drowsiness after overnight abstinence, has been identified as a central mechanism underlying the reinforcing effects of caffeine.

Anxiety and Caffeine

Studies have shown that high dietary doses of caffeine (200 mg or more) increase anxiety ratings and induce panic attacks in the general population. Individuals with panic and anxiety disorders are especially sensitive to the effects of caffeine. Although highly anxious individuals tend to be more likely to limit their caffeine use, not all individuals with anxiety problems naturally avoid caffeine, and some may fail to recognize the role that caffeine is playing in their anxiety symptoms.

Sleep and Caffeine

Studies have demonstrated that caffeine disrupts sleep. When caffeine is consumed immediately before bedtime or continuously throughout the day, sleep onset may be delayed, total sleep time reduced, normal stages of sleep altered, and the quality of sleep decreased. Because of its ability to cause insomnia, sleep researchers have used caffeine as a challenge agent in order to study insomnia in healthy volunteers. Caffeine's effects on sleep appear to be determined by a variety of factors including dose, the time between caffeine ingestion and attempted sleep, and individual differences in sensitivity and tolerance to caffeine. The effects of caffeine on sleep are dose-dependent, with higher doses showing greater disruption on a number of sleep quality measures. Caffeine administered immediately prior to bedtime or throughout the day has been shown to delay sleep onset, reduce total sleep time, alter the normal stages of sleep, and decrease the reported quality of sleep. There is some evidence to suggest that caffeine taken early in the day also negatively affects nighttime sleep. Caffeine-induced sleep disturbance is greatest among individuals who are not regular caffeine users. Although there is evidence for some tolerance to the sleep-disrupting effects of caffeine, complete tolerance may not occur and thus habitual caffeine consumers are still vulnerable to caffeine-induced sleep problems.

Section 32.4

Medications that Can Interfere with Sleep

Reprinted from "Don't Lose Any Sleep Over It: Medications That Interfere With Sleep," by David A. Cooke, MD, FACP, © 2009 Omnigraphics.

Sleep seems like a very simple, effortless process until you have difficulty falling asleep. In reality, it requires a very complex interplay of brain chemicals and hormones in order to allow a smooth transition from consciousness to sleep. Not surprisingly, a large number of medications can affect sleep by altering brain chemistry.

This section will review the most common medication culprits in sleep problems, but this is by no means an all-inclusive list. Additionally, some individuals react differently than most to certain medications, probably due to genetic differences in how their bodies process them, or variations in the parts the drugs work on. Therefore, almost any drug may affect sleep in at least a few people.

If you suspect that a medication is affecting your sleep, definitely raise the issue with your physician. Your doctor may be able to better determine whether the drug is actually responsible.

Amphetamines

Amphetamines raise levels of adrenaline, dopamine, and related chemicals in the nervous system, which activate the "fight or flight" response in dangerous situations. This produces a sense of high alertness, focus, and energy. By the same token, they can cause severe insomnia and restlessness, and the timing of doses can be very important.

In the past, amphetamines were often used for these stimulating effects to treat depression, fatigue, or obesity. However, their use has become increasingly restricted due to recognition that they are highly addictive and can have dangerous side effects. Currently, they are mostly used for attention-deficit disorder or narcolepsy, most commonly dextroamphetamine (Ritalin®, Concerta®) or a mixture of dextroamphetamine and amphetamine (Adderall®).

Amphetamines have strong potential for addiction and abuse, as some find their stimulating effects pleasurable, and they can cause euphoria. Diversion of prescription amphetamines for recreational use is a significant issue, and there is a black market in illegal amphetamines such as MDMA (Ecstasy) and methamphetamine (crystal meth). The illegal drugs share the basic characteristics of prescription amphetamines, but are generally regarded as more addictive and dangerous. In addition to addiction, abuse of these drugs may trigger severely elevated blood pressure, seizures, and fatal heart rhythm disturbances.

Antidepressants

These medications improve mood by altering the levels of various chemicals that control communication among nerve cells in the brain. Therefore, it should not be surprising that these drugs may affect sleep.

Serotonin-specific reuptake inhibitors (SSRIs) are the most commonly used antidepressant medications, and work by raising levels of serotonin, an important brain chemical. This group includes fluoxetine (Prozac®, Sarafem®, Pexeva®), paroxetine (Paxil®), sertraline (Zoloft®), citalopram (Celexa®), escitalopram (Lexapro®), and fluvoxamine (Luvox®). They are frequently used to treat depression, anxiety, and obsessive-compulsive disorder, among other medical conditions.

Most types of antidepressants cause drowsiness, and this can be quite severe in some. A major advantage of the SSRIs is that they have no effect on sleep for most people. However, a minority do find SSRIs make them drowsy or cause insomnia. In most cases, this can be dealt with by changing the time of day the medication is taken. Unusually vivid dreams or nightmares are also sometimes reported with SSRIs.

Serotonin-norepinephrine reuptake inhibitors (SNRIs) are a related class of antidepressants, currently represented by venlafaxine

(Effexor®), desvenlafaxine (Pristiq®), and duloxetine (Cymbalta®). Like SSRIs, they boost levels of serotonin in the brain, but they differ by also increasing norepinephrine levels. They are similar to the SSRIs in uses and side effects, and also tend to be neutral with regard to sleep. However, as with SSRIs, some people may have drowsiness, insomnia, and dream changes with SNRIs.

Bupropion (Wellbutrin®, Zyban®) works quite differently from the SSRIs and SNRIs, mainly affecting levels of dopamine, another important brain hormone. In addition to treating depression, bupropion is also frequently used to help with quitting smoking.

Bupropion has a stimulating effect in most people, and may be useful for depressed patients who sleep excessively. However, this can also cause insomnia. When this is a problem, taking medication doses earlier in the day often helps. Alternatively, bupropion is made in several formulations that differ in how quickly the drug is released from the pill. In some cases, switching to a shorter- or longer-acting form of the drug may eliminate sleep problems.

Tricyclic (sometimes called heterocyclic) antidepressants are an older class, used less frequently now due to worse side effect profiles than the newer drugs. Examples include amitriptyline (Elavil®), imipramine (Tofranil®), and nortriptyline (Pamelor®). Tricyclics merit mention because they are sometimes useful when poor sleep is a problem. In addition to promoting sleep when taken before bed, they also have beneficial effects on the structure of sleep, and may be used in low doses for this purpose.

Antihistamines

Histamine is a natural chemical produced in many parts of the body, and plays important roles in brain function, immune response, and stomach acid production. Antihistamines interfere with the effects of histamine. They are mostly used to treat allergic conditions, but are also frequently found in cold remedies and nonprescription sleeping pills. There are two basic varieties of antihistamines.

First-generation (also called sedating) antihistamines have been in use for many years. They enter brain tissue and typically cause severe drowsiness. Commonly used first-generation antihistamines include diphenhydramine (Benadryl®), chlorpheniramine (Chlor-Trimeton®), clemastine (Tavist®), hydroxyzine (Atarax®, Vistaril®), and meclizine (Antivert®, Bonine®).

Second-generation (also called nonsedating) antihistamines include loratadine (Claritin®), fexofenadine (Allegra®), cetirizine (Zyrtec®),

319

desloratadine (Clarinex®), and levocetirizine (Xyzal®). These drugs don't enter the brain very well, so they don't typically cause drowsiness. However, some individuals complain of sleepiness, especially if more than the recommended dose is taken. This may also be more common with cetirizine than other second-generation antihistamines, as it penetrates the nervous system more than the other drugs.

First-generation antihistamines are frequently marketed as over-the-counter sleep medications; common formulations include Tylenol PM®, Excedrin PM®, and Advil PM®. The ingredients vary from brand to brand, but they generally consist of diphenhydramine (a first-generation antihistamine) and a pain reliever. They can be useful for people who sleep poorly due to aches and pains, but they can also be problematic. The sleep they cause is not entirely normal or restful, and they can also cause significant drowsiness the following day.

A small percentage of people will have "paradoxical" reactions to antihistamines. Instead of becoming drowsy, they may feel anxious, sleepless, and uncomfortable. In the elderly, this may be more severe, and can cause hallucinations, confusion, and agitation. It is unknown why this occurs, but it may recur if they take the medication again.

Caffeine and Other Methylxanthines

Methylxanthines are a type of drug with widespread and complex actions in the body. They alter levels of a signaling molecule within cells called cAMP, which has a major role in regulating cell activities. They have modest generalized stimulating effects on the central nervous system, but they work differently than amphetamines and other stimulants.

Caffeine is the most familiar member of this drug class, and most people are familiar with its ability to increase alertness, decrease fatigue, and offset the need for sleep. Many consider themselves psychologically, if not physically, dependent on caffeine for their daily activities. Caffeine is present in many beverages such as coffee, tea, and most soda brands, and is also present in some foods, such as chocolate. In recent years, "energy drinks" and "energy tablets" have become popular; high doses of caffeine are their major active ingredients.

Theophylline and aminophylline are two prescription drugs related to caffeine. They are primarily used in treatment of asthma, but are prescribed less commonly now as better medications have been developed. They share the stimulating effects of caffeine, and if taken close to bedtime, they can cause severe insomnia.

Cocaine

Cocaine is primarily a drug of abuse, and has only a handful of medical uses. Like amphetamines, it boosts levels of adrenaline and related chemicals in the nervous system, but it is considerably more powerful, and carries a high risk of dangerous or fatal side effects. Profound insomnia is common after cocaine use, and will persist until the drug is cleared from the bloodstream.

Corticosteroids

Corticosteroids are potent anti-inflammatory medications, which mimic the effects of cortisol, a natural hormone. These medications are used to treat many conditions, including allergic reactions, auto-immune disorders, certain cancers, and in organ transplantation. The most commonly used drugs of this class are prednisone, prednisolone (Solu-Medrol®), and dexamethasone (Decadron®).

Corticosteroids are often given in "bursts," where a high dose of the medication is prescribed for a period of days or weeks. Sudden exposures to high doses frequently cause insomnia; the degree of sleep disturbance varies from person to person, but tends to be dose-related. Fortunately, these problems resolve soon after the dose is reduced or the drug is stopped. Corticosteroids prescribed at low to moderate doses on a chronic basis do not usually cause sleep problems.

Opiates

Opiates are widely used for control of pain. They quiet the activity of nerve cells responsible for pain perception, and this tends to be sedating. Common examples include morphine, hydrocodone (present in Vicodin® and many others), oxycodone (present in Percocet® and OxyContin®), and propoxyphene (Darvon®, Darvocet®).

Opiates are often called "narcotics," due to their tendency to cause drowsiness and sleep. However, a significant minority of patients will develop insomnia with these medications. Some people using these medications complain they feel extremely drowsy, yet they are unable to fall asleep.

Tramadol (Ultram®) is chemically unrelated to the opiates, and is technically not considered a narcotic. However, it works very much like an opiate in the brain, so it shares their potential to cause drowsiness or insomnia.

Nicotine

Nicotine is very widely used, but mainly in nonprescription forms. Cigarettes, cigars, chewing tobacco, and all other tobacco products

321

contain nicotine, which is the source of their appeal. Nicotine is also available as patches absorbed through the skin, chewing gum, lozenges, nasal sprays, and oral inhalers. The latter forms are normally used to assist with overcoming tobacco addiction.

Nicotine acts on receptors in the central nervous system involved in normal transmission of nerve impulses. When taken from external sources, nicotine has complex effects on the brain, including promoting alertness and wakefulness. For this reason, smoking before bed may interfere with sleep. Similarly, use of nicotine-containing products for smoking cessation also can cause sleeplessness in some cases.

Sedative-Hypnotics

Sedative-hypnotics, usually referred to as sleeping pills, suppress brain activity in a generalized way, which leads to sleep. Several distinct types exist, but the irony is that these "sleeping pills" can also cause significant sleep problems.

Benzodiazepines are common prescription medications for sleeplessness; examples include alprazolam (Xanax®), clonazepam (Klonopin®), diazepam (Valium®), lorazepam (Ativan®), and temazepam (Restoril®). They can be quite effective when used occasionally, but dependence can develop if they are taken frequently. This may cause inability to fall asleep without the medication. Additionally, if these medications are stopped abruptly, they can cause withdrawal effects similar to alcohol withdrawal, which also severely impairs sleep. Mixing these medications with alcohol or other sedatives can be quite dangerous, as this can be sedating to the point of stopping breathing.

Barbiturates are used far less frequently today as sleeping medications, as they can kill if taken in overdose or mixed with alcohol. The most commonly used example is secobarbital (Seconal®). Barbiturates have the same hazards as benzodiazepines; benzodiazepines are preferred only because they are somewhat less lethal than the barbiturates if misused.

In the past decade or so, yet another class of sleep medications has been introduced. These medications act very similarly to benzodiazepines and barbiturates, but they are chemically quite different, and appear to have subtle differences in how they affect the brain. Members of this class include zolpidem (Ambien®), zaleplon (Sonata®), and eszopiclone (Lunesta®). It appears that dependence and withdrawal are less common with these medications than with benzodiazepines, although they may still occur.

While most people fall asleep promptly with these medications, bizarre sleep behavior can emerge, most commonly if the medication is taken with alcohol. While rare, sleepwalking, sleep eating, and hallucinations are well documented, and there are reports of performing complex behaviors such as cooking meals and driving cars while asleep.

Stimulants

Amphetamines, caffeine, and cocaine are all stimulants, and they have already been discussed separately. The following additional miscellaneous stimulants also are worth mentioning.

Atomoxetine (Strattera®) is a non-amphetamine stimulant used in treatment of attention-deficit disorder. It is chemically different from amphetamines and does not appear to have their addictive potential. However, it shares their potential to cause insomnia.

Modafinil (Provigil®) and armodafinil (Nuvigil®) are wakefulness-promoting agents used to treat excessive drowsiness in conditions such as narcolepsy, and may also be used for sleep apnea and some other disorders. It remains unclear exactly how they work, but it appears to be different than other stimulants. They can be very useful for management of daytime sleepiness, but the effect is not always limited to the daytime, and can be problematic at night.

Varenicline

Varenicline (Chantix®) is a medication used to promote smoking cessation. The drug has effects resembling nicotine in the brain, but also blocks the action of nicotine from other sources. As a result, it tends to reduce nicotine withdrawal symptoms and eliminate the pleasure of smoking.

While it is quite effective, its use can be limited due to psychiatric effects seen in a minority of patients. Some people report extremely vivid and intense dreams while on the medication, and in some cases the dreams can be quite violent or disturbing. It can also cause anxiety or depression in certain individuals, which may also change sleep habits.

Section 32.5

Smoking Linked to Sleep Disturbances

New research shows that cigarette smokers are four times as likely
as nonsmokers to report feeling unrested after a night's sleep. The study,
appearing in the February 2008 issue of *CHEST*, the peer-reviewed
journal of the American College of Chest Physicians (ACCP), also reveals
that smokers spend less time in deep sleep and more time in light sleep
than nonsmokers, with the greatest differences in sleep patterns seen
in the early stages of sleep. Researchers speculate that the stimulating
effects of nicotine could cause smokers to experience nicotine withdrawal
each night, which may contribute to disturbances in sleep.

"It is possible that smoking has time-dependent effects across the
sleep period," said study author Naresh M. Punjabi, MD, PhD, FCCP,
Johns Hopkins University School of Medicine, Baltimore, Maryland.
"Smokers commonly experience difficulty falling asleep due to the
stimulating effects of nicotine. As night evolves, withdrawal from nicotine may further contribute to sleep disturbance."

Dr. Punjabi and colleagues from Johns Hopkins University School
of Medicine compared the sleep architecture of forty smokers with that
of a matched group of forty nonsmokers, all of whom underwent home
polysomnography. Previous studies comparing smokers and nonsmokers have primarily used subjective measures of sleep; what makes
this recent study unique is the study population, the use of objective
measure of sleep, and the quantitative nature of the analysis. Unlike
most studies on sleep comparing smokers and nonsmokers, Dr. Punjabi's study included smoking and nonsmoking subjects who were free
of most medical comorbidities and medication use.

"Finding smokers with no health conditions was challenging. But in
order to isolate the effects of smoking on sleep architecture, we needed
to remove all factors that could potentially affect sleep, in particular,
coexisting medical conditions," said Dr. Punjabi. "In the absence of
several medical conditions, sleep abnormalities in smokers could then
be directly associated with cigarette use."

An additional strength of this study was that sleep architecture was analyzed using both the conventional method of visual classification of electroencephalogram (EEG) patterns and through power spectral analysis of the EEG, which relies on a mathematical analysis of different frequencies contained within the sleep EEG.

"Previous sleep studies have relied on visual scoring of sleep stages, which is time-consuming and subject to misclassification," said Dr. Punjabi. "Spectral analysis allows us to more objectively classify the sleep EEG signals and helps detect subtle changes that may have been overlooked with visual scoring."

Visual scoring of sleep staging showed similar results between smokers and nonsmokers. However, spectral analysis showed that smokers had a lower percentage of delta power, or deep sleep, and a higher percentage of alpha power, or light sleep. When asked about sleep quality, 22.5 percent of smokers reported lack of restful sleep compared with 5.0 percent of nonsmokers. Spectral analysis also showed that the largest difference in sleep architecture occurred at the onset of sleep, which supports the premise that nicotine's effects are strongest in the early stages of sleep and potentially decrease throughout the sleep cycle. The researchers speculate the results of their study may have significant future implications in the area of smoking cessation.

"Many smokers have difficulty with smoking cessation partly because of the sleep disturbances as a result of nicotine withdrawal," said Dr. Punjabi. "By understanding the temporal effects of nicotine on sleep, we may be able to better tailor nicotine replacement to minimize the withdrawal effects that smokers experience, particularly during sleep." Smokers also reported more caffeine use than nonsmokers. However, caffeine consumption was not associated with the results of the EEG spectral analysis or lack of restful sleep.

"The long-term effects of smoking on respiratory and cardiovascular health are well known," said Alvin V. Thomas Jr., MD, FCCP, and president of the ACCP. "However, this study is significant because it suggests that smokers may also be deprived of the much-needed restorative effects of sleep. This study provides yet one more reason to stop smoking or to never start."

Chapter 33

Stress and Sleep

Chapter Contents

Section 33.1

Stress Can Negatively Impact Sleep

New research suggests anxiety from stressful life situations may disturb an individual's sleep for at least the first six months after the event. And, for people sensitive to anxiety, the chances for sleep disturbances after a stressful event were two to three times greater than among individuals not as liable to anxiety.

In the new study, Finnish researchers focused on a population sample of 16,627 men and women with undisturbed sleep and 2,572 with disturbed sleep, all of whom participated in a five-year longitudinal observational cohort study.

A measurement of each person's liability to anxiety, as determined by a general feeling of stressfulness and symptoms of hyperactivity, was assessed at the onset. The occurrence of post-onset life events (i.e., death or illness in the family, divorce, financial difficulty, and violence) and sleep disturbances was measured at follow-up five years later.

The study is published in the November 1, 2007, issue of the journal *SLEEP*.

According to the results, both liability to anxiety and exposure to negative life events were strongly associated with sleep disturbances.

Among the men liable to anxiety, the odds of sleep disturbances were 3.11 times higher for those who had experienced a severe life event within six months than for the others. The men not liable to anxiety had odds of only 1.13 for sleep disturbances.

For the men and women liable to anxiety, the odds ratio for sleep disturbance zero to six months after divorce was 2.05, with the corresponding ratio being 1.47 for those not liable to anxiety.

"This five-year follow-up showed that exposure to severe stressful events can trigger sleep disturbances in people with undisturbed sleep before the event. Those liable to anxiety before the event seemed to be at a higher risk of post-event sleep disturbances compared with those not liable to anxiety.

"The strength of this study is a study design that allowed the timing of pre-event predisposing traits and the occurrence of specific stressful events precipitating the onset of sleep disturbances. Control for a large number of potential confounding factors suggest that the observed associations were not explained by socioeconomic position, obesity, high alcohol intake, or chronic medical conditions at study entry," said Dr. Vahtera.

Experts recommend that adults get seven to eight hours of sleep each night for good health and optimum performance. Adolescents should sleep about nine hours a night, school-aged children between ten and eleven hours a night, and children in preschool between eleven and thirteen hours a night.

Those who think they might have a sleep disorder are urged to discuss their problem with their primary care physician or a sleep specialist.

Section 33.2

Stress-Related Sleep Problems Increasing in America

"Stress Keeping More Americans Up at Night," reprinted with permission from www.bettersleep.org. Copyright © 2003 The Better Sleep Council. All rights reserved. Reviewed by David A. Cooke, MD, FACP, April 2010.

According to the second annual Better Sleep Council Stress Survey, 66 percent of Americans are losing sleep due to stress, up from 51 percent last year. The number one source of stress that keeps Americans tossing and turning? Family matters, with 22 percent of survey respondents citing issues close to home as the reason they are kept awake at night. Job-related concerns and financial matters were also a source for worry among 19 percent and 13 percent of individuals surveyed, respectively, and only 5 percent of Americans are kept awake by current events in the news.

The 2003 Better Sleep Council Stress Survey found that 17 percent of Americans are losing sleep at least three nights a week, with most (49 percent) losing sleep only a few nights a month. According to Dr. Louis Libby, pulmonologist and medical director of the Sleep

Disorders Center at Providence Portland Medical Center, losing sleep due to stress one or two nights a week generally will not impact an individual's ability to perform. However, loss of sleep three or four days in a row will impact performance.

"With all the forces on our life competing for time and attention, it's important to recognize what we can control—like getting an adequate amount of sleep each night. A good night's sleep improves an individual's energy level, enhances their ability to think clearly, and strengthens their capacity to deal with life's daily challenges, " says Nancy Shark, executive director at The Better Sleep Council.

The Better Sleep Council (BSC) reminds sleep-deprived Americans that starting each day with a good night's sleep and taking control of their sleep environment can effectively reduce stress and improve their quality of life. And while there's much that Americans are not able to control when it comes to causing stress, the BSC reminds consumers what they can do to control their sleep environment and increase their chances of getting a better night sleep.

Five Tips to Control Your Sleep Environment

Determine your sleep requirement: Determining the amount of sleep you need each night to be fully alert the next day is a big step toward sleep environment control. You should try to get at least your minimum sleep requirement each night, if not more. Most adults need between seven and nine hours of sleep each night.

Reduce noise: Keeping your bedroom noise level at a minimum creates an ideal, relaxed sleep environment. Consider removing your television and/or radio from the bedroom.

Create a comfortable bed: Evaluating your mattress is important—is it giving you the support and comfort you need to get a good night's sleep?

Engage in pre-bedtime relaxation: Engaging in a relaxing, non-alerting activity at bedtime such as reading or listening to music will help you sleep better. Avoid activities that are mentally and physically stimulating that might keep you awake.

Develop a sleep ritual: Keeping the same routine each night just before bed signals your body to settle down for the night. Set a regular schedule that takes you from dusk to dawn.

"These tips will help empower consumers to make decisions that improve their sleep environment," Shark added. "After all, everyone deserves to start their day with a good night sleep."

Section 33.3

Mindfulness Training Improves Sleep Quality

"Mindfulness Training Improves Sleep Quality; Lessens Need for
Sleep Medicines," June 25, 2009. © 2009 Duke University Health
System. Reprinted with permission.

Stressed-out people sleep better and take sleep medication less
often when they learn to let go of intrusive thoughts, according to
researchers at Duke Integrative Medicine.

Their data shows participants who took an eight-week mindfulness-
based stress reduction (MBSR)course reported less trouble sleeping
through the night, and also less sleepiness during the day. This is the
first study to document several positive effects of mindfulness training on
sleep quality in a group of generally healthy, but stressed, individuals.

"When we don't know what to do with intrusive and persistent
thoughts, the mind and body feel threatened," says Jeff Greeson, PhD,
MS, a clinical health psychologist at Duke who presented his preliminary results at the North American Research Conference on Complementary and Integrative Medicine.

"That signals the 'fight or flight' response which starts a cascade of
sleep-robbing emotions like agitation and anxiety."

Greeson's study followed 151 adults, three-quarters of whom were
women, who underwent eight weeks of MBSR training. He validated
improvements in sleep quality using a nationally recognized sleep
quality scale—the Pittsburgh Sleep Quality Index (PSQI).

Statistically significant improvements were noted in overall sleep
quality (26 percent), sleep disturbances, i.e., waking up at night and
feeling uncomfortable (16 percent), frequency of using prescription or
over-the-counter sleep medications (25 percent), and improvements in
experiencing sleepiness during the day (28 percent).

"Before beginning the MBSR program, 70 percent of the study participants met the clinical cutoff for poor sleep quality," Greeson said.
"After MBSR, 50 percent of participants reported clinically significant
sleep disturbances. That's a 20 percent improvement rate."

"When people become more mindful," he explained, "they learn to
look at life through a new lens. They learn how to accept the presence

331

of thoughts and feelings that may keep them up at night. They begin to understand that they don't have to react to them. As a result, they experience greater emotional balance and less sleep disturbances."

The findings are particularly relevant as they come at a time when stress in the general population is at an all-time high. More people are worrying about the economy, jobs, their financial situation, and the strain of coping with it all in their daily lives.

"All that worrying, obsessing, and ruminating can increase risk of illness and disease," says Greeson. "When the mind worries, the body responds." The key, he says, is not to push those thoughts away, but to acknowledge them. "That helps people manage their reaction to stress and anxiety and helps them remain calm."

Greeson's research is part of a larger study on mindfulness funded by the National Center for Complementary and Alternative Medicine. His work will continue to research the effects of the MBSR program first developed by Jon Kabat-Zinn at the University of Massachusetts thirty years ago. That program is now taught by trained professionals throughout the country.

Chapter 34

Shift Work and Sleep

Overview

Shift work definitely has its rewards—like the extra income, the lack of interruptions, the sense of freedom you get working nontraditional hours, and the ability to be home with the kids during the day. But working night or rotating shifts also has its drawbacks—and one of the biggest is not getting enough restful sleep. That can make you feel tired and grumpy. It can make it hard to get through work. And worst of all, it can cause you to fall asleep behind the wheel while driving home.

Your Body Clock Was Set by Nature

The human body is governed by an internal clock known as the circadian rhythm. In each twenty-four-hour cycle, it makes you want to sleep when it's dark and be awake when it's light. It causes periods of sleepiness between midnight and 6 a.m.—the "natural" time for humans to sleep—then again in the midafternoon.

"Overview" is excerpted from "Sick and Tired of Waking Up Sick and Tired," National Highway Traffic Safety Administration. The full text of this document is available online at http://www.nhtsa.gov/people/injury/drowsy_driving1/human/drows_driving/wbroch/wbrochure.pdf; accessed August 2010. "Tips for Families of Shift Workers" is excerpted from "A Wake-Up Call for the Whole Family," National Highway Traffic Safety Administration. The full text of this document is available online at http://www.nhtsa.gov/people/injury/drowsy_driving1/human/drows_driving/fbroch/FamilyBrochure.pdf; accessed August 2010.

But as a shift worker, you have to try to sleep when your body is telling you to be awake, and be awake during those dips in your alertness level when your body is telling you to sleep. And as you get sleepier, you begin to miss things you would normally respond to, resulting in careless and even dangerous errors.

Additionally, sleeping during the day can make it difficult to get the amount of sleep your body needs. Some research shows shift workers average five hours of sleep per day, at least one to one-and-a-half hours less than non-shift workers.

Regularly getting less than seven or eight hours of sleep in a twenty-four-hour period can lead to chronic problem sleepiness and cause irritability, crankiness, and depression. It also makes it more likely that you might fall asleep while driving. And the only way to correct the problem is to get more or better sleep.

Don't Learn about Drowsy Driving by Accident

Perhaps one of the most dangerous consequences associated with shift work is sleepiness behind the wheel. The late night and early morning drive times are the most hazardous, with the majority of crashes occurring between the hours of midnight and 6 a.m. when the body naturally experiences sleepiness. This contributes to the high rate of serious injuries and fatalities for several reasons:

- Crashes involving drivers who fall asleep occur more often on highways and roadways where speed limits are higher.

- The driver's eyes are closed so there is no attempt to avoid the crash.

- The driver is usually alone in the vehicle so there's no one to alert the driver to danger.

The National Highway Traffic Safety Administration (NHTSA) estimates that more than 100,000 crashes each year are the result of drowsy driving. Some studies have proven that roughly one-quarter of shift workers report having at least one crash or close call within the last year. In fact, research shows that drivers are just as impaired when they're sleepy as when they've consumed alcohol.

Drowsiness and Drinking Don't Mix

Drinking alcohol when you're sleepy only serves to increase your drowsiness and further impair your judgment, perception, and ability to react to road conditions and other drivers. It's a hazardous combination.

How dangerous? NHTSA has found that nearly 20 percent of all sleepiness-related, single-vehicle crashes involve alcohol. Even if you've had just a small amount to drink and are feeling just a little sleepy, the effects of one are intensified by the other.

There Are Other Driving Forces

The use of certain medications and drugs can also compound sleepiness. And the risk increases for people taking higher doses or more than one sedating medication simultaneously. Another factor to consider is your driving pattern—longer trips in terms of miles or minutes put you at a higher risk.

The Best Thing to Do Is "Sleep on It."

The single most important key to eliminating most problems caused by shift work is to make sleep a number one priority. Set a specific bedtime for yourself. Get good, uninterrupted sleep at the same time every day, even on your days off. And even if you can't sleep more, there are things you can do to make sure you sleep better.

Steps You Can Take to Improve Your Sleep

Create a restful, comfortable sleeping place—and set aside time for uninterrupted sleep:

- **Make your room dark—the darker, the better:** As a shift worker, you're waking and sleeping against the natural rhythms of lightness and darkness—the most powerful regulators of our internal clocks. Your body wants to be active when it's light, and craves rest when it's dark. Try using special room darkening shades, lined drapes, or a sleep mask to simulate nighttime. Sleep without a night light, block the light that comes from your doorway, and if your alarm clock is illuminated, cover it up.

- **Block outside sounds:** Sleep can be easily interrupted by sudden, unexpected sounds—the screech of a passing siren, a plane flying overhead, construction work, or a barking dog, to name a few. Use ear plugs, a fan, or turn the FM radio or TV to in between stations so the "shhhh" blocks out other noises and lulls you to sleep. (Just be sure to turn off the brightness on your TV or cover the screen.) You might even want to consider a "white noise" machine, which plays a steady stream of lulling sounds such as ocean waves.

- **Adjust your thermostat before going to bed:** A room that is too hot or too cold can disturb your sleep. Some research shows that 60 to 65 degrees Fahrenheit or 16 to 18 degrees Celsius is ideal.

- **Keep a regular schedule:** Go to bed and get up at the same time every day. The best way to ensure a good night's sleep is to stick to a regular schedule, even on your days off, holidays, or when traveling.

Improve other habits and routines that can help improve your sleep habits:

- **Maintain or improve your overall health:** Eat well and establish a regular exercise routine. It can be as simple as a twenty- to thirty-minute walk, jog, swim, or bicycle ride three times a week. Exercising too close to bedtime may actually keep you awake because your body has not had a chance to unwind. Allow at least three hours between working out and going to bed.

- **Avoid caffeine several hours before bedtime:** Its stimulating effects will peak two to four hours later and may linger for several hours more. The result is diminished deep sleep and increased awakenings.

- **Avoid alcohol before going to sleep:** It may initially make you fall asleep faster, but it can make it much harder to stay asleep. As the immediate effects of the alcohol wear off, it deprives your body of deep rest and you end up sleeping in fragments and waking often.

- **Know the side effects of medications:** Some medications can increase sleepiness and make it dangerous to drive. Other medications can cause sleeping difficulties as a side effect.

- **Change the time you go to sleep:** After driving home from work, don't go right to bed. Take a few hours to unwind and relax.

- **Develop a relaxing sleep ritual:** Before going to sleep, try taking a warm bath, listening to soothing music, or reading until you feel sleepy—but don't read anything exciting or stimulating.

- **Don't make bedtime the time to solve the day's problems:** Try to clear your mind. Make a list of things you are concerned about or need to do the next day so you don't worry about them when you're trying to sleep.

Work with your family members and friends so they can understand your sleep schedule:

- **Set house rules:** Speak with your family about your sleep schedule and why your sleep time is so important. Establish guidelines for everyone in your household to help maintain a peaceful sleeping environment—such as wearing headphones to listen to music or watch TV and avoiding vacuuming, dishwashing, and noisy games.

- **Keep a sleep schedule:** Let family and friends know your sleep schedule and ask them to call or visit at times that are convenient for you. Plan ahead for activities together.

- **Unplug the phone:** Be sure unimportant calls don't wake you up. Unplug the phone in your bedroom and, if necessary, get a beeper so your family can reach you in an emergency.

- **Hang a "do not disturb" sign on your door:** Make sure your family understands the conditions under which they should wake you. Make a deal with them. If they let you sleep, you will be less grumpy! And make sure delivery people and solicitors understand your sleeping rules by hanging a "do not disturb" sign on your front door, too.

When You Sleep Better, You Feel Better

By following as many tips as possible, you should start to experience improvements in the quality of your sleep. It won't happen right away, but if you stick with it for a week or two, you'll begin to notice positive changes. Staying alert on the job will be much easier. Drowsy driving will no longer be a problem. And you'll be able to enjoy more quality time with your family—and they'll enjoy you!

Let's Set the Record Straight

Even getting one hour less sleep per day than your body needs can impair your ability to function. And contrary to popular belief, you usually can't tell when you're about to fall asleep. What's more, when it comes to staying awake behind the wheel, many common remedies just don't work.

These *won't* keep you awake while driving:

- Turning up the volume of your radio

- Singing loudly

- Chewing gum or eating food

- Getting out of the car and running around

- Slapping yourself

- Sticking your head out the window

The key is to learn to recognize the warning signs of drowsiness and to take corrective action.

Warning signs of drowsy driving:

- You can't stop yawning.

- You have trouble keeping your eyes open and focused, especially at stoplights.

- Your mind wanders or you have disconnected thoughts.

- You can't remember driving the last few miles.

- Your driving becomes sloppy—you weave between lanes, tailgate, or miss traffic signals.

- You find yourself hitting the grooves or rumble strips on the side of the road.

Tips for getting home safely:

- Avoid driving home from work if you're drowsy. Some experts recommend drinking two cups of coffee, then taking a short fifteen- to twenty-minute nap. You'll get some sleep before the caffeine takes effect, and when it does, you'll wake up and be alert for your drive home.

- Avoid alcohol or any medications that could make you drowsy.

- Carpool if possible, so that you're driving with someone else awake in the car, or get a ride from a family member.

- Take a taxi or public transportation.

- If you hit a rumble strip, it's a sure sign that you need to pull off to a safe place, take a nap, or get some coffee.

If You're Still Having Problems

Sometimes making changes in your lifestyle isn't enough. If you continue to have trouble falling asleep, staying asleep, or waking too early, or if you or your significant other is a chronic snorer, see your doctor. Nonprescription sleep aids won't help you get better sleep. But rest assured, your doctor or a sleep specialist can prescribe treatment that can make quality sleep more than just a dream.

Tips for Families of Shift Workers

Living with Shift Work

When you live with a shift worker, you're a shift worker too. Their schedule interrupts your schedule. When they're up, you're up. When they're driving home late at night, you're up worried in bed. Or on the sofa. Chances are, you could use better quality sleep as much as your shift worker.

So What's Wrong with Losing Sleep?

If you and your shift worker don't get enough sleep, it can result in everything from grumpiness to lowered immune systems, and even depression. It can also lead to something very dangerous—drowsy driving.

Make Sure You and Your Loved One Crash in the Right Spot

Research shows that when you're driving under the strain of sleep deprivation, you're not going to react to situations as quickly as when you're rested and alert. The effect is almost like driving while impaired by alcohol or drugs. And there isn't a big warning sign that flashes every time you're about to fall asleep. Drowsiness creeps up on you. It's almost impossible to predict when you might doze off.

The National Highway Traffic Safety Administration estimates that more than 100,000 crashes each year are the result of drowsy driving. Some studies reveal that roughly one-quarter of shift workers reported having at least one crash or close call within the last year. So you can see why it's so critical for everyone to get quality sleep. People's lives are at stake.

When the Shift Worker Loses Sleep, It's a Family Affair

It's not easy getting quality sleep when the shift worker in the family is coming home from work in the middle of the night or unwinding from a hard shift at three in the morning. Everybody's day (and night) is disturbed. And the whole household must work its schedule around the shift worker's waking and sleeping hours.

It's important that everybody gets the best quality sleep possible. It's also vital to talk on a regular basis about the challenges, frustrations and issues that come with being a shift work family.

The Better the Communication, the Happier the Household

The goal is to make the most of the time you spend together as a shift work family. So here are some tips everyone in the house can follow.

Hold regular family meetings, once or twice a week:

- Discuss problems or concerns about the shift worker's schedule, or anything else that comes up. Open up the lines of communication.
- Try to deal with minor problems early on, before they become major problems.
- Determine solutions together as a family. Listen, and think about all ideas.

Keep household members in touch with the shift worker, and each other:

- Set up a bulletin board in your house where everybody can leave notes, school work, drawings, photographs, cartoons, reminders, or anything else to help keep the family connected.
- Rent or purchase a camcorder to capture special moments the shift worker may miss, such as birthday parties, Little League games, and school recitals.
- Select a time each week to relax and talk with your partner.
- Plan a "family day" once a month.
- Schedule family events and get-togethers on the shift worker's days off when he or she is normally awake, such as breakfast or early lunch.

Ensure your family feels safe at night. Some research suggests that the safer people feel in their home environment, the better they sleep. Here are some ideas:

- Install a home security system.
- Get a dog.
- Keep emergency phone numbers (i.e., 911, fire, police) handy by your bedside telephone.

Here's to Better Sleep

The benefits to getting better sleep include more patience with loved ones, better performance on the job and at school—and most critical of all— safer driving on the road. So get together regularly, talk about what works, and commit to making as many changes as possible.

The key is to be persistent, and to try as many tips as you can, for at least several weeks. Changing habits doesn't work overnight. It takes time.

Everything you've read about here will lead to one common goal: achieving a better quality of life for the whole family.

Chapter 35

Bedding and Sleep Environment

Chapter Contents

Section 35.1

Choosing the Right Mattress

The right mattress for a great night's sleep is the one that meets your personal needs for comfort and support. But before you start shopping for a new mattress, you will need to know some bedding basics. With some general mattress information on the variety of choices available, it will be easier to choose the right bed for you—and get a great night's sleep.

Innerspring: The most widely purchased type of bedding uses the support of tempered steel coils in a variety of configurations. Varying types and layers of upholstery provide insulation and cushioning between your body and the spring unit, resulting in a range of comfort choices.

Foam: Solid foam mattresses also offer a wide choice of sleeping sensations or "feels." They can be made of a solid core or of several layers of different types of foam laminated together. Advanced technology in polyurethane foams, refinements to traditional latex, and the new viscoelastic ("memory") foams have added to the choice of comfort, support, and performance.

Airbeds: Airbeds are now designed to look like the familiar mattress/ foundation (box spring) combination, with an air-filled core providing the support instead of an innerspring unit or foam core. These designs also offer a range of "feels" and typically are adjustable to suit individual sleeper's needs.

Other sleep options: There are many popular mattress alternatives to address individuals' comfort, support, and space needs, including futons, adjustable beds, and waterbeds. Futons are a popular alternative for those who need a sofa by day and a mattress by night. Electrically adjustable beds enable sleepers to adjust the head and foot of the bed to the most comfortable position. And most waterbeds are now designed to look like the familiar mattress/foundation, with a water-filled core providing support, coupled with layers of upholstery for insulation and surface comfort.

Regardless of the type of sleep system you decide to purchase, always evaluate a mattress for comfort, support, durability, and space. The mattress that best addresses these needs is the mattress for you.

Comfort: Today's top quality mattress/foundation ensembles are built for superior comfort. Luxurious new cushioning materials and extra-soft surface treatments create a plusher, more comfortable feel.

Support: A good mattress and foundation will gently support your body at all points and keep your spine in the same shape as a person with good standing posture. Pay special attention to your shoulders, hips, and lower back—the heaviest parts of the body.

Durability: It's the quality of the materials used and how they're put together that determines how long a mattress and foundation will provide comfort and support.

Space: Cramped quarters can turn sleeping into a nightly wrestling match. A healthy person moves anywhere from forty to sixty times a night, including dozens of full body turns. You need freedom of motion while you sleep and to help you relax while getting to sleep. Make sure that your mattress gives you room to move around comfortably throughout the night.

Size Matters

Two people sleeping on a full sized ("double") mattress only have as much personal sleeping space as a baby in a crib. It is recommended that bed partners buy a mattress no smaller than a queen mattress:

- California King 72" x 84"
- King 76" x 80"
- Queen 60" x 80"
- Full (Double) 53" x 75"
- Twin 38" x 75"

Deciding between a queen or king size mattress really boils down to personal choice. A queen bed is 60 inches wide by approximately 80 inches long, perfect for couples who prefer close quarters. King beds are 76 inches wide by 80 inches long, the best choice for couples that want maximum personal sleeping space. Both twin and full sizes are approximately 75 inches long, which may be too short for some adults, especially men. Full size allows only enough space for a single sleeper shorter than 5 feet 5 inches tall.

Section 35.2

Caring for Your Mattress

Consider your new mattress and foundation as "sleep equipment" that needs to be cared for in order to assure the best hygiene and performance. It's important to follow mattress care instructions from the maker of your mattress as products vary greatly. However in general it's important to know about the following:

- **Proper installation:** Make sure your new mattress and foundation are properly installed in your home. Improper installation can damage your new sleep set. If you choose to transport and install on your own, ask the store personnel to give you some tips to help you avoid problems.

- **Use a protective pad:** A good quality, washable mattress pad (and one for the foundation, too, if you like) is a must to keep your set fresh and free from stains.

- **Let it breathe:** If you detect a slight "new product" odor, leave the mattress and foundation uncovered and well ventilated for a few hours. A breath of fresh air should do the trick!

- **Give it good support:** Use a sturdy bed frame. If it's a queen or king size set, make sure your frame has the adequate center support that will prevent bowing or breakage.

- **Don't dry clean:** The chemicals in dry cleaning agents/spot removers may be harmful to the fabric or underlying materials. Vacuuming is the only recommended cleaning method. But if you're determined to tackle a stain, use mild soap with cold water and apply lightly. Do not ever soak a mattress or foundation.

- **Don't remove the tag:** Contrary to popular belief, it's not illegal to remove the law tag, but the information on the label will serve as a means of identification should you have a warranty claim.

- **It's not a trampoline:** Don't let the kids jump on your sleep set. Their rough-housing could do damage to the interior construction, as well as to themselves!

- **No boards, please:** Never put a board between the mattress and foundation. It may enhance the sense of support for a while, but it will only make the problem worse over time. When any bed in your home has reached the "board stage," get rid of it.

- **Out with the old:** Now that you've treated yourself to a new sleep set, arrange to have your old bed removed and disposed of. Don't give it to the kids, relatives, guests, or neighbors. If it wasn't good enough for you, it isn't good enough for anyone else. Throw it out!

Section 35.3

Choosing the Right Pillow

"Picking the Perfect Pillow," © 2007 Somerset Medical Center Sleep for Life Program (www.smcsleepforlife.com). Reprinted with permission.

When it comes to picking the right pillow, it is important to understand there are two distinct types of sleepers:

- Individuals with no anatomical abnormalities or sleep disorders.

- People who have atypical anatomy of the head and neck, which leads to a diagnosable sleep disorder. The National Sleep Foundation estimates that nearly forty million Americans have sleep disorders with at least estimated eighteen million falling into the group with anatomical abnormalities.

For "normal" sleepers, the type of pillow is a personal preference and a matter of picking pillow materials that are comfortable and soothing so that the right environment is created for sleep. For those people with a sleep disorder, such as obstructive sleep apnea, underlying muscle and skeletal abnormalities and medical conditions that contribute to sleep disorders may make getting a restful night's sleep difficult even with the right pillow.

With all the pillow choices, how is it possible to know which one to pick? There is little available in the medical research to guide the process of pillow selection. However, for both groups there are some tips you can follow that might improve your chances of finally securing that night of dreams.

Options for Those without Sleep Disorders

- Cosmetic choices and comfort are key. The focus should be on creating a relaxing environment that will help a person transition into sleep as well as choosing soothing materials that would help limit sleep disruption.

- Choose materials that are soft and comfortable. Higher thread count means the pillow will be softer. Anything that is irritating to the skin can disrupt sleep.

- Pillows with silk or organic materials such as cotton are not only hypoallergenic but can be kinder to the skin, which can make for a more restful night.

- Wool pillow covers discourage mold and mildew growth and are flame resistant.

- Some will also prefer the softness provided by down or other organic fill.

- Although research in the medical literature is limited, one study has shown that a cooler pillow can help maintain deeper sleep. This could be accomplished with a water pillow or by simply making sure the environment in the room is a slightly cooler temperature.

- Choose soothing colors and peaceful graphics, as this will help create a relaxing environment conducive to sleep. This is not just about aesthetics; anything that stimulates that brain can limit the ability to get a good night's rest.

- A pillow that maintains its shape or responds to adjustments in your position may mean you will not have to fluff your pillow as often to accommodate the change in body contour.

- Pillows with special materials, such as goose down, buckwheat pillows, or Dux pillows, are worth the expense if you feel they are more comfortable and allow for a more restful night.

Options for Those with Sleep Disorders

Cosmetic choices and comfort also are important. However there are some additional considerations in this group.

For People Who Snore

Snoring can be benign; however, it can be a sign of a more serious disorder called obstructive sleep apnea, which can be lethal for some. Sleep apnea is believed to affect thirty million Americans, with 85 percent having yet to be diagnosed:

- Traditional pillows do not alleviate snoring. However, pillows are available that promote side sleeping. These pillows help keep a person off their back and on their side. Side sleeping maintains the jaw and tongue in a more forward position and stops the tongue from falling into the throat, which can contribute to snoring and positional sleep apnea.

- Pillows that allow the individual to sleep on an incline also can help. However, none of these pillows would resolve more serious sleep apnea. Whether these pillows would be appropriate for a snorer or sleep apnea could only be determined after medical evaluation and a sleep study to rule out a more serious concern.

For People with Arthritis or Chronic Pain

- Review of the available literature indicates for these individuals the ideal pillow should have good shape and consistency with firm support for cervical lordosis. This means pillows with a special shape or ones able to conform and cradle the neck, such as "memory pillows," might be the best bet. The ideal pillow should be soft and not too high. Pillows that included supporting cores for neck lordosis received the best rating.

- Also for this group, a study done at Johns Hopkins demonstrated that patients had better ratings for sleep quality with water pillows, which allowed the pillow to contour to the neck.

- Roll pillows were found to be too difficult to maintain their shape, remain in place, or provide adequate support.

- Pillow studies in patients with fibromyalgia were inconclusive to be of any benefit and here personal preference would be the best.

For People with Asthma or Allergies

- Hypoallergenic pillows are available for people with chemical sensitivities or allergies and have successfully improved sleep quality. Studies have shown that these pillows may improve the subjective quality of sleep but may not improve the overall condition.

- Despite down's softness and comfort, it was traditionally believed that people with asthma and allergies may need to avoid this material or choose a variety of hypoallergenic down which is available in some pillows. Pillows made of latex, silk, or down were considered other options. Newer studies, however, are showing that synthetic fillers and not feathers are more likely to cause wheeze and that feathers may actually reduce the sensitivity to house dust mite allergens. Organic choices are then likely the best for allergy sufferers.

- For those with dust mite allergies, pillowcases that limit exposure to dust mites are suggested. The pillow otherwise would be personal preference. Choosing cases with a higher thread count will not only mean the case is soft and comfortable but that the dust mites will have a harder time getting access to the fill material and breeding in your pillow. Of course you will need cases with zippers, or dust mites will still get into your pillow. Cases that limit dust mite exposure will reduce allergy symptoms such as wheeze and nasal congestion that may disrupt the quality of your sleep. Latex pillows also limit dust mites. Some cases are little more than plastic covers that make noise every time the person rolls over, disrupting sleep. Plastic cases would also make it difficult for those who like to scrunch up their pillows. Although more expensive, organic material or high thread count materials would likely be a better choice. Research published in the *New England Journal of Medicine* concluded that despite the effectiveness in reducing exposure to dust mite allergies, there was no reduction in symptoms in patients with allergic rhinitis with these casings.

Chapter 36

Exercise and Sleep

Can Exercise Help Me Sleep Better?

Yes, there is growing scientific evidence that regular exercise will help you sleep better. But let me emphasize that a good night's sleep is linked to many other factors to which you should pay attention.

The National Sleep Foundation reports that 74 percent of adults in the United States experience a sleeping problem a few nights a week or more, 39 percent get less than seven hours of sleep each weeknight, and 37 percent are so sleepy during the day that it interferes with daily activities.[1]

According to a report issued by the National Commission on Sleep Disorders Research, 30 to 40 percent of people in the United States have insomnia within any given year, defined by the National Institutes of Health as "an experience of inadequate or poor quality sleep."[2] Characteristics of insomnia include the following:

- Difficulty falling asleep
- Difficulty maintaining sleep
- Waking up too early in the morning
- Nonrefreshing sleep
- Daytime tiredness, lack of energy, difficulty concentrating, and irritability

"Can Exercise Help Me Sleep Better?" David C. Nieman, Dr.PH, FACS, ACSM's *Health and Fitness Journal*, May/June 2005, 9(3): 6–7. © 2005 Lippincott Williams and Wilkins, Inc. Reprinted with permission. Reviewed by David A. Cooke, MD, FACP, April 2010.

Lack of sleep leads to problems completing a task, concentrating, making decisions, and working with and getting along with other people, as well as unsafe actions.[1] Sleep duration is related to length of life, with a greater risk of death in those sleeping fewer than six hours a night.[3] Sleep deprivation is linked to approximately 100,000 vehicle crashes and 1,500 deaths each year.[1] Insomnia early in adult life is a risk factor for the development of clinical depression and mental health disorders.[1]

A night's sleep consists of four or five cycles, each of which progresses through several stages.[1] During each night, a person alternates between non–rapid eye movement (NREM) sleep and rapid eye movement (REM) sleep. The entire cycle of NREM and REM sleep takes approximately ninety minutes. The average adult sleeps 7.5 hours (five full cycles), with 25 percent of that in REM. By age seventy, total sleep time decreases to approximately six hours (four sleep cycles), but the proportion of REM stays at approximately 25 percent. Sleep efficiency is reduced in elderly individuals with an increased number of awakenings during the night.

In NREM sleep, brain activity, heart rate, respiration, blood pressure, and metabolism (vital signs) slow down and body temperature falls as a deep, restful state is reached. The brain waves slow in NREM, a state termed "slow-wave sleep" by sleep researchers. Slow-wave sleep usually terminates with the sleeper changing position. The brain waves now reverse their course as the sleeper heads for the active REM stage.

In REM sleep, the eyes dart about under closed eyelids, and vivid dreams transpire that often can be remembered. The even breathing of NREM gives way to halting uncertainty, and the heart rhythm speeds or slows unaccountably. The brain is highly active during REM sleep, and overall brain metabolism may be increased above the level experienced when awake.

Getting a good night's sleep has proven to be a difficult goal for many people in this modern era. The National Sleep Foundation has published several guidelines for better sleep. Here are ten guidelines for better sleep[1]:

- Maintain a regular bed and wake time schedule, including weekends.

- Establish a regular, relaxing bedtime routine such as soaking in a hot bath or hot tub and then reading a book or listening to soothing music.

- Create a sleep-conducive environment that is dark, quiet, comfortable, and cool.

- Sleep on a comfortable mattress and pillows.

- Use your bedroom only for sleep and sex. It is best to take work materials, computers, and televisions out of the sleeping environment.

- Finish eating at least two to three hours before your regular bedtime.

- Avoid nicotine (e.g., cigarettes and other tobacco products). Used close to bedtime, it can lead to poor sleep.

- Avoid caffeine (e.g., coffee, tea, soft drinks, or chocolate) close to bedtime. It can keep you awake.

- Avoid alcohol close to bedtime. It can lead to disrupted sleep later in the night.

- Exercise regularly. It is best to complete your workout at least a few hours before bedtime.

Compared with those who avoid exercise, physically fit people claim that they fall asleep more rapidly, sleep better, and feel less tired during the day. These beliefs have been confirmed, and scientists have shown that people who exercise regularly do indeed spend more time in slow-wave sleep.[4-6]

In a study conducted at Stanford University, physically inactive older adults were assigned to exercise or nonexercise groups for sixteen weeks.[5] Subjects in the exercise group engaged in low-impact aerobics and brisk walking for thirty to forty minutes, four days per week. Exercise training led to improved sleep quality, longer sleep, and a shorter time to fall asleep. A yearlong study of postmenopausal women showed that those exercising moderately in the morning for three to four hours per week had less trouble falling asleep compared with those exercising less.[6]

So yes, exercise should help you sleep better. There is some evidence, however, that exercising and sweating close to bedtime can have an adverse effect on sleep quality for both fit and sedentary subjects.[1,5,6] This is why the National Sleep Foundation recommends avoiding heavy exercise late in the day.

References

1. National Sleep Foundation. Sleep Facts and Stats; Healthy Sleep Tips. http://www. sleepfoundation.org/. Accessed December 15, 2004.

2. National Center on Sleep Disorders Research and Office of Prevention, Education, and Control, National Institutes of Health. Insomnia: Assessment and Management in Primary Care. Bethesda, MD: National Institutes of Health, NIH Publication No. 98-4088, 1998.

3. Patel, S. R., N. T. Ayas, M. R. Malhotra, et al. A prospective study of sleep duration and mortality risk in women. *Sleep* 27: 440–44, 2004.

4. Kubitz, K. A., D. M. Landers, S. J. Petruzzello, and M. Han. The effects of acute and chronic exercise on sleep: a meta-analytic review. *Sports Medicine* 21:277–91, 1996.

5. King, A. C., R. F. Oman, G. S. Brassington, et al. Moderate-intensity exercise and self-related quality of sleep in older adults. *Journal of the American Medical Association* 277:32–37, 1997.

6. Tworoger, S. S., Y. Yasui, M. V. Vitiello, et al. Effects of a year-long moderate intensity exercise and a stretching intervention on sleep quality in postmenopausal women. *Sleep* 26:830–36, 2003.

Chapter 37

Recognizing Sleep Disorders

Chapter Contents

Section 37.1

What Are the Common Symptoms of a Sleep Disorder?

Excerpted from "Recognize Symptoms for Sleep Disorders,"
Centers for Disease Control and Prevention, February 2009.

Sleep. Like the weather, that's one topic on which everyone has an opinion. How often do you hear friends and family complaining they don't get enough sleep? Or talking about what a hard time they had falling asleep the night before? Maybe you're one of those people who has trouble staying asleep, or perhaps you get a full night's sleep but you just don't feel refreshed when you get up in the morning. These complaints may signal a treatable sleep disorder or simply reflect not getting enough sleep. Either can cause serious health problems.

You won't be surprised to learn that a recent Centers for Disease Control and Prevention (CDC) study found that many people have trouble staying awake during the day. The real news is that 16 percent of those surveyed experience persistent problems staying awake during the day, but only 10 percent reported having been diagnosed with a sleep disorder.

This study analyzed interview data from almost seven thousand randomly selected adults who participated in the Georgia Chronic Fatigue Syndrome (CFS) surveillance study. Because people with CFS may complain of problems sleeping, the study also evaluated sleep.

In addition to problems staying awake, the study also found the following:

- 33 percent report that they snore
- 25 percent complain that they have problems falling asleep
- 31 percent cannot sleep through the night
- 35 percent wake up in the morning feeling unrefreshed

It's well understood that your quality of life decreases when you're sleepy. Excessive daytime sleepiness can also greatly increase the risk of accidents on the highways and at work. Insufficient sleep and primary sleep disorders are associated with many serious chronic diseases such as diabetes, hypertension, cardiovascular disease, and stroke.

Know the Signs and Symptoms of Sleep Disorders

Daytime sleepiness is one of the most common signs of a sleep-related disorder. People often attribute daytime sleepiness to aging, lack of exercise, or being overworked. For these and many other reasons, people live with persistent daytime sleepiness without realizing that it may be a symptom of a sleep disorder. Other signs and symptoms of sleep-related disorders include the following:

- Snoring that is accompanied by pauses in breathing

- Loud or disruptive snoring

- Difficulty falling asleep or staying asleep

- Awakening from sleep and feeling unrefreshed or with a headache

- Creepy crawling sensations in the legs or arms during evening hours

- Physically acting out dreams during sleep

What Can You Do?

A sleep disorder can exist for weeks to years before a person recognizes it. It's not normal to always feel sleepy during the daytime or have problems falling asleep, staying asleep, or awakening unrefreshed. These are signs to as talk about with your doctor.

Be prepared with information about your sleep patterns and provide your doctor with as much supporting information as possible. You may need to ask your bed partner to find out if you snore or kick during the night. Tell your doctor if you're waking up with a dry mouth, snore, experience morning headaches, can't sleep, awaken in the middle of the night, or experience a tingling in your legs during the evening.

Many people are predisposed to developing sleep disorders. If you think that your bed partner has signs of sleep disorder, then let him or her know, as he or she may be unaware of it. Sleep disorders also exist in children. A parent with a sleep disorder often passes along those genes or traits that increase the likelihood that their children may also develop the same disorder.

Section 37.2

Keeping a Sleep Diary

Excerpted from "A Good Night's Sleep," © 2005 Department of Health, Government of Western Australia. Reproduced with permission from the Prevention Branch, Drug and Alcohol Office, Western Australia. Reviewed by David A. Cooke, MD, FACP, April 2010.

Improving the length or quality of your sleep will take time and patience, but the results will be worth the effort. Don't expect instant results, especially if your insomnia has been a problem for months or years.

The first step in managing your sleep is to find out what might be stopping you from getting a good night's sleep. You will need to chart your sleeping patterns every night for two weeks.

Keeping records this long may seem difficult, but it will help you work out the factors causing your particular insomnia.

You could keep your diary next to your bed or the kettle, so you are reminded to fill it in straight away or as you drink your first cup of tea or coffee in the morning.

How to Fill in Your Diary

You should record the following "pre-sleep" details:

- How many naps you had during the day and the approximate time and length of the naps.

- Pre-bed activities, including the time you ate your last full meal. If you follow a regular routine you may want to just record an "r" in the box. If it was different, for example, you stayed up late watching television or had a relaxing bath, you should jot that down.

- In-bed activities. Note what you did just before turning out the light, for example, reading or watching television.

- Record any caffeine or alcohol you drank or the number of cigarettes you smoked for the day within five hours of going to bed. Also include any medication you took, including sleeping pills.

- Any tension or worrying experienced when in bed.

- The time you turned the light out to go to sleep.

- Any physical activity done during the day and at what time.

Bed/sleep patterns should be filled in the next morning. Record:

- the time it took you to fall asleep;
- the number of times you woke and the approximate time in minutes awake;
- the number of hours slept;
- the type of sleep;
- a "rest score."

Make a brief comment if sleep was disturbed. That is, if it took a while to fall asleep, if you woke during the night or early in the morning, and the causes (for example, was it due to worry, or noise, or being too hot?)

Table 37.1. Sleep Diary

Pre-Sleep Information								
Day Date	Naps	Dinner time	Caffeine Alcohol Nicotine	Medications	Pre-bed activities	Day* fatigue level (1–5)	** Tension in bed (1–5)	In-bed activities
Bed/Sleep Pattern							
Day Date	Lights out	Minutes to fall asleep	Waking time	Hours slept	No. of times woke up (+min.)	*** Type of sleep (1–5)	**** Rest score (1–5)

Notes:

*Day fatigue is how energetic or fatigued you feel during the day (1: extreme fatigue; 2: some fatigue; 3: OK; 4: fairly energetic; 5: very energetic).

** For tension in bed, rate how tense or calm you feel in bed (1: extreme tension; 2: some tension; 3: OK; 4: fairly calm; 5: very calm).

***For type of sleep, rate the type of sleep you have had (1: very restless; 2: restless; 3: OK; 4: sound; 5: very sound sleep).

****Rest score is how refreshed or exhausted you feel on wakening (1: extreme exhaustion; 2: exhaustion; 3: OK; 4: pretty good; 5: really refreshed).

Section 37.3

Self-Test: The Epworth Sleepiness Scale

"Self-Test," © 2009 American Academy of Dental Sleep Medicine
(www.aadsm.org). Reprinted with permission.

The only way to be sure if you have obstructive sleep apnea is to have a sleep test either at home from a qualified sleep physician or in a hospital sleep center, but a score of 9 or above on this test is an indication that you should see your doctor.

Fill out this test and take with you to your physician.

The Epworth Sleepiness Scale

How likely are you to doze off or fall asleep in the following situations? Choose the most appropriate number for each situation:

0 = would never doze   2 = moderate chance of dozing

1 = slight chance of dozing   3 = high chance of dozing

	Activity:
	Sitting and reading
	Watching TV
	Sitting, inactive in a public place (theater, meeting, etc.)
	As a passenger in a car for an hour without a break
	Lying down to rest in the afternoon when circumstances permit
	Sitting and talking to someone
	Sitting quietly after lunch without alcohol
	In a car, while stopped for a few minutes in traffic
	Total

A score of 9 or above indicates you may be having a problem with daytime sleepiness but below 9 does not necessarily mean that you don't have a problem. See your healthcare professional for advice if you snore, have been told that you awake gasping for breath, or if you are sleepy during the day.

Chapter 38

What You Need to Know about Sleep Studies

Chapter Contents

Section 38.1

Understanding the Different Types of Sleep Studies

"Sleep Studies," National Heart Lung and Blood Institute,
National Institutes of Health, December 2009.

What Are Sleep Studies?

Sleep studies allow doctors to measure how much and how well you sleep. They also help show whether you have sleep problems and how severe they are.

Sleep studies are important because untreated sleep disorders can increase your risk of high blood pressure, heart attack, stroke, and other medical conditions. Sleep disorders also have been linked to an increased risk of injury due to falls and car accidents.

People usually aren't aware of their breathing and movements while sleeping. They may never think to talk to their doctors about sleep- and health-related issues that may be linked to sleep problems.

Doctors can diagnose and treat sleep disorders. Talk with your doctor if you snore regularly or feel very tired while at work or school most days of the week.

You also may want to talk with your doctor if you often have trouble falling or staying asleep, or if you wake up too early and aren't able to go back to sleep. These are common signs of a sleep disorder.

Doctors can diagnose some sleep disorders by asking questions about your sleep schedule and habits and by getting information from sleep partners or parents. To diagnose other sleep disorders, doctors also use the results from sleep studies and other medical tests.

Sleep studies can help doctors diagnose the following:

- Sleep-related breathing disorders (such as sleep apnea)

- Sleep-related seizure disorders

- Narcolepsy

Types of Sleep Studies

To diagnose sleep-related problems, doctors may use one or more of the following sleep studies:

- Polysomnogram, or PSG

- Multiple sleep latency test, or MSLT

- Maintenance of wakefulness test, or MWT

- Home-based portable monitor (PM)

Your doctor may use actigraphy if he or she thinks you have a circadian rhythm disorder.

Polysomnogram

A PSG usually is done while you stay overnight at a sleep center. A PSG records brain activity, eye movements, heart rate, and blood pressure.

A PSG also records the amount of oxygen in your blood, how much air is moving through your nose while you breathe, snoring, and chest movements. The chest movements show whether you're making an effort to breathe.

PSG results are used to help diagnose the following:

- Sleep-related breathing disorders (such as sleep apnea)

- Narcolepsy (PSG and MSLT results will be reviewed together)

- Sleep-related seizure disorders

Your doctor also may use a PSG to find the right setting for you on a continuous positive airway pressure (CPAP) machine. CPAP is the most common treatment for sleep apnea.

Sleep apnea is a common disorder in which you have one or more pauses in breathing or shallow breaths while you sleep. In obstructive sleep apnea, the airway collapses or is blocked during sleep. A CPAP machine uses mild air pressure to keep your airway open while you sleep.

If your doctor thinks that you have sleep apnea, he or she may schedule a split-night sleep study. During the first half of the night, your sleep is checked without a CPAP machine. This will show whether you have sleep apnea and how severe it is.

If the PSG shows that you have sleep apnea, you may use a CPAP machine during the second half of the split-night study. A technician will help you select a CPAP mask that fits and is comfortable.

While you sleep, the technician will check the amount of oxygen in your blood and whether your airway stays open. He or she will adjust the flow of air through the mask to find the setting that's right for you. This process is called CPAP titration.

In some cases, this isn't done all in the same night. Some people need to go back to the sleep center for the CPAP titration study.

Your doctor may recommend a follow-up PSG to do the following things:

- Adjust your CPAP settings after weight loss or weight gain

- Recheck your sleep if symptoms return despite treatment with CPAP

- Find out how well surgery has worked to correct a sleep-related breathing disorder

Multiple Sleep Latency Test

This daytime sleep study measures how sleepy you are. It's typically done the day after a PSG. You relax in a quiet room for about thirty minutes while a technician checks your brain activity.

The MSLT records whether you fall asleep during the test and what types and stages of sleep you're having. Sleep has two basic types: rapid eye movement (REM) and non-REM. Non-REM sleep has three distinct stages. REM sleep and the three stages of non-REM sleep occur in regular cycles throughout the night.

The types and stages of sleep you have during the day can help your doctor diagnose sleep disorders such as narcolepsy and idiopathic hypersomnia.

An MSLT is repeated four or five times throughout the day. This is because your ability to fall asleep also changes throughout the day.

Maintenance of Wakefulness Test

This daytime sleep study measures your ability to stay awake and alert. It's usually done the day after a PSG and takes most of the day.

Results may be used to show whether your inability to stay awake is a public or personal safety concern or to check your response to treatment.

Home-Based Portable Monitor

Your doctor may recommend a home-based sleep test with a PM. The PM will record some of the same information as a PSG. For example, it may record the following:

- The amount of oxygen in your blood
- How much air is moving through your nose while you breathe
- Your heart rate
- Chest movements that show whether you're making an effort to breathe

A sleep specialist may use the results from a home-based sleep test to help diagnose sleep apnea. He or she also may use the results to see how well some treatments for sleep apnea are working.

Home-based testing is appropriate for only some people. Talk with your doctor to find out whether a PM is an option for you. If your doctor recommends this test, you'll need to visit a sleep center or your doctor's office to pick up the equipment and learn how to use it.

If you're diagnosed with sleep apnea, your doctor may prescribe treatment with CPAP. If so, he or she will need to find the correct airflow setting for your CPAP machine. To do this, you may have a PSG, or you may be able to find the correct setting at home with an autotitrating CPAP machine.

An autotitrating CPAP machine automatically finds the right airflow setting for you. These machines work well for some people who have sleep apnea. A technician or a doctor will help you learn how to use the machine.

Actigraphy

Actigraphy is a test that's done while you go about your normal routine. It's useful for all age groups and doesn't require an overnight stay at a sleep center.

An Actigraph is a simple device that's usually worn like a wristwatch. Your doctor may ask you to wear the device for several days and nights, except when bathing or swimming.

Actigraphy gives your doctor a better idea about your sleep schedule, such as when you sleep or nap and whether the lights are on while you sleep.

Doctors can use actigraphy to help diagnose a number of sleep disorders, including those related to jet lag and shift work. The test also may be used to check how well sleep treatments are working.

Who Needs a Sleep Study?

If you often feel very sleepy, even though you've spent enough time in bed to be well rested, talk with your doctor about whether you might benefit from a sleep study.

Doctors can diagnose some sleep disorders by asking questions about your sleep schedule and habits and by getting information from sleep partners or parents. To diagnose other sleep disorders, doctors also use the results from sleep studies and other medical tests.

Sleep studies often are used to diagnose sleep-related breathing disorders. Signs of these disorders include loud snoring, gasping, or choking sounds while you sleep or pauses in breathing during sleep.

Other common signs and symptoms of sleep disorders include the following:

- It takes you more than thirty minutes to fall asleep at night.

- You often wake up during the night and then have trouble falling back to sleep, or you wake up too early and aren't able to go back to sleep.

- You feel sleepy during the day and fall asleep within five minutes if you have a chance to nap, or you fall asleep at inappropriate times during the day.

- You have creeping, tingling, or crawling feelings in your legs that are relieved by moving or massaging them, especially in the evening and when you try to fall asleep.

- You have vivid, dreamlike experiences while falling asleep or dozing.

- You have episodes of sudden muscle weakness when you're angry, fearful, or when you laugh.

- You feel as though you can't move when you first wake up.

- Your bed partner notes that your legs or arms jerk often during sleep.

- You regularly feel the need to use stimulants, such as caffeine, to stay awake during the day.

Talk with your doctor if you have any signs or symptoms of a sleep disorder. It's important to note how tired you feel and whether your signs and symptoms affect your daily routine.

In infants and children, many of the same signs and symptoms of sleep disorders can occur. If your child has persistent snoring or other signs or symptoms of sleep problems, talk with his or her doctor.

If you've had a sleep disorder for a long time, it may be hard for you to notice how it affects your daily routine. Using a sleep diary may be helpful.

Your doctor will work with you to help decide whether you need a sleep study. A sleep study allows your doctor to observe sleep patterns and diagnose a sleep disorder, which can then be treated.

Certain medical conditions have been linked to sleep disorders. These include heart failure, coronary heart disease (also called coronary artery disease), obesity, diabetes, high blood pressure, and stroke or transient ischemic attack (TIA, or "mini-stroke").

If you have or have had one of these conditions, talk with your doctor about whether it would be helpful to have a sleep study.

What to Expect Before a Sleep Study

Before a sleep study, your doctor may ask you about your sleep habits and whether you feel well rested and alert during the day.

You may be asked to keep a sleep diary or sleep log. You'll record information such as when you went to bed, when you woke up, how many times you woke up during the night, and more.

What to Bring with You

Depending on what type of sleep study you're having, you may need to bring the following things:

- Notes from your sleep diary or sleep log. These may be helpful to your doctor.

- Pajamas and a toothbrush for overnight sleep studies.

- A book or something to do between testing periods if you're having a maintenance of wakefulness test (MWT) or multiple sleep latency test (MSLT).

How to Prepare

You may need to stop or limit the use of tobacco, caffeine, and other stimulants, and some medicines before having a sleep study.

Your doctor may ask you about alcohol, medicines, or other substances that you take. Make sure you tell your doctor about all of the medicines you take, including over-the-counter products. Your doctor also may ask about any allergies you have.

Talk with your doctor before the sleep study and never stop taking your medicines unless the doctor who prescribed them tells you to do so.

You should try to sleep well the night before you have an MWT because you'll have to try to stay awake during the test. If you're being tested as a requirement for a transportation- or safety-related job, you may be asked to take a drug-screening test.

You also should try to sleep well for a night or two before you have an MSLT because the results will be more accurate.

If you're going to have a home-based sleep test with a portable monitor, you'll need to visit a sleep center or your doctor's office to pick up the equipment. Your doctor or a technician will tell you how to use the equipment.

What to Expect During a Sleep Study

Sleep studies are painless. The polysomnogram (PSG), multiple sleep latency test (MSLT), and maintenance of wakefulness test (MWT) usually are done at a sleep center.

The room the sleep study is done in may look like a hotel room. A technician makes the room comfortable for you and sets the temperature to your liking.

Most of your contact at the sleep center will be with nurses or technicians. You can ask them questions about the sleep study. They can answer questions about the test itself, but they usually can't give you the test results.

During a Polysomnogram

Sticky patches and sensors called electrodes are placed on your scalp, face, chest, limbs, and a finger. While you sleep, these sensors record your brain activity, eye movements, heart rate and rhythm, blood pressure, and the amount of oxygen in your blood.

Elastic belts are placed around your chest and abdomen. They measure chest movements and the strength and duration of inhaled and exhaled breaths.

Wires attached to the sensors transmit the data to a computer in the next room. The wires are very thin and flexible and are bundled together so they don't restrict movement, disrupt your sleep, or cause other discomfort.

If you have signs of sleep apnea, you may have a split-night sleep study. During the first half of the night, the technician records your sleep patterns. At the start of the second half of the night, he or she wakes you to fit a CPAP (continuous positive airway pressure) mask over your nose and/or mouth.

The mask is connected to a small machine that gently blows air through the mask. This creates mild pressure that keeps your airway open while you sleep.

The technician checks how you sleep with the CPAP machine. He or she adjusts the flow of air through the mask to find the setting that's right for you.

At the end of the PSG, the technician removes the sensors. If you're having a daytime sleep study, such as an MSLT, some of the sensors may be left on for that test.

Parents usually are required to spend the night with their child during the child's PSG.

During a Multiple Sleep Latency Test

The MSLT is a daytime sleep study that's usually done after a PSG. Sensors on your scalp, face, and chin usually are used for this test. These sensors record brain activity. They show various stages of sleep and how long it takes you to fall asleep. Sometimes your breathing also is checked during an MSLT.

A technician in another room watches these recordings as you sleep. He or she fixes any problems with the recordings that occur.

About 1.5 to 3 hours after you wake from the PSG, you're asked to relax in a quiet room for about thirty minutes. The test is repeated four or five times throughout the day. This is because your ability to fall asleep changes throughout the day.

You get two-hour breaks between tests. You need to stay awake during the breaks.

The MSLT records whether you fall asleep during the test and what types and stages of sleep you have. Sleep has two basic types: rapid eye movement (REM) and non-REM. Non-REM sleep has three distinct stages. REM sleep and the three stages of non-REM sleep occur in patterns throughout the night.

The types and stages of sleep you have during the day can help your doctor diagnose sleep disorders such as narcolepsy and idiopathic hypersomnia.

During a Maintenance of Wakefulness Test

This sleep study occurs during the day. It's usually done after a PSG and takes most of the day. Sensors on your scalp, face, and chin are used to measure when you're awake or asleep.

You sit quietly on a bed in a comfortable position and look straight ahead. Then you simply try to stay awake for a period of time.

An MWT typically includes four trials lasting about forty minutes each. If you fall asleep, the technician will wake you after about ninety seconds. There usually are two-hour breaks between trials. During these breaks, you can read, watch television, and so on.

367

If you're being tested as a requirement for a transportation- or safety-related job, you may need a drug-screening test before a MWT.

During a Home-Based Portable Monitor Test

If you're having a home-based portable monitor test, you'll need to set up the equipment at home before you go to sleep. When you pick up the equipment at the sleep center or your doctor's office, someone will tell you how to use it.

During Actigraphy

You don't have to go to a sleep center for this test. An Actigraph is a small device that's usually worn like a wristwatch. You can go about your normal routine while you wear it. You remove it while bathing or swimming.

The Actigraph measures your sleep-wake behavior over three to seven days and nights. Results give your doctor a better idea about your sleep habits, such as when you sleep or nap and whether the lights are on while you sleep.

You may be asked to keep a sleep diary while you wear an Actigraph.

What to Expect After a Sleep Study

Once the sensors are removed after a polysomnogram (PSG), multiple sleep latency test, or maintenance of wakefulness test, you can go home. If you used an Actigraph or a home-based portable monitor, you'll return the equipment to a sleep center or your doctor's office.

You won't receive a diagnosis right away. Your primary care doctor or sleep specialist will review the results of your sleep study or sleep studies. He or she will use your medical history, your sleep history, and the test results to make a diagnosis.

It may take a couple of weeks to get the sleep study results. Usually, your doctor, nurse, or sleep specialist will explain the test results and work with you and your family to develop a treatment plan.

What Do Sleep Studies Show?

Sleep studies allow doctors to watch sleep patterns and note sleep-related problems that patients don't know or can't describe during routine office visits. These studies are needed to diagnose certain sleep disorders, such as narcolepsy and sleep apnea.

After your sleep study, your doctor will get the results. The results may include information about sleep and wake times, sleep stages, abnormal breathing, the amount of oxygen in your blood, and any movement during sleep.

Your doctor will use your sleep study results and your medical and sleep histories to make a diagnosis and create a treatment plan.

Results from a Polysomnogram

Polysomnogram (PSG) results are used to help diagnose the following things:

- Sleep-related breathing disorders, such as sleep apnea

- Narcolepsy (PSG and multiple sleep latency test (MSLT) results will be reviewed together)

- Sleep-related seizure disorders

If you have sleep apnea, your doctor also may use a PSG to find the correct setting for you on a CPAP (continuous positive airway pressure) machine.

A CPAP machine gently supplies air to your nose and/or mouth through a special mask. Finding the right setting involves adding just enough extra air to create mild pressure that keeps your airway open while you sleep.

Your doctor may recommend a follow-up PSG to do the following things:

- Adjust your CPAP settings after weight loss or weight gain

- Recheck your sleep if symptoms return despite treatment with CPAP

- Find out how well surgery has worked to correct a sleep-related breathing disorder

Technicians also use PSGs to record the number of abnormal breathing events that occur with sleep-related breathing disorders, such as sleep apnea. These events include either pauses in breathing or dips in the level of oxygen in your blood.

In adults, when the number of events is ten or more per hour, treatment may be needed. Children who have one to three events per hour also may need treatment.

Results from a Multiple Sleep Latency Test

MSLT results are used to help diagnose narcolepsy and idiopathic hypersomnia.

For narcolepsy, technicians study how quickly you fall asleep. The MSLT also shows how long it takes you to reach different types and stages of sleep.

Sleep has two basic types: rapid eye movement (REM) and non-REM. Non-REM sleep has three distinct stages. REM sleep and the three stages of non-REM sleep occur in patterns throughout the night.

People who fall asleep in less than five minutes or quickly reach REM sleep may need treatment for a sleep disorder.

Results from a Maintenance of Wakefulness Test

Maintenance of wakefulness test (MWT) results may be used to show whether your inability to stay awake is a public or personal safety concern. This study also is used to show how well treatment for a sleep disorder is working.

Results from a Home-Based Portable Monitor Test

Home-based portable monitors (PMs) may be used to help diagnose sleep apnea. PMs also can show how well some treatments for sleep apnea are working.

Sometimes, home-based PMs don't record enough information for doctors to make accurate diagnoses. If this happens, you may be asked to take the PM home again and repeat the test, or your sleep specialist may ask you to have a PSG.

Results from Actigraphy

Actigraphy results give your doctor a better idea about your sleep habits, such as when you sleep or nap and whether the lights are on while you sleep. This test also is used to help diagnose circadian rhythm disorders.

What Are the Risks of Sleep Studies?

Sleep studies are painless. There's a small risk of skin irritation from the sensors. The irritation will go away once the sensors are removed.

Although the risks of sleep studies are minimal, these studies take time (at least several hours). If you're having a daytime sleep study, bring a book or something to do during the test.

Key Points

- Sleep studies allow doctors to measure how much and how well you sleep. They also help show whether you have sleep problems and how severe they are.

- Sleep studies are important because untreated sleep disorders can increase your risk of high blood pressure, heart attack, stroke, and other medical conditions. Sleep disorders also have been linked to an increased risk of injury due to falls and car accidents.

- People usually aren't aware of their breathing and movements while sleeping. They may never think to talk to their doctors about sleep- and health-related issues that may be linked to sleep problems.

- Sleep studies can help doctors diagnose sleep-related breathing disorders (such as sleep apnea), sleep-related seizure disorders, and narcolepsy.

- To diagnose sleep-related problems, doctors may use one or more of the following sleep studies:

  - A polysomnogram (PSG) is an overnight sleep study that records brain activity, eye movements, heart rate, and blood pressure. It also records the amount of oxygen in your blood, how much air is moving through your nose while you breathe, snoring, and chest movements that show whether you're making an effort to breathe. Your doctor also may use a PSG to find the correct setting for you on a CPAP (continuous positive airway pressure) machine.

  - A multiple sleep latency test (MSLT) is a daytime sleep study that measures how sleepy you are. It records brain activity to show various stages of sleep. It also shows how long it takes you to fall asleep.

  - A maintenance of wakefulness test (MWT) is a daytime sleep study that measures your ability to stay awake. Results may be used to show whether your inability to stay awake is a public or personal safety concern or to check your response to treatment.

  - A home-based portable monitor (PM) records some of the same information as a PSG. Results may help your doctor diagnose sleep apnea. Results also can show how well some treatments for sleep apnea are working.

- Your doctor may use a test called actigraphy if he or she thinks you have a circadian rhythm disorder. Actigraphy measures sleep-wake behavior while you go about your normal routine. Results give your doctor a better idea about your sleep habits, such as when you sleep or nap and whether the lights are on while you sleep. An Actigraph is a small device that's usually worn like a wristwatch.

- If you often feel very sleepy, even though you've spent enough time in bed to be well rested, talk with your doctor about whether you might benefit from a sleep study.

- Sleep studies often are used to diagnose and treat sleep-related breathing disorders. Signs of these disorders include loud snoring, gasping, or choking sounds while you sleep or pauses in breathing during sleep.

- Certain medical conditions have been linked to sleep disorders. These include heart failure, coronary heart disease, obesity, diabetes, high blood pressure, and stroke or transient ischemic attack (TIA, or "mini-stroke"). If you have one of these conditions, talk with your doctor about whether it would be helpful to have a sleep study.

- Before a sleep study, your doctor may ask you to keep a sleep diary or sleep log. You'll record information such as when you went to bed, when you woke up, how many times you woke up during the night, and more.

- You also may need to stop or limit the use of tobacco, caffeine and other stimulants, and some medicines before having a sleep study. Talk with your doctor before the sleep study and never stop taking your medicines unless the doctor who prescribed them tells you to do so.

- Sleep studies are painless. The PSG, MSLT, and MWT usually are done in a sleep center. The room the study is done in may look like a hotel room. Some people may be able to use home-based PMs to do sleep studies in their own homes.

- If you're having actigraphy, you'll go about your normal daily routine while you wear an Actigraph on your wrist. An Actigraph is a device that records data about your sleep habits.

- After a sleep study, your doctor will get the results. The results may include information about sleep and wake times, sleep stages, abnormal breathing, the amount of oxygen in your blood, and any movement during sleep.

- Your doctor will study the results and use them and your medical and sleep histories to make a diagnosis and help develop a treatment plan. You may not get the diagnosis until a few weeks after the sleep study.

- The risks of sleep studies are minimal. There is a small risk of skin irritation from the sensors. The irritation will go away once the sensors are removed.

Section 38.2

Who Should Be Evaluated for Obstructive Sleep Apnea?

Excerpted from "Sleep Apnea Evaluations" and "How to Select a Sleep Center," © 2008 Scottsdale Sleep Center. Reprinted with permission.

Sleep Apnea Evaluations

Evaluation for Obstructive Sleep Apnea

Sleep is a very personal time. We are unaware of our surroundings and are unprotected. We don't know if we move, talk, or snore. We are unable to present the best image of ourselves. We are vulnerable and helpless. Those we let into our personal lives, family, friends, and loved ones, may tell us things about what we do during sleep, things we do not believe. Other times, we experience things that our loved ones do not see or have trouble believing. There may be no one to tell us if we are doing something unusual during our sleep.

We are reluctant to seek help for sleep problems. Sleep is a time when we are not consciously aware of our actions. We dislike having someone outside our inner circle involved in such a personal problem. In the past, it was not unusual for physicians to tell patients that a sleep problem was all in their heads. Now, the medical profession is more enlightened and knowledgeable. There are professionals who specialize in sleep problems.

This section is designed to help you answer questions you may have regarding the evaluation of sleep. Who should be evaluated? Who should do the evaluation? What kinds of tests are performed? Where should the tests be performed?

Who Should Be Evaluated?

Anyone who has symptoms or signs that suggest sleep apnea should discuss them with their physician. There are a few things that are absolute indicators of the need for a thorough evaluation—sleep testing. So how do you decide? When is your complaint an indicator of a serious medical condition?

373

Let's start with the absolute indicators: those things that strongly suggest the presence of a significant breathing problem during sleep. The first is loud snoring. A sleep evaluation and testing are indicated if your snoring "rattles the rafters," "shakes the walls," can be heard at the other end of the house, is loud enough that it is easily heard outside the room, or consistently drives your mate to another room to sleep.

If you are observed to have periods during your sleep when your breathing is seen to stop, sleep evaluation and testing are indicated. While normal individuals can have an occasional obstructive event associated with cession of breathing, repeated observations strongly indicate a problem.

If you are extremely sleepy, sleep evaluation and testing are indicated. Normal individuals sleep eight to nine hours a night and feel rested. It is abnormal to sleep ten to twelve hours and be sleepy during the waking hours. Sleeping more than ten hours a day means you should seek help. If you are sleeping seven to eight hours per night and falling asleep during normal activities, you should seek help. Falling asleep while doing dangerous activities such as driving or working with machinery is an absolute indication that sleep evaluation and testing are indicated.

When someone exhibits more than one of these three absolute indicators—loud snoring, observed cessation of breathing during sleep, and excessive sleepiness—the question is not, "Does that person have apnea?" but, "How bad is it?" However, most people who suffer from significant obstructive sleep apnea, even many of those with severe apnea, do not report such extreme symptoms.

How to Select a Sleep Center

What to Look for in a Sleep Facility

- Is the center certified by the American Academy of Sleep Medicine?

- Is the ownership of the facility clear and easy to establish?

- Is the center listed in the phone book?

- If you call the phone number, does the person answering work at the facility?

- Can you visit the center during the daytime to see the facility and meet the daytime staff?

- When you visit, is the facility clean?

- Is the facility designed and used just for sleep testing?

- Does it have private baths for each sleep room?

- Does each technician care for no more than two patients each night?

- Is the staff friendly, professional, and competent?

Sleep Center Ownership

It is important to identify the ownership of the sleep center. All centers operate to make money. A business cannot survive without income. The reasons for ownership may give you insight into the center's operations. There are three types of owners:

- **Sleep physicians:** Sleep physicians own sleep centers to provide a service and control the quality of testing.

- **Hospitals and healthcare systems:** Hospitals own centers to provide a service and direct patients to their other facilities and services.

- **Corporate, multi-location, multi-state systems, non-sleep physicians, and those of unclear ownership:** These centers are operated primarily to make a profit. The majority of their business is selling equipment needed to treat obstructive sleep apnea.

What to Look for in a Sleep Center's Physicians

- Is the medical director a certified sleep physician?

- Does the physician medical director practice medicine?

- Can you make an appointment to see the physician medical director?

- Can you see a physician sleep specialist before any testing?

- Are patients who require testing seen in follow-up by a physician sleep specialist?

- Is the interpreting physician a certified sleep specialist?

- Will the interpreting physician be available to see you as a patient?

The answer to each of the questions should be yes. If all the answers are yes, you have found an ideal sleep center.

Section 38.3

Home Sleep Studies

Home Sleep Testing: Benefits to Patients

In 2008, Medicare and Aetna, who together provide insurance coverage for nearly sixty million Americans, decided that patients could now be tested for obstructive sleep apnea (OSA) with a simple at-home test. Prior to this, home testing was only covered in limited situations by very few insurers.

"Medicare beneficiaries who have obstructive sleep apnea face significant risks for cardiovascular disease and other ailments," said Centers for Medicare and Medicaid Services (CMS) acting administrator Charlene Frizzera in announcing this landmark policy change. "This coverage decision establishes nationally consistent coverage and assures that beneficiaries who have sleep apnea can be appropriately diagnosed and referred for treatment."

Now, other insurance companies are starting to modify policies to allow this simpler, home-based approach for all patients suspected of having sleep apnea. Many others will now consider payment on a case-by-case basis.

This is great news for patients suspected of having sleep apnea, as well as those that have already been diagnosed and may need repeat testing. The cost of a home study can be anywhere from one-third to one-tenth the cost of an in-lab study, depending on the provider. Since employers are shifting healthcare costs to their employees, many patients are now facing higher co-pays and deductibles.

Not all home sleep testing options are the same. In some cases, you may go to a lab or other diagnostic service center to pick up a device and have someone explain how to use it. You will then need to bring it back the next day. Depending on how far away the center is, this may or may not be a great option for patients.

Table 38.1. In-Lab versus Home Sleep Testing

	Testing Option	
	In-Lab PSG	**Home Sleep Test**
Process	Spend the night at a lab with numerous electrodes on	Device delivered, you apply a few simple sensors before bedtime
Time from Referral to Treatment	3–12 weeks[a]	1–2 weeks
Key Difference	Ideal for sicker, more complicated patients	Easier, less expensive option to rule out obstructive sleep apnea
Billed Cost	$1,600–5,000[a]	$300
Patient Cost (depends on plan)	$320–1,000	$25–30

[a]Lab studies often involve seeing a specialist first, waiting for insurance approval, an initial diagnostic study in a lab, waiting for results, and then a second in-lab study to determine continuous positive airway pressure.

Other companies are bundling home sleep testing within an online or facility-based sleep management program, which may have additional costs associated with them. For example, you may be asked to fill out some questionnaires that are reviewed by a sleep professional, and the cost of this is added to your bill. Or, you may still be directed to more expensive and unnecessary testing by someone at the company who tries to make your case seem more complicated than it is.

"When I was told I might have sleep apnea, I was forced to go to a sleep lab by my insurance company, even though I asked to have a home test," says Chuck Makarov, who was diagnosed with sleep apnea last year. "I had trouble working it into my schedule, missed work the next day, and had to pay $350 for my portion. And, it was really difficult to sleep at the lab with all of those sensors on. I would have much rather taken the test at home and the results would have been exactly the same."

Home sleep testing has been commonly used in countries like Europe, Australia, and Canada for many years with excellent results. As Americans struggle with higher costs for healthcare and less money in their pockets, home sleep testing could not have arrived at a better time!

If you know someone who has been avoiding a sleep study because of the cost, inconvenience, or inability to sleep in new places, let them know about this new option.

Hooking Up at Home: Not All Agree on Its Usefulness

"Hooking Up at Home," © 2008 American Sleep Apnea Association (www.sleepapnea.org). Reprinted with permission.

Countless snorers have no doubt thought, as they packed up their jammies and headed to the sleep lab for an overnight study, "Boy, it sure would be nice if I could do this at home in my own bed." In fact, home studies—also known as portable monitoring—have been around as long as continuous positive airway pressure (CPAP). But persistent questions about their reliability, and the consequent refusal of most insurers to pay for them, have kept them out of the mainstream of practice.

That's all changing. In March 2008, the Centers for Medicare and Medicaid Services (CMS), whose reimbursement rules are generally adopted by private insurers, dropped its long-standing opposition to home studies. According to the National Coverage Determination (NCD) that was released that month, a diagnosis of obstructive sleep apnea can be made—and CPAP therapy covered—on the basis of a clinical evaluation coupled with a home study using a device that measures, at a minimum, airflow, heart rate, and oxygen saturation.

A positive diagnosis is established if: The apnea-hypopnea index (AHI) as measured by the portable device is 15 or more (15 apneas an hour) or the AHI is between 5 and 14 and the patient has documented symptoms of excessive daytime sleepiness, impaired cognition, mood disorders, hypertension, ischemic heart disease, or history of stroke. The NCD specifies that the home study must be ordered and supervised by the treating physician. It also limits the initial coverage of CPAP to a twelve-week trial period.

Previous to its 2008 decision, the CMS had considered—and rejected—home studies on four occasions. In its last rejection, in 2005, the government body declared that there was insufficient evidence to support the contention that portable monitoring was a valid diagnostic tool.

It was asked to revisit the issue by the American Academy of Otolaryngology—Head and Neck Surgery (AAO-HNS). An association of specialists who treat conditions of the ear, nose, and throat, the AAO-HNS in its petition to the CMS maintained that the prevalence of sleep disordered breathing, combined with a paucity of laboratories that could perform the required polysomnographic studies, resulted in unacceptable delays in diagnosis and treatment. Citing a number of studies, the organization stated that "home sleep testing is a validated alternative" to lab testing, and declared that "it is incumbent upon CMS to lead the way to improve diagnostic and treatment paradigms" by covering portable monitoring.

Clearly, the CMS found the AAO-HNS argument—which was buttressed by testimony from numerous individuals and organizations, among them the American Sleep Apnea Association (ASAA)—compelling. But the change in CMS policy does not reflect a consensus among practitioners. During the deliberative process, the CMS heard objections, some strenuous, from medical professionals and organizations (including the American Academy of Sleep Medicine) unconvinced that change was called for and that the new policy will prove to be in the best interest of patients.

Some of the disagreement revolves around how difficult it actually is for patients to access in-lab studies and consequent care. Another dispute has to do with how much data is needed to make a diagnosis. (Some doctors will tell you, off the record, that most of the time they don't really need a sleep study of any sort—they can look around their waiting rooms and pick out the people with sleep apnea. They're the ones who, rather than impatiently leafing through a magazine or talking on a cell phone, are taking a nap.)

But some physicians' qualms about home studies go to the fundamental nature of sleep disorders, and of sleep itself. Dr. Steven Feinsilver, a specialist in sleep medicine who teaches at New York University, points out that while a portable device that measures airflow can detect disordered breathing, it can't diagnose sleep-disordered breathing, since it can't tell whether a person is, in fact, asleep.

"You can't monitor sleep at home," Dr. Feinsilver says flatly. "Without an EEG [an electroencephalogram, which measures brainwave activity], you have no way of knowing if somebody is asleep or awake.

"A home study doesn't take the place of a laboratory sleep study," he continues. "Spending a night in a sleep lab has enormous benefits for relatively little cost. But the sleep community has not voiced that view. It's just rolled over and played dead. It's terrible."

On the other hand, physician Michael Coppola, a board member of the ASAA, is delighted with the CMS decision. He himself, frustrated with the long waits his patients endured before they could schedule a lab study, and sympathetic with their anxieties about traveling long distances to sleep in a strange place, was using portable monitoring twenty years ago, as part of a collaboration with a health maintenance organization (HMO).

"It was my preferred methodology at the time," he says. "I'd do a home test, and give the patient a CPAP set at the lowest pressure. I'd ask the wife if her husband was still snoring, and raise the pressure until he stopped. Lo and behold, it worked. I very quickly ended up with a lot of healthy, happy patients."

Such a low-tech approach—which admittedly has the drawback of requiring a bed partner—is not likely to be the future of obstructive sleep apnea (OSA) therapy. At this point, however, it's not possible to say what that future will be. It may be that portable monitoring will be used in appropriate, selected populations of comparatively healthy patients with relatively simple sleep disordered breathing (SDB), with laboratory studies reserved for more complex situations, increasing access to care for all. Or it may be that financial considerations—a lab study costs about three times as much as a home study—will become paramount, making polysomnography a luxury item for those who can afford Cadillac care. Or, in an even worse-case scenario, the market may be flooded with shoddy home devices that make proper diagnosis and treatment more elusive.

As mentioned earlier, the American Academy of Sleep Medicine is on record opposing the CMS coverage expansion. However, the Academy, anticipating the rule change, convened a task force in 2007 to develop guidelines for the use of portable monitoring. These were published in the *Journal of Clinical Sleep Medicine*, Vol. 3, No. 7, 2007.

The guidelines, which are highly nuanced and complex, cannot be summarized in this brief article. But one of the major points can serve as the conclusion here: Portable monitoring "should be integrated into a comprehensive program of patient evaluation and treatment under the direction of a sleep specialist board certified in sleep medicine."

Or perhaps we'll give Dr. Coppola the last word. "One doesn't get a test [i.e., a sleep study] the way one gets an x-ray," he points out. "Success isn't about the test, it's how the patient is managed before, during, and after the test."

Chapter 39

Sleeping Medication

Chapter Contents

Section 39.1

Sleeping Pills: Many Options

Insomnia is a common affliction: About a third of Americans report trouble sleeping. More and more, people are resorting to prescription sleep aids to combat insomnia. Prescriptions for sleep aids nearly doubled between 2001 and 2005, from twenty-nine million to forty-nine million.

Before even considering medication for a sleep problem, consider taking some basic steps to make your home and daily routine more sleep friendly. This includes making sure your bedroom environment is comfortable, dark, and quiet at night, sticking to a regular sleep-wake schedule, exercising regularly, and avoiding alcohol, food, and stimulating mental activities in the evening close to bedtime. For some people, a form of counseling called cognitive-behavioral therapy (CBT) may be as effective for treating insomnia as sleeping pills.

There are many medical causes of disturbed sleep, among them chronic heartburn, depression, congestive heart failure, arthritis pain, sleep apnea that interferes with night-time breathing, and urinary tract infections, uncontrolled diabetes, or prostate trouble that rouses one from bed to bathroom. In these cases, sleeping pills are not the medications to use. But used appropriately, prescription sleep aids help many people get the sleep they want.

When an otherwise healthy person suffers from chronic insomnia (difficulty sleeping three or more times per week for an extended period), one step people can easily take is occasional use of over-the-counter sleeping pills that contain an antihistamine, which causes drowsiness as a side effect.

If the problem persists, doctors may prescribe a "hypnotic" medication to induce sleep. The hypnotics produce sleep by suppressing brain activity. Common older-generation hypnotics are benzodiazepines, including diazepam (Valium®), triazolam (Halcion®), alprazolam (Xanax®), and temazepam (Restoril®). These drugs act by enhancing the activity of a brain chemical called gamma aminobutyric acid (GABA), which reduces arousal, thereby helping you to fall asleep.

Older hypnotics are widely available in affordable generic versions. On the downside, their effects may persist into the following day, leaving you with a groggy sleeping-pill "hangover" or, more rarely, amnesia or confusion. Among older people, hypnotics raise the risk of injurious falls. Also, over time your brain can habituate to the effects of hypnotics, causing you to need higher doses for the same effect. In addition, it is possible to become addicted to them. For these reasons, hypnotics are recommended only for short-term or occasional use.

In the past decade, pharmaceutical companies have developed new hypnotics. They have a similar mechanism of action in the central nervous system but are in a different chemical class than the older drugs. They are reputed to reduce the frequency of side effects such as next-day grogginess, unsteadiness, and memory impairment. The new sleeping pills are also reported to have less potential for addiction than older hypnotics.

The new-generation hypnotics, which include zolpidem (Ambien®), zaleplon (Sonata®), and eszopiclone (Lunesta®), are heavily advertised and widely prescribed. Ambien remains the market leader, at least recently. Another new hypnotic, called ramelteon (Rozerem®), works in a unique way by simulating the effect of melatonin, a natural brain chemical that regulates the daily sleep-wake cycle.

Some research suggests that people can use these new sleeping medications long term with less risk of adverse effects than the older generations of hypnotics. However, there are reports and warnings of addiction, withdrawal symptoms when people stop them suddenly after prolonged use (for example, for a surgical procedure or hospitalization for an acute illness), and mental impairment. They are also more expensive.

Which sleeping pill is right for you? It depends on many factors and should be a matter of discussion and evaluation with your physician.

Whenever you take sleeping pills, don't mix them with alcohol.

Take care if you rise during the night; you may feel unsteady on your feet and could fall and hurt yourself.

Make sure you and your family tell your doctor if you develop any unusual behaviors or symptoms while taking sleeping pills.

Section 39.2

Side Effects of Sleep Drugs

"Side Effects of Sleep Drugs," U.S. Food and Drug Administration,
November 10, 2009.

Eating a little bit of chocolate was a treat that Teresa Wood looked forward to after work. The Fairfax Station, Virginia, resident allowed herself two small pieces of chocolate candy a day.

But after taking a drug to help her sleep at night, Wood awoke in the morning to find an empty box on the table in place of a pound of chocolates that had been there the night before.

"I couldn't believe it," says Wood. "I started looking all around the house—I even looked under the bed. I thought for sure someone came into the house during the night and ate them." But she was alone.

A few weeks later, Wood awoke to find a near-full box of chocolates gone again. "I just don't remember eating all that candy," she says.

Complex Sleep-Related Behaviors

Wood and her doctor determined that she had been getting up during the night and "sleep eating," an occurrence known as a complex sleep-related behavior. Other behaviors include making phone calls, having sex, and getting into the car and driving while not fully awake. Most people do not remember these events later.

Complex behaviors are a potential side effect of sedative-hypnotic products—a class of drugs used to help a person fall asleep and stay asleep.

"Complex behaviors, such as sleep-driving, could be potentially dangerous to both the patients and to others," says Russell Katz, M.D., director of the Food and Drug Administration's (FDA's) Division of Neurology Products.

Allergic Reactions

Other rare but potential side effects of sedative-hypnotic drugs are a severe allergic reaction (anaphylaxis) and severe facial swelling (angioedema), which can occur as early as the first time the product is taken.

"Severe allergic reactions can affect a patient's ability to breathe and can affect other body systems as well, and can even be fatal at times," says Katz. "Although these allergic reactions are probably very rare, people should be aware that they can occur, because these reactions may be difficult to notice as people are falling asleep."

Stronger Warnings

To make known the risks of these products, FDA requested in early 2007 that all manufacturers of sedative-hypnotic drug products strengthen their product labeling to include warnings about complex sleep-related behaviors and anaphylaxis and angioedema.

"There are a number of prescription sleep aids available that are well tolerated and effective for many people," says Steven Galson, M.D., M.P.H., director of FDA's Center for Drug Evaluation and Research. However, after reviewing the available information on adverse events that occurred after the sedative-hypnotic drugs were on the market, FDA concluded that labeling changes were necessary to inform healthcare providers and consumers about risks, says Galson.

In addition to the labeling changes, FDA has requested that manufacturers of sedative-hypnotic products do the following:

- Send letters to healthcare providers to notify them about the new warnings (manufacturers sent these letters beginning in March 2007)

- Develop patient medication guides for the products to inform consumers about risks and advise them of precautions that can be taken (patient medication guides are handouts given to patients, families, and caregivers when a medicine is dispensed containing FDA-approved information, such as proper use and the recommendation to avoid ingesting alcohol or other central nervous system depressants)

- Conduct clinical studies to investigate the frequency with which sleep-driving and other complex behaviors occur in association with individual drug products

The revised labeling and other actions to make risks known affect these sedative-hypnotic products:

- Ambien®, Ambien CR ® (zolpidem tartrate)
- Butisol sodium

- Carbitol® (pentobarbital and carbromal)
- Dalmane® (flurazepam hydrochloride)
- Doral® (quazepam)
- Halcion® (triazolam)
- Lunesta® (eszopiclone)
- Placidyl® (ethchlorvynol)
- ProSom® (estazolam)
- Restoril® (temazepam)
- Rozerem® (ramelteon)
- Seconal® (secobarbital sodium)
- Sonata® (zaleplon)

Precautions

FDA advises people who are treated with any of these products to take the following precautions:

- Talk to your healthcare provider before you start these medications and if you have any questions or concerns.
- Read the medication guide, when available, before taking the product.
- Do not increase the dose prescribed by your healthcare provider. Complex sleep-related behaviors are more likely to occur with higher than appropriate doses.
- Do not drink alcohol or take other drugs that depress the nervous system.
- Do not discontinue the use of these medications without first talking to your healthcare provider.

Over-the-Counter Sleep Aids

Not all sleep medications are prescription. FDA has approved over-the-counter (OTC) medications for use for up to two weeks to help relieve occasional sleepiness in people ages twelve and older. "If you continue to have sleeping problems beyond two weeks, you should see a doctor," says Marina Chang, R.Ph., pharmacist and team leader in FDA's Division of Nonprescription Regulation Development.

OTC sleep aids are non-habit-forming and do not present the risk of allergic reactions and complex sleep-related behaviors that are known to occur with sedative-hypnotic drugs.

But just because they're available over-the-counter doesn't mean they don't have side effects, says Chang. "They don't have the same level of precision as the prescription drugs. They don't completely stop working after eight hours—many people feel drowsy for longer than eight hours after taking them."

Chang advises reading the product label and exercising caution when taking OTC sleep aids until you learn how they will affect you. "They affect people differently," she says. "They are not for everybody."

Chapter 40

Dietary Supplements and Complementary and Alternative Medicine for Sleep Disorders

Chapter Contents

Section 40.1

Melatonin

Background

Melatonin is a hormone produced in the brain by the pineal gland, from the amino acid tryptophan. The synthesis and release of melatonin are stimulated by darkness and suppressed by light, suggesting the involvement of melatonin in circadian rhythm and regulation of diverse body functions. Levels of melatonin in the blood are highest prior to bedtime.

Synthetic melatonin supplements have been used for a variety of medical conditions, most notably for disorders related to sleep.

Melatonin possesses antioxidant activity, and many of its proposed therapeutic or preventive uses are based on this property.

New drugs that block the effects of melatonin are in development, such as BMS-214778 or luzindole, and may have uses in various disorders.

Synonyms

5-Methoxy-N-acetyltryptamine, acetamide, beta-methyl-6-chloromelatonin, BMS-214778, luzindole, mel, MEL, melatonine, MLT, N-acetyl-5-methoxytryptamine, N-2-(5-methoxyindol-3-ethyl)-acetamide, Ramelteon ((TAK-375) a selective MT1/MT2-receptor agonist).

Evidence

These uses have been tested in humans or animals. Safety and effectiveness have not always been proven. Some of these conditions are potentially serious, and should be evaluated by a qualified healthcare provider.

Uses of Melatonin Based on Scientific Evidence

Key to grades is as follows: A—Strong scientific evidence for this use; B—Good scientific evidence for this use; C—Unclear scientific evidence for this use; D—Fair scientific evidence against this use; F—Strong scientific evidence against this use.

Jet Lag (Grade: A)

Several human trials suggest that melatonin taken by mouth, started on the day of travel (close to the target bedtime at the destination) and continued for several days, reduces the number of days required to establish a normal sleep pattern, diminishes the time it takes to fall asleep ("sleep latency"), improves alertness, and reduces daytime fatigue. Although these results are compelling, the majority of studies have had problems with their designs and reporting, and some trials have not found benefits. Overall, the scientific evidence does suggest benefits of melatonin in up to half of people who take it for jet-lag. More trials are needed to confirm these findings, to determine optimal dosing, and to evaluate use in combination with prescription sleep aids.

Delayed Sleep Phase Syndrome (DSPS) (Grade: B)

Delayed sleep phase syndrome is a condition that results in delayed sleep onset, despite normal sleep architecture and sleep duration. Although these results are promising, additional research with larger studies is needed before a stronger recommendation can be made.

Insomnia in the Elderly (Grade: B)

Several human studies report that melatonin taken by mouth before bedtime decreases the amount of time it takes to fall asleep ("sleep latency") in elderly individuals with insomnia. However, most studies have not been high quality in their designs and some research has found limited or no benefits. The majority of trials have been brief in duration (several days long), and long-term effects are not known.

Sleep Disturbances in Children with Neuropsychiatric Disorders (Grade: B)

There are multiple trials investigating melatonin use in children with various neuropsychiatric disorders, including mental retardation, autism, psychiatric disorders, visual impairment, or epilepsy. Studies have demonstrated reduced time to fall asleep (sleep latency) and increased sleep duration. Well-designed controlled trials in select patient populations are needed before a stronger or more specific recommendation can be made.

Sleep Enhancement in Healthy People (Grade: B)

Multiple human studies have measured the effects of melatonin supplements on sleep in healthy individuals. A wide range of doses has been used often taken by mouth thirty to sixty minutes prior to sleep time. Most trials have been small, brief in duration, and have not been rigorously designed or reported. However, the weight of scientific evidence does suggest that melatonin decreases the time it takes to fall asleep ("sleep latency"), increases the feeling of "sleepiness," and may increase the duration of sleep. Better research is needed in this area.

Alzheimer Disease (Sleep Disorders) (Grade: C)

There is limited study of melatonin for improving sleep disorders associated with Alzheimer disease (including nighttime agitation or poor sleep quality in patients with dementia). It has been reported that natural melatonin levels are altered in people with Alzheimer disease, although it remains unclear if supplementation with melatonin is beneficial. Further research is needed in this area before a firm conclusion can be reached.

Antioxidant (Free Radical Scavenging) (Grade: C)

There are well over one hundred laboratory and animal studies of the antioxidant (free radical scavenging) properties of melatonin. As a result, melatonin has been proposed as a supplement to prevent or treat many conditions that are associated with oxidative damage. However, well-designed trials in humans are lacking.

Attention Deficit Hyperactivity Disorder (ADHD) (Grade: C)

There is limited research of the use of melatonin in children with ADHD both on the treatment of ADHD and insomnia in ADHD children. A clear conclusion cannot be made at this time.

Benzodiazepine Tapering (Grade: C)

A small amount of research has examined the use of melatonin to assist with tapering or cessation of benzodiazepines such as diazepam (Valium®) or lorazepam (Ativan®). Although preliminary results are promising, further study is necessary before a firm conclusion can be reached.

Bipolar Disorder (Sleep Disturbances) (Grade: C)

There is limited study of melatonin given to patients with sleep disturbances associated with bipolar disorder (such as insomnia or irregular sleep patterns). No clear benefits have been reported. Further research is needed in this area before a clear conclusion can be reached.

Cancer Treatment (Grade: C)

There are several early-phase and controlled human trials of melatonin in patients with various advanced stage malignancies, including brain, breast, colorectal, gastric, liver, lung, pancreatic, and testicular cancer, as well as lymphoma, melanoma, renal cell carcinoma, and soft-tissue sarcoma. Currently, no clear conclusion can be drawn in this area. There is not enough definitive scientific evidence to discern if melatonin is beneficial against any type of cancer, whether it increases (or decreases) the effectiveness of other cancer therapies, or if it safely reduces chemotherapy side effects.

Chemotherapy Side Effects (Grade: C)

Several human trials have examined the effects of melatonin on side effects associated with various cancer chemotherapies. Although these early reported benefits are promising, high-quality controlled trials are necessary before a clear conclusion can be reached in this area. It remains unclear if melatonin safely reduces side effects of various chemotherapies without altering effectiveness.

Circadian Rhythm Entraining (in Blind Persons) (Grade: C)

Limited human study is available in this area. Present studies and individual cases suggest that melatonin, administered in the evening, may correct circadian rhythm. Large, well-designed controlled trials are needed before a stronger recommendation can be made.

Depression (Sleep Disturbances) (Grade: C)

Depression can be associated with neuroendocrine and sleep abnormalities, such as reduced time before dream sleep (REM latency). Melatonin has been suggested for the improvement of sleep patterns in patients with depression, although research is limited in this area. Further studies are needed before a clear conclusion can be reached.

393

Glaucoma (Grade: C)

It has been theorized that high doses of melatonin may increase intraocular pressure and the risk of glaucoma, age-related maculopathy and myopia, or retinal damage. However, there is preliminary evidence that melatonin may actually decrease intraocular pressure in the eye, and it has been suggested as a possible therapy for glaucoma. Additional study is necessary in this area. Patients with glaucoma taking melatonin should be monitored by a healthcare professional.

Headache Prevention (Grade: C)

Several small studies have examined the possible role of melatonin in preventing various forms of headache, including migraine, cluster, and tension-type headache (in people who suffer from regular headaches). Limited initial research suggests possible benefits in all three types of headache, although well-designed controlled studies are needed before a firm conclusion can be drawn.

High Blood Pressure (Hypertension) (Grade: C)

Several controlled studies in patients with high blood pressure report small reductions in blood pressure when taking melatonin by mouth (orally) or inhaled through the nose (intranasally). Better-designed research is necessary before a firm conclusion can be reached.

Human Immunodeficiency Virus (HIV)/Acquired Immunodeficiency Syndrome (AIDS) (Grade: C)

There is a lack of well-designed scientific evidence to recommend for or against the use of melatonin as a treatment for AIDS. Melatonin should not be used in place of more proven therapies, and patients with HIV/AIDS should be treated under the supervision of a medical doctor.

Inflammatory Bowel Disease (IBS) (Grade: C)

Based on preliminary study, melatonin is a promising therapeutic agent for IBS. Further research is needed before a recommendation can be made.

Insomnia (of Unknown Origin in the Non-Elderly) (Grade: C)

Study results have been inconsistent, with some studies reporting benefits on sleep latency and subjective sleep quality, and other research finding no benefits. Most studies have been small and not rigorously designed or reported. Better research is needed before a firm conclusion can be drawn. Notably, several studies in elderly individuals with insomnia provide preliminary evidence of benefits on sleep latency (discussed above).

Parkinson Disease (Grade: C)

Due to very limited study to date, a recommendation cannot be made for or against the use of melatonin in Parkinsonism or Parkinson disease. Better-designed research is needed before a firm conclusion can be reached in this area.

Periodic Limb Movement Disorder (Grade: C)

There is very limited study to date for the use of melatonin as a treatment in periodic limb movement disorder. Better-designed research is needed before a recommendation can be made in this area.

Preoperative Sedation/Anxiolysis (Grade: C)

Results are promising, with similar results reported for melatonin as for benzodiazepines such as midazolam (Versed®), and superiority to placebo. There are also promising reports using melatonin for sedation/anxiolysis prior to magnetic resonance imaging (MRI). However, due to weaknesses in the design and reporting of the available research, better studies are needed before a clear conclusion can be drawn. Melatonin has also been suggested as a treatment for delirium following surgery, although there is little evidence in this area.

Rapid Eye Movement (REM) Sleep Behavior Disorder (Grade: C)

Limited case reports describe benefits in patients with REM sleep behavior disorder who receive melatonin. However, better research is needed before a clear conclusion can be drawn.

Rett Syndrome (Grade: C)

Rett syndrome is a presumed genetic disorder that affects female children, characterized by decelerated head growth and global developmental regression. There is limited study of the possible role of melatonin in improving sleep disturbance associated with Rett syndrome. Further research is needed before a recommendation can be made in this area.

Schizophrenia (Sleep Disorders) (Grade: C)

There is limited study of melatonin for improving sleep latency (time to fall asleep) in patients with schizophrenia. Further research is needed in this area before a clear conclusion can be reached.

Seasonal Affective Disorder (SAD) (Grade: C)

There are several small, brief studies of melatonin in patients with SAD. This research is not well designed or reported, and further study is necessary before a clear conclusion can be reached.

Seizure Disorder (Children) (Grade: C)

The role of melatonin in seizure disorder is controversial. Better evidence is needed in this area before a clear conclusion can be drawn regarding the safety or effectiveness of melatonin in seizure disorder.

Sleep Disturbances Due to Pineal Region Brain Damage (Grade: C)

Several published cases report improvements in sleep patterns in young people with damage to the pineal gland area of the brain due to tumors or surgery. Due to the rarity of such disorders, controlled trials may not be possible. Consideration of melatonin in such patients should be under the direction of a qualified healthcare provider.

Sleep in Asthma (Grade: C)

Based on preliminary study, melatonin may improve sleep in patients with asthma. Further studies looking into long-term effects of melatonin on airway inflammation and bronchial hyper-responsiveness are needed before melatonin can be recommended.

Smoking Cessation (Grade: C)

Although preliminary results are promising, due to weaknesses in the design and reporting of this research, further study is necessary before a firm conclusion can be reached.

Stroke (Grade: C)

At this time, the effects of melatonin supplements immediately after stroke are not clear.

Tardive Dyskinesia (Grade: C)

Tardive dyskinesia (TD) is a serious potential side effect of antipsychotic medications, characterized by involuntary muscle movements. Limited small studies of melatonin use in patients with TD report mixed findings. Additional research is necessary before a clear conclusion can be drawn.

Thrombocytopenia (Low Platelets) (Grade: C)

Increased platelet counts after melatonin use have been observed in patients with decreased platelets due to cancer therapies (several studies reported by the same author). Stimulation of platelet production (thrombopoiesis) has been suggested but not clearly demonstrated. Additional research is necessary in this area before a clear conclusion can be drawn.

Ultraviolet Light Skin Damage Protection (Grade: C)

It has been proposed that antioxidant properties of melatonin may be protective. Further study is necessary before a clear conclusion can be drawn about clinical effectiveness in humans.

Work Shift Sleep Disorder (Grade: C)

There are several studies of melatonin use in people who work irregular shifts, such as emergency room personnel. Results are mixed. Additional research is necessary before a clear conclusion can be drawn.

Uses Based on Tradition or Theory

The below uses are based on tradition or scientific theories. They often have not been thoroughly tested in humans, and safety and effectiveness have not always been proven. Some of these conditions are potentially serious, and should be evaluated by a qualified healthcare provider: Acetaminophen toxicity, acute respiratory distress syndrome (ARDS), aging, aluminum toxicity, asthma, beta-blocker sleep disturbance, cancer prevention, cardiac syndrome X, cognitive enhancement, colitis, contraception, critical illness/ICU sleep disturbance, depression, edema (swelling), duodenal ulcer, erectile dysfunction, fibromyalgia, gastroesophageal reflux disease (GERD), gentamicin-induced kidney damage, glaucoma, heart attack prevention, heart disease, hyperpigmentation, immunostimulant, interstitial cystitis, intestinal motility disorders, itching, kidney damage (amikacin-induced, cyclosporin-induced), lead toxicity, liver damage, melatonin deficiency, memory enhancement, multiple sclerosis, neurodegenerative disorders, noise-induced hearing loss, pancreatitis, polycystic ovarian syndrome (PCOS), postmenopausal osteoporosis, post-operative adjunct, post-operative delirium, prevention of post-lung transplant ischemia-reperfusion injury, rheumatoid arthritis, sarcoidosis, sedation, sexual activity enhancement, schistosomiasis, sudden infant death syndrome (SIDS) prevention, tachycardia, tinnitus (ringing in the ears), tuberculosis, tuberous sclerosis, ulcerative colitis, wasting, withdrawal from narcotics, wound healing.

Dosing

The below doses are based on scientific research, publications, traditional use, or expert opinion. Many herbs and supplements have not been thoroughly tested, and safety and effectiveness may not be proven. Brands may be made differently, with variable ingredients, even within the same brand. The below doses may not apply to all products. You should read product labels, and discuss doses with a qualified healthcare provider before starting therapy.

Adults (Eighteen Years and Older)

Studies have evaluated 0.5–50 milligrams of melatonin taken nightly by mouth. Research suggests that quick-release melatonin may be more effective than sustained-release formulations for sleep related conditions. Intramuscular injections of 20 milligrams of melatonin have also been studied.

In studies of patients with melanoma, melatonin preparations have been applied to the skin. Patients are advised to discuss cancer treatment plans with an oncologist and pharmacist before considering use of melatonin either alone or with other therapies.

Intranasal melatonin (1 percent solution in ethanol) at a dose of 2 milligrams daily for one week has also been studied for high blood pressure.

There are other uses with limited study and unclear effectiveness or safety. Use of melatonin for any condition should be discussed with a primary healthcare provider, appropriate specialist, and pharmacist prior to starting and should not be substituted for more proven therapies.

Children (Younger than Eighteen Years)

There is limited study of melatonin supplements in children, and safety is not established. Use of melatonin should be discussed with the child's physician and pharmacist prior to starting.

Safety

The U.S. Food and Drug Administration does not strictly regulate herbs and supplements. There is no guarantee of strength, purity, or safety of products, and effects may vary. You should always read product labels. If you have a medical condition, or are taking other drugs, herbs, or supplements, you should speak with a qualified healthcare provider before starting a new therapy. Consult a healthcare provider immediately if you experience side effects.

Allergies

There are rare reports of allergic skin reactions after taking melatonin by mouth. Melatonin has been linked to a case of autoimmune hepatitis.

Side Effects and Warnings

Based on available studies and clinical use, melatonin is generally regarded as safe in recommended doses for short-term use. Available trials report that overall adverse effects are not significantly more common with melatonin than placebo. However, case reports raise concerns about risks of blood clotting abnormalities (particularly in patients taking warfarin), increased risk of seizure, and disorientation with overdose.

Commonly reported adverse effects include fatigue, dizziness, headache, irritability, and sleepiness, although these effects may occur due to jet-lag and not to melatonin itself. Fatigue may particularly occur with morning use or high doses, and irregular sleep-wake cycles may occur. Disorientation, confusion, sleepwalking, vivid dreams, and nightmares have also been noted, with effects often resolving after cessation of melatonin. Due to risk of daytime sleepiness, those driving or operating heavy machinery should take caution. Headache has been reported. Ataxia (difficulties with walking and balance) may occur following overdose.

It has been suggested that melatonin may lower seizure threshold and increase the risk of seizure, particularly in children with severe neurologic disorders. However, multiple other studies actually report reduced incidence of seizure with regular melatonin use. This remains an area of controversy. Patients with seizure disorder taking melatonin should be monitored closely by a healthcare professional.

Mood changes have been reported, including giddiness and dysphoria (sadness). Psychotic symptoms have been reported, including hallucinations and paranoia, possibly due to overdose. Patients with underlying major depression or psychotic disorders taking melatonin should be monitored closely by a healthcare professional.

Melatonin should be avoided in patients using warfarin, and possibly in patients taking other blood-thinning medications or with clotting disorders.

Melatonin may cause drops in blood pressure. Caution is advised in patients taking medications that may also lower blood pressure. Based on preliminary evidence, increases in cholesterol levels may occur. Caution is therefore advised in patients with high cholesterol levels, atherosclerosis, or at risk for cardiovascular disease. Abnormal heart rhythms have been associated with melatonin.

Elevated blood sugar levels (hyperglycemia) have been reported in patients with type 1 diabetes (insulin-dependent diabetes), and low doses of melatonin have reduced glucose tolerance and insulin sensitivity. Caution is advised in patients with diabetes or hypoglycemia, and in those taking drugs, herbs, or supplements that affect blood sugar. Serum glucose levels may need to be monitored by a healthcare provider, and medication adjustments may be necessary.

Hormonal effects are reported, including decreases or increases in levels of luteinizing hormone, progesterone, estradiol, thyroid hormone (T4 and T3), growth hormone, prolactin, cortisol, oxytocin, and vasopressin. Gynecomastia (increased breast size) has been reported in men, as well as decreased sperm count (both which resolved with cessation of melatonin). Decreased sperm motility has been reported in rats and humans.

Mild gastrointestinal distress commonly occurs, including nausea, vomiting, or cramping. Melatonin has been linked to a case of autoimmune hepatitis and with triggering of Crohn disease symptoms.

It has been theorized that high doses of melatonin may increase intraocular pressure and the risk of glaucoma, age-related maculopathy and myopia, or retinal damage. However, there is preliminary evidence that melatonin may actually decrease intraocular pressure in the eye, and it has been suggested as a possible therapy for glaucoma. Patients with glaucoma taking melatonin should be monitored by a healthcare professional.

Pregnancy and Breastfeeding

Melatonin supplementation should be avoided in women who are pregnant or attempting to become pregnant, based on possible hormonal effects. High levels of melatonin during pregnancy may increase the risk of developmental disorders. In animal studies, melatonin is detected in breast milk and therefore should be avoided during breastfeeding. In men, decreased sperm motility and decreased sperm count are reported with use of melatonin.

Interactions

Most herbs and supplements have not been thoroughly tested for interactions with other herbs, supplements, drugs, or foods. The interactions listed below are based on reports in scientific publications, laboratory experiments, or traditional use. You should always read product labels. If you have a medical condition, or are taking other drugs, herbs, or supplements, you should speak with a qualified healthcare provider before starting a new therapy.

Interactions with Drugs

Melatonin is broken down (metabolized) in the body by liver enzymes. As a result, drugs that alter the activity of these enzymes may increase or decrease the effects of melatonin supplements.

Increased daytime drowsiness is reported when melatonin is used at the same time as the prescription sleep aid zolpidem (Ambien®), although it is not clear that effects are greater than with the use of zolpidem alone. In theory, based on possible risk of daytime sleepiness, melatonin may increase the amount of drowsiness caused by some other drugs, for example benzodiazepines such as lorazepam (Ativan®) or diazepam (Valium®), barbiturates such as phenobarbital, narcotics such as codeine, some antidepressants, and alcohol. Caution is advised while driving or operating machinery.

Based on preliminary evidence, melatonin should be avoided in patients taking the blood-thinning medication warfarin (Coumadin®), and possibly in patients using other blood thinners (anticoagulants) such as aspirin or heparin.

Multiple drugs are reported to lower natural levels of melatonin in the body. It is not clear that there are any health hazards of lowered melatonin levels, or if replacing melatonin with supplements is beneficial. Examples of drugs that may reduce production or secretion of melatonin include non-steroidal anti-inflammatory drugs (NSAIDs) such as ibuprofen (Motrin®, Advil®) or naproxen (Naprosyn®, Aleve®); beta-blocker blood pressure medications such as atenolol (Tenormin®) or metoprolol (Lopressor®, Toprol®); and medications that reduce levels of vitamin B_6 in the body (such as oral contraceptives, hormone replacement therapy, loop diuretics, hydralazine, theophylline). Other agents that may alter synthesis or release of melatonin include diazepam, vitamin B_{12}, verapamil, temazepam, and somatostatin.

Based on preliminary evidence, melatonin should be avoided in patients taking anti-seizure medications. It has been suggested that melatonin may lower seizure threshold and increase the risk of seizure. However, multiple other studies actually report reduced incidence of seizure with regular melatonin use. This remains an area of controversy. Patients with seizure disorder taking melatonin should be monitored closely by a healthcare professional.

Melatonin may increase or decrease blood pressure; study results conflict. Therefore it may interact with heart or blood pressure medications making close monitoring necessary.

It is not clear if caffeine alters the effects of melatonin supplements in humans. Caffeine is reported to raise natural melatonin levels in the body, possibly due to effects on liver enzymes. However, caffeine may also alter circadian rhythms in the body, with effects on melatonin secretion.

Elevated blood sugar levels (hyperglycemia) have been reported in patients with type 1 diabetes (insulin-dependent diabetes), and low doses of melatonin have reduced glucose tolerance and insulin sensitivity. Caution is advised in patients taking drugs for diabetes by mouth or insulin. Serum glucose levels may need to be monitored by a healthcare provider, and medication adjustments may be necessary.

Alcohol consumption seems to affect melatonin secretion at night.

Preliminary reports suggest that melatonin may aid in reversing symptoms of tardive dyskinesia associated with haloperidol use.

Based on preliminary evidence, melatonin may increase the effects of isoniazid against *Mycobacterium tuberculosis*.

Based on animal research, melatonin may increase the adverse effects of methamphetamine on the nervous system.

Based on laboratory study, melatonin may increase the neuromuscular blocking effect of the muscle relaxant succinylcholine, but not vecuronium.

Interactions with Herbs and Dietary Supplements

Melatonin may increase daytime sleepiness or sedation when taken with herbs or supplements that may cause sedation.

Elevated blood sugar levels (hyperglycemia) have been reported in patients with type 1 diabetes (insulin-dependent diabetes), and low doses of melatonin have reduced glucose tolerance and insulin sensitivity. Caution is advised when using herbs or supplements that may also raise blood sugar levels, such as arginine, cocoa, dehydroepiandrosterone (DHEA), and ephedra (when combined with caffeine).

Based on preliminary evidence of an interaction with the blood thinning drug warfarin, and isolated reports of minor bleeding, melatonin may increase the risk of bleeding when taken with herbs and supplements that are believed to increase the risk of bleeding.

It is not clear if caffeine alters the effects of melatonin supplements in humans. Caffeine is reported to raise natural melatonin levels in the body, possibly due to effects on liver enzymes. However, caffeine may also alter circadian rhythms in the body, with effects on melatonin secretion.

Chasteberry (*Vitex agnus-castus*) may increase natural secretion of melatonin in the body, based on preliminary research.

In animal study, DHEA and melatonin have been noted to stimulate immune function, with slight additive effects when used together. Effects of this combination in humans are not clear.

Based on animal study, a combination of echinacea and melatonin may reduce immune function. Effects of this combination in humans are not clear.

Severe folate deficiency may reduce the body's natural levels of melatonin, based on preliminary study.

Methodology

This information is based on a professional level monograph edited and peer-reviewed by contributors to the Natural Standard Research Collaboration (www.naturalstandard.com).

Selected References

Arendt J, Aldhous M, Wright J. Synchronisation of a disturbed sleep-wake cycle in a blind man by melatonin treatment. *Lancet.* 4-2-1988;1(8588):772–73.

Almeida Montes LG, Ontiveros Uribe MP, Cortes Sotres J, et al. Treatment of primary insomnia with melatonin: a double-blind, placebo-controlled, crossover study. *J Psychiatry Neurosci.* 2003;28(3):191–96.

Andrade C, Srihari BS, Reddy KP, et al. Melatonin in medically ill patients with insomnia: a double-blind, placebo-controlled study. *J Clin Psychiatry.* 2001;62(1):41–45.

Campos FL, Silva-Junior FP, de Bruin VM, et al. Melatonin improves sleep in asthma: a randomized, double-blind, placebo-controlled study. *Am J Respir Crit Care Med.* 11-1-2004;170(9):947–51.

Coppola G, Iervolino G, Mastrosimone M, et al. Melatonin in wake-sleep disorders in children, adolescents and young adults with mental retardation with or without epilepsy: a double-blind, cross-over, placebo-controlled trial. *Brain Dev.* 2004 Sep;26(6):373–76.

Dowling GA, Mastick J, Colling E, et al. Melatonin for sleep disturbances in Parkinson's disease. *Sleep Med.* 2005 Sep;6(5):459–66.

Gupta M, Gupta YK, Agarwal S, et al. A randomized, double-blind, placebo controlled trial of melatonin add-on therapy in epileptic children on valproate monotherapy: effect on glutathione peroxidase and glutathione reductase enzymes. *Br J Clin Pharmacol.* 2004 Nov;58(5):542–47.

Lewy AJ, Lefler BJ, Emens JS, et al. The circadian basis of winter depression. *Proc Natl Acad Sci U S A.* 2006 May 9;103(19):7414–19.

Lu WZ, Gwee KA, Moochhalla S, et al. Melatonin improves bowel symptoms in female patients with irritable bowel syndrome: a double-blind placebo-controlled study. *Aliment Pharmacol Ther.* 2005 Nov 15;22(10):927–34.

Peres MF, Zukerman E, da Cunha Tanuri F, et al. Melatonin, 3 mg, is effective for migraine prevention. *Neurology.* 2004 Aug 24;63(4):757.

Samarkandi A, Naguib M, Riad W, et al. Melatonin vs. midazolam premedication in children: a double-blind, placebo-controlled study. *Eur J Anaesthesiol.* 2005 Mar;22(3):189–96.

Shamir E, Barak Y, Shalman I, et al. Melatonin treatment for tardive dyskinesia: a double-blind, placebo- controlled, crossover study. *Arch Gen Psychiatry.* 2001;58(11):1049–52.

Shamir EZ, Barak Y, Shalman I, et al. Melatonin treatment for tardive dyskinesia: a double-blind, placebo-controlled, cross-over study. Annual Meeting of the American Psychiatric Association, May 5–10 2001.

Weiss MD, Wasdell MB, Bomben MM, et al. Sleep hygiene and melatonin treatment for children and adolescents with ADHD and initial insomnia. *J Am Acad Child Adolesc Psychiatry.* 2006 May;45(5):512–19.

Zemlan FP, Mulchahey JJ, Scharf MB, et al. The efficacy and safety of the melatonin agonist beta-methyl-6-chloromelatonin in primary insomnia: a randomized, placebo-controlled, crossover clinical trial. *J Clin Psychiatry.* 2005 Mar;66(3):384–90.

Section 40.2

Valerian

Excerpted from "Valerian," Office of Dietary Supplements,
National Institutes of Health, January 16, 2008.

What is valerian?

Valerian (*Valeriana officinalis*), a member of the Valerianaceae family,
is a perennial plant native to Europe and Asia and naturalized in North
America.[1] It has a distinctive odor that many find unpleasant.[2,3] Other
names include setwall (English), *Valerianae radix* (Latin), *Baldrianwur-
zel* (German), and *phu* (Greek). The genus *Valerian* includes over 250
species, but *V. officinalis* is the species most often used in the United
States and Europe and is the only species discussed in this section.[3,4]

What are common valerian preparations?

Preparations of valerian marketed as dietary supplements are made
from its roots, rhizomes (underground stems), and stolons (horizontal
stems). Dried roots are prepared as teas or tinctures, and dried plant materials and extracts are put into capsules or incorporated into tablets.[5]

There is no scientific agreement as to the active constituents of
valerian, and its activity may result from interactions among multiple
constituents rather than any one compound or class of compounds.[6]
The content of volatile oils, including valerenic acids; the less volatile
sesquiterpenes; or the valepotriates (esters of short-chain fatty acids) is
sometimes used to standardize valerian extracts. As with most herbal
preparations, many other compounds are also present.

Valerian is sometimes combined with other botanicals.[5] Because
this section focuses on valerian as a single ingredient, only clinical
studies evaluating valerian as a single agent are included.

What are the historical uses of valerian?

Valerian has been used as a medicinal herb since at least the time
of ancient Greece and Rome. Its therapeutic uses were described by
Hippocrates, and in the second century, Galen prescribed valerian for

insomnia.[5,7] In the sixteenth century, it was used to treat nervousness, trembling, headaches, and heart palpitations.[8] In the mid-nineteenth century, valerian was considered a stimulant that caused some of the same complaints it is thought to treat and was generally held in low esteem as a medicinal herb.[2] During World War II, it was used in England to relieve the stress of air raids.[9]

In addition to sleep disorders, valerian has been used for gastrointestinal spasms and distress, epileptic seizures, and attention deficit hyperactivity disorder. However, scientific evidence is not sufficient to support the use of valerian for these conditions.[10]

What clinical studies have been done on valerian and sleep disorders?

In a systematic review of the scientific literature, nine randomized, placebo-controlled, double-blind clinical trials of valerian and sleep disorders were identified and evaluated for evidence of efficacy of valerian as a treatment for insomnia.[11] Reviewers rated the studies with a standard scoring system to quantify the likelihood of bias inherent in the study design.[12] Although all nine trials had flaws, three earned the highest rating (5 on a scale of 1 to 5) and are described below. Unlike the six lower-rated studies, these three studies described the randomization procedure and blinding method that were used and reported rates of participant withdrawal.

The first study used a repeated-measures design; 128 volunteers were given 400 mg of an aqueous extract of valerian, a commercial preparation containing 60 mg valerian and 30 mg hops, and a placebo.[13] Participants took each one of the three preparations three times in random order on nine nonconsecutive nights and filled out a questionnaire the morning after each treatment. Compared with the placebo, the valerian extract resulted in a statistically significant subjective improvement in time required to fall asleep (more or less difficult than usual), sleep quality (better or worse than usual), and number of nighttime awakenings (more or less than usual).This result was more pronounced in a subgroup of 61 participants who identified themselves as poor sleepers on a questionnaire administered at the beginning of the study. The commercial preparation did not produce a statistically significant improvement in these three measures. The clinical significance of the use of valerian for insomnia cannot be determined from the results of this study because having insomnia was not a requirement for participation. In addition, the study had a participant withdrawal rate of 22.9 percent, which may have influenced the results.

In the second study, eight volunteers with mild insomnia (usually had problems falling asleep) were evaluated for the effect of valerian on sleep latency (defined as the first five-minute period without movement).[14] Results were based on nighttime motion measured by activity meters worn on the wrist and on responses to questionnaires about sleep quality, latency, depth, and morning sleepiness filled out the morning after each treatment. The test samples were 450 or 900 mg of an aqueous valerian extract and a placebo. Each volunteer was randomly assigned to receive one test sample each night, Monday through Thursday, for three weeks for a total of twelve nights of evaluation. The 450-mg test sample of valerian extract reduced average sleep latency from about sixteen to nine minutes, which is similar to the activity of prescription benzodiazepine medication (used as a sedative or tranquilizer). No statistically significant shortening of sleep latency was seen with the 900-mg test sample. Evaluation of the questionnaires showed a statistically significant improvement in subjectively measured sleep. On a 9-point scale, participants rated sleep latency as 4.3 after the 450-mg test sample and 4.9 after the placebo. The 900-mg test sample increased the sleep improvement but participants noted an increase in sleepiness the next morning. Although statistically significant, this seven-minute reduction in sleep latency and the improvement in subjective sleep rating are probably not clinically significant. The small sample size makes it difficult to generalize the results to a broader population.

The third study examined longer-term effects in 121 participants with documented nonorganic insomnia.[15] Participants received either 600 mg of a standardized commercial preparation of dried valerian root (LI 156, Sedonium®) or placebo for twenty-eight days. Several assessment tools were used to evaluate the effectiveness and tolerance of the interventions, including questionnaires on therapeutic effect (given on days 14 and 28), change in sleep patterns (given on day 28), and changes in sleep quality and well-being (given on days 0, 14, and 28). After twenty-eight days, the group receiving the valerian extract showed a decrease in insomnia symptoms on all the assessment tools compared with the placebo group. The differences in improvement between valerian and placebo increased between the assessments done on days 14 and 28.

The reviewers concluded that these nine studies are not sufficient for determining the effectiveness of valerian to treat sleep disorders.[11] For example, none of the studies checked the success of the blinding, none calculated the sample size necessary for seeing a statistical effect, only one partially controlled pre-bedtime variables,[15] and only one validated outcome measures.[13]

Two other randomized, controlled trials published after the systematic review described above[11] are presented below.

In a randomized, double-blind study, seventy-five participants with documented nonorganic insomnia were randomly assigned to receive 600 mg of a standardized commercial valerian extract (LI 156) or 10 mg oxazepam (a benzodiazepine medication) for twenty-eight days.[16] Assessment tools used to evaluate the effectiveness and tolerance of the interventions included validated sleep, mood scale, and anxiety questionnaires as well as sleep rating by a physician (on days 0, 14, and 28). Treatment result was determined via a four-step rating scale at the end of the study (day 28). Both groups had the same improvement in sleep quality but the valerian group reported fewer side effects than did the oxazepam group. However, this study was designed to show superiority, if any, of valerian over oxazepam and its results cannot be used to show equivalence.

In a randomized, double-blind, placebo-controlled crossover study, researchers evaluated sleep parameters with polysomnographic techniques that monitored sleep stages, sleep latency, and total sleep time to objectively measure sleep quality and stages.[17] Questionnaires were used for subjective measurement of sleep parameters. Sixteen participants with medically documented nonorganic insomnia were randomly assigned to receive either a single dose and a fourteen-day administration of 600 mg of a standardized commercial preparation of valerian (LI 156) or placebo. Valerian had no effect on any of the fifteen objective or subjective measurements except for a decrease in slow-wave sleep onset (13.5 minutes) compared with placebo (21.3 minutes). During slow-wave sleep, arousability, skeletal muscle tone, heart rate, blood pressure, and respiratory frequency decreased. Increased time spent in slow-wave sleep may decrease insomnia symptoms. However, because all but one of the fifteen endpoints showed no difference between placebo and valerian, the possibility that the single endpoint showing a difference was the result of chance must be considered. The valerian group reported fewer adverse events than did the placebo group.

Although the results of some studies suggest that valerian may be useful for insomnia and other sleep disorders, results of other studies do not. Interpretation of these studies is complicated by the fact the studies had small sample sizes, used different amounts and sources of valerian, measured different outcomes, or did not consider potential bias resulting from high participant withdrawal rates. Overall, the evidence from these trials for the sleep-promoting effects of valerian is inconclusive.

How does valerian work?

Many chemical constituents of valerian have been identified, but it is not known which may be responsible for its sleep-promoting effects in animals and in in vitro studies. It is likely that there is no single active compound and that valerian's effects result from multiple constituents acting independently or synergistically.[18,19]

Two categories of constituents have been proposed as the major source of valerian's sedative effects. The first category comprises the major constituents of its volatile oil including valerenic acid and its derivatives, which have demonstrated sedative properties in animal studies.[6,20] However, valerian extracts with very little of these components also have sedative properties, making it probable that other components are responsible for these effects or that multiple constituents contribute to them.[21] The second category comprises the iridoids, which include the valepotriates. Valepotriates and their derivatives are active as sedatives in vivo but are unstable and break down during storage or in an aqueous environment, making their activity difficult to assess.[6,20,22]

A possible mechanism by which a valerian extract may cause sedation is by increasing the amount of gamma aminobutyric acid (GABA, an inhibitory neurotransmitter) available in the synaptic cleft. Results from an in vitro study using synaptosomes suggest that a valerian extract may cause GABA to be released from brain nerve endings and then block GABA from being taken back into nerve cells.[23] In addition, valerenic acid inhibits an enzyme that destroys GABA.[24] Valerian extracts contain GABA in quantities sufficient to cause a sedative effect, but whether GABA can cross the blood-brain barrier to contribute to valerian's sedative effects is not known. Glutamine is present in aqueous but not in alcohol extracts and may cross the blood-brain barrier and be converted to GABA.[25] Levels of these constituents vary significantly among plants depending on when the plants are harvested, resulting in marked variability in the amounts found in valerian preparations.[26]

What is the regulatory status of valerian in the United States?

In the United States, valerian is sold as a dietary supplement, and dietary supplements are regulated as foods, not drugs. Therefore, premarket evaluation and approval by the Food and Drug Administration are not required unless claims are made for specific disease prevention or treatment. Because dietary supplements are not always tested for manufacturing consistency, the composition may vary considerably between manufacturing lots.

Can valerian be harmful?

Few adverse events attributable to valerian have been reported for clinical study participants. Headaches, dizziness, pruritus, and gastrointestinal disturbances are the most common effects reported in clinical trials but similar effects were also reported for the placebo.[14–17] In one study an increase in sleepiness was noted the morning after 900 mg of valerian was taken.[14] Investigators from another study concluded that 600 mg of valerian (LI 156) did not have a clinically significant effect on reaction time, alertness, and concentration the morning after ingestion.[27] Several case reports described adverse effects, but in one case where suicide was attempted with a massive overdose it is not possible to clearly attribute the symptoms to valerian.[28–31]

Valepotriates, which are a component of valerian but are not necessarily present in commercial preparations, had cytotoxic activity in vitro but were not carcinogenic in animal studies.[32–35]

Who should not take valerian?

- Women who are pregnant or nursing should not take valerian without medical advice because the possible risks to the fetus or infant have not been evaluated.[36]

- Children younger than three years old should not take valerian because the possible risks to children of this age have not been evaluated.[36]

- Individuals taking valerian should be aware of the theoretical possibility of additive sedative effects from alcohol or sedative drugs, such as barbiturates and benzodiazepines.[10,37,38]

Does valerian interact with any drugs or affect laboratory tests?

Although valerian has not been reported to interact with any drugs or to influence laboratory tests, this has not been rigorously studied.[5,10,36]

References

1. Wichtl M, ed.: Valerianae radix. In: Bisset NG, trans-ed. *Herbal Drugs and Phytopharmaceuticals: A Handbook for Practice on a Scientific Basis.* Boca Raton, FL: CRC Press, 1994: 513–16.

2. Pereira J: Valeriana officinalis: common valerian. In: Carson J, ed. *The Elements of Materia Medica and Therapeutics.* 3rd ed. Philadelphia: Blanchard and Lea, 1854: 609–16.

3. Schulz V, Hansel R, Tyler VE: Valerian. In: *Rational Phytotherapy*. 3rd ed. Berlin: Springer, 1998: 73–81.

4. Davidson JRT, Connor KM: Valerian. In: *Herbs for the Mind: Depression, Stress, Memory Loss, and Insomnia*. New York: Guilford Press, 2000: 214–33.

5. Blumenthal M, Goldberg A, Brinckmann J, eds.: Valerian root. In: *Herbal Medicine: Expanded Commission E Monographs*. Newton, MA: Integrative Medicine Communications, 2000: 394–400.

6. Hendriks H, Bos R, Allersma DP, Malingre M, Koster AS: Pharmacological screening of valerenal and some other components of essential oil of Valeriana officinalis. *Planta Medica* 42: 62–68, 1981

7. Turner W: Of Valerianae. In: Chapman GTL, McCombie F, Wesencraft A, eds. *A New Herbal, Parts II and III*. Cambridge: Cambridge University Press, 1995: 464–66, 499–500, 764–65. [Republication of parts II and III of *A New Herbal*, by William Turner, originally published in 1562 and 1568, respectively.]

8. Culpeper N: Garden valerian. In: *Culpeper's Complete Herbal*. New York: W. Foulsham, 1994: 295–97. [Republication of *The English Physician*, by Nicholas Culpeper, originally published in 1652.]

9. Grieve M: Valerian. In: *A Modern Herbal*. New York: Hafner Press, 1974: 824–30.

10. Jellin JM, Gregory P, Batz F, et al.: Valerian In: *Pharmacist's Letter/Prescriber's Letter Natural Medicines Comprehensive Database*. 3rd ed. Stockton, CA: Therapeutic Research Faculty, 2000: 1052–54.

11. Stevinson C, Ernst E: Valerian for insomnia: a systematic review of randomized clinical trials. *Sleep Medicine* 1: 91–99, 2000.

12. Jadad AR, Moore RA, Carroll D, et al.: Assessing the quality of reports of randomized clinical trials: is blinding necessary? *Controlled Clinical Trials* 17: 1–12, 1996.

13. Leathwood PD, Chauffard F, Heck E, Munoz-Box R: Aqueous extract of valerian root (Valeriana officinalis L.) improves sleep quality in man. *Pharmacology, Biochemistry and Behavior* 17: 65–71, 1982.

14. Leathwood PD, Chauffard F: Aqueous extract of valerian reduces latency to fall asleep in man. *Planta Medica* 2: 144–48, 1985.

15. Vorbach EU, Gortelmeyer R, Bruning J: Treatment of insomnia: effectiveness and tolerance of a valerian extract [in German]. *Psychopharmakotherapie* 3: 109–15, 1996.

16. Dorn M: Valerian versus oxazepam: efficacy and tolerability in nonorganic and nonpsychiatric insomniacs: a randomized, double-blind, clinical comparative study [in German]. *Forschende Komplementärmedizin und Klassische Naturheilkunde* 7: 79–84, 2000.

17. Donath F, Quispe S, Diefenbach K, Maurer A, Fietze I, Roots I: Critical evaluation of the effect of valerian extract on sleep structure and sleep quality. *Pharmacopsychiatry* 33: 47–53, 2000.

18. Russo EB: Valerian. In: *Handbook of Psychotropic Herbs: A Scientific Analysis of Herbal Remedies in Psychiatric Conditions.* Binghamton, NY: Haworth Press, 2001: 95–106.

19. Houghton PJ: The scientific basis for the reputed activity of valerian. *Journal of Pharmacy and Pharmacology* 51: 505–12, 1999.

20. Hendriks H, Bos R, Woerdenbag HJ, Koster AS. Central nervous depressant activity of valerenic acid in the mouse. *Planta Medica* 1: 28–31, 1985.

21. Krieglstein VJ, Grusla D. Central depressing components in Valerian: Valepotriates, valeric acid, valerone, and essential oil are inactive, however [in German]. *Deutsche Apotheker Zeitung* 128:2041–46, 1988.

22. Bos R, Woerdenbag HJ, Hendriks H, et al.: Analytical aspects of phytotherapeutic valerian preparations. *Phytochemical Analysis* 7: 143–51, 1996.

23. Santos MS, Ferreira F, Cunha AP, Carvalho AP, Macedo T: An aqueous extract of valerian influences the transport of GABA in synaptosomes. *Planta Medica* 60: 278–79, 1994.

24. Morazzoni P, Bombardelli E: Valeriana officinalis: traditional use and recent evaluation of activity. *Fitoterapia* 66: 99–112, 1995.

25. Cavadas C, Araujo I, Cotrim MD, et al.: In vitro study on the interaction of Valeriana officinalis L. extracts and their amino acids on GABAA receptor in rat brain. *Arzneimittel-Forschung Drug Research* 45: 753–55, 1995.

26. Bos R, Woerdenbag HJ, van Putten FMS, Hendriks H, Scheffer JJC: Seasonal variation of the essential oil, valerenic acid and derivatives, and valepotriates in Valeriana officinalis roots and rhizomes, and the selection of plants suitable for phytomedicines. *Planta Medica* 64:143–47, 1998.

27. Kuhlmann J, Berger W, Podzuweit H, Schmidt U: The influence of valerian treatment on "reaction time, alertness and concentration" in volunteers. *Pharmacopsychiatry* 32: 235–41, 1999.

28. MacGregor FB, Abernethy VE, Dahabra S, Cobden I, Hayes PC: Hepatotoxicity of herbal remedies. *British Medical Journal* 299: 1156–57, 1989.

29. Mullins ME, Horowitz BZ: The case of the salad shooters: intravenous injection of wild lettuce extract. *Veterinary and Human Toxicology* 40: 290–91, 1998.

30. Garges HP, Varia I, Doraiswamy PM: Cardiac complications and delirium associated with valerian root withdrawal. *Journal of the American Medical Association* 280: 1566–67, 1998.

31. Willey LB, Mady SP, Cobaugh DJ, Wax PM: Valerian overdose: a case report. *Veterinary and Human Toxicology* 37: 364–65, 1995.

32. Bounthanh, C, Bergmann C, Beck JP, Haag-Berrurier M, Anton R. Valepotriates, a new class of cytotoxic and antitumor agents. *Planta Medica* 41: 21–28, 1981.

33. Bounthanh, C, Richert L, Beck JP, Haag-Berrurier M, Anton R: The action of valepotriates on the synthesis of DNA and proteins of cultured hepatoma cells. *Journal of Medicinal Plant Research* 49: 138–42, 1983.

34. Tufik S, Fuhita K, Seabra ML, Lobo LL: Effects of a prolonged administration of valepotriates in rats on the mothers and their offspring. *Journal of Ethnopharmacology* 41: 39–44, 1996.

35. Bos R, Hendriks H, Scheffer JJC, Woerdenbag HJ: Cytotoxic potential of valerian constituents and valerian tinctures. *Phytomedicine* 5: 219–25, 1998.

36. European Scientific Cooperative on Phytotherapy: Valerianae radix: valerian root. In: *Monographs on the Medicinal Uses of Plant Drugs*. Exeter, UK: ESCOP, 1997: 1–10.

37. Rotblatt M, Ziment I. Valerian (Valeriana officinalis). In: *Evidence-Based Herbal Medicine*. Philadelphia: Hanley & Belfus, Inc., 2002: 355–59.

38. Givens M, Cupp MJ: Valerian. In: Cupps MJ, ed. *Toxicology and Clinical Pharmacology of Herbal Products*. Totowa, NJ: Humana Press, 2000: 53–66.

Section 40.3

Complementary and Alternative Medicine

Excerpted from "Sleep Disorders and CAM: At a Glance,"
National Center for Complementary and Alternative Medicine,
National Institutes of Health, July 2009.

Chronic, long-term sleep disorders affect millions of Americans each year. These disorders and the sleep deprivation they cause can interfere with work, driving, social activities, and overall quality of life, and can have serious health implications. Sleep disorders account for an estimated $16 billion in medical costs each year, plus indirect costs due to lost productivity and other factors.

Complementary and Alternative Medicine (CAM) Use for Insomnia

In 2002 and 2007, the National Health Interview Survey (NHIS) asked participants about CAM use. In 2002, 2.2 percent of respondents who used some form of CAM in the past twelve months said they used it for insomnia or trouble sleeping; in 2007, that figure was 1.4 percent.

An analysis of data from the 2002 NHIS found that 17.4 percent of all participants said they regularly had insomnia or trouble sleeping in the past twelve months; most who reported insomnia also reported other medical/psychiatric conditions, such as anxiety or depression, chronic heart failure, diabetes, hypertension, and obesity. Among participants with insomnia, 4.5 percent (which translates to a total of 1.6 million U.S. adults) used some form of CAM to treat their condition—primarily biological/herbal therapies (64.8 percent) or mind-body/relaxation therapies (39.1 percent). Most found these therapies helpful.

Among the CAM approaches that people use for insomnia are the following:

- Herbs, including aromatherapy, chamomile tea, and herbal supplements such as valerian and various "sleep formula" products

- Melatonin and related dietary supplements

- Other CAM modalities, such as acupuncture, music therapy, and relaxation techniques

What the Science Says about CAM and Insomnia

Research on CAM and insomnia has produced promising results for some CAM therapies. However, evidence of effectiveness is still limited for most therapies, and additional research is needed. This section summarizes what is known about some of the CAM approaches that people use for insomnia.

Herbs

Aromatherapy using essential oils from herbs such as lavender or chamomile is a popular sleep aid; preliminary research suggests some sleep-inducing effects, but more studies are needed.

The herb chamomile is commonly used as a bedtime tea, but scientific evidence of its effectiveness for insomnia is lacking.

The herb kava has been used for insomnia, but there is no evidence of its efficacy. The U.S. Food and Drug Administration has issued a warning that kava supplements have been linked to a risk of severe liver damage.

The herbal supplement valerian is one of the most popular CAM therapies for insomnia. Several studies suggest that valerian (for up to four to six weeks) can improve the quality of sleep and slightly reduce the time it takes to fall asleep. However, not all of the evidence is positive. One systematic review of the research concluded that although valerian is commonly used as a sleep aid, the scientific evidence does not support its efficacy for insomnia. Researchers have concluded that valerian appears to be safe at recommended doses for short-term use. Some "sleep formula" products combine valerian with other herbs such as hops, lavender, lemon balm, and skullcap. Although many of these other herbs have sedative properties, there is no reliable evidence that they improve insomnia or that combination products are more effective than valerian alone.

Melatonin and Related Supplements

Like valerian, melatonin supplements (melatonin is a naturally occurring hormone associated with sleep) are widely used and researched for insomnia. Although more research is still needed, studies suggest that melatonin can help elderly people with insomnia fall asleep faster, and may also be beneficial for other people with insomnia; however, effects are generally small, with larger effects observed in patients whose sleep problems are caused by a circadian rhythm abnormality (disruption of the body's internal "clock"). Studies indicate that melatonin also appears to be safe at recommended doses for short-term use.

Dietary supplements containing melatonin "precursors"—L-tryptophan and 5-HTP—are also used as sleep aids. (The amino acid L-tryptophan is converted to 5-HTP, which is converted to serotonin and then melatonin.) However, these supplements have not been proven effective in treating insomnia, and there are concerns that they may be linked to eosinophilia-myalgia syndrome (EMS), a complex and debilitating systemic condition with multiple symptoms including severe muscle pain.

Other CAM Approaches

Traditional Chinese medicine commonly uses acupuncture to treat insomnia. A review of available studies found some evidence of benefits, but many studies had design flaws that make it difficult to draw firm conclusions.

There is scientific evidence that music therapy can have sleep benefits for older adults and children.

Studies suggest that relaxation techniques may help people with insomnia, although the effects appear to be short-lived. Cognitive forms of relaxation (such as meditation) have had slightly better results than somatic forms (such as progressive muscle relaxation). Preliminary studies suggest that yoga may also improve sleep quality. In addition, when these forms of relaxation are combined with other components of cognitive-behavioral therapy (e.g., sleep restriction and stimulus control), lasting improvements in sleep have been observed. Again, additional research is needed in these areas.

If You Are Considering CAM for Sleep Problems

Talk to your healthcare providers. Tell them about the therapy you are considering and ask any questions you may have. They may know about the therapy and be able to advise you on its safety, use, and likely effectiveness in relieving your sleep problems. Because trouble sleeping can be an indication of a more serious condition, it is especially important to discuss any sleep-related symptoms (such as snoring or daytime fatigue) with your healthcare providers before trying a CAM approach.

Be cautious about using any sleep product—prescription medications, over-the-counter drugs, or CAM dietary supplements. Find out about potential side effects and the effects of long-term use and use of more than one product at a time.

If you are considering herbal or other dietary supplements, keep in mind that "natural" does not always mean safe. For example, the herbs comfrey and kava can cause serious harm to the liver. Also, a manufacturer's use of the term "standardized" (or "verified" or "certified") does not necessarily guarantee product quality or consistency. Herbal or other dietary supplements can act in the same way as drugs. They can cause medical problems if not used correctly, and some may interact with medications you are already taking. The healthcare providers you see about your sleep problems can advise you. It is especially important to consult your healthcare provider if you are pregnant or nursing a child, or if you are considering giving a child a dietary supplement.

If you are considering a practitioner-provided CAM therapy such as acupuncture, check with your insurer to see if the services will be covered, and ask a trusted source (such as your doctor or a nearby hospital or medical school) to recommend a practitioner.

Tell your health care providers about any complementary and alternative practices you use. Give them a full picture of what you do to manage your health. This will help ensure coordinated and safe care.

Chapter 41

Cognitive Behavioral Therapy for Sleep Disorders

Sleep is a fundamental function of the body, and critically important to neurologic health. However, in addition to its important biological purposes, sleep is also very much a behavior. We structure our daily schedules and our social activities around our sleep time. As children, we are tucked into bed by our parents, and even as adults, most of us have sleep rituals of one sort or another. Therefore, it should not come as a surprise that interventions to change behaviors are very relevant to sleep.

As discussed in other sections of this book, there are a variety of medical disorders that can affect sleep. Behavioral sleep problems are probably at least as common. Cognitive behavioral therapy (CBT) is frequently the cornerstone of treatment for these issues.

What is cognitive behavioral therapy?

Cognitive behavioral therapy is a widely used form of psychological therapy, aimed at correcting problem behaviors. It is used to treat a number of disorders, including depression, anxiety, obsessive-compulsive disorder, and eating disorders. It can also be helpful in the treatment of some sleep disorders.

CBT is based on the idea that many psychological problems are the result of deeply ingrained mental habits. These habits reinforce and perpetuate problematic behaviors. Identifying and changing these habits can lead to improvement.

"Cognitive Behavioral Therapy and Sleep," by David A. Cooke, MD, FACP, © 2010 Omnigraphics.

How does cognitive behavioral therapy work?

CBT involves working with a therapist trained in the technique. Most often, therapists are psychologists or social workers, but psychiatrists, clergy, and other professionals may also learn to perform CBT. CBT may be done one-on-one, but CBT group sessions are also common. Computer software designed to promote CBT techniques have also been used for therapy.

The first stage of CBT is learning to recognize the internal mental processes that are unconscious for most people. Over a lifetime, people develop automatic ways of responding to outside events and internal thoughts, and these responses may vary from person to person.

For example, being complimented may lead one person to react with the thought "I have done well," while another may believe "I don't deserve the compliment, and that person is just being polite." These differences in responses may have divergent results. The first person may develop appropriate self-esteem, while the other may be very self-critical.

A therapist helps the patient identify thought patterns and "self-talk," and to consider how this may be coloring their outlook and reactions. This may take some time, as the patterns feel very "natural" to the patient. With practice, however, the participant can begin to identify their internal thoughts during their daily interactions.

Once a level of awareness has developed, the therapist guides the patient toward developing new responses and mental habits. For example, the patient who does not believe praise is warranted may be encouraged to tell him or herself "the compliment was genuine." With repetition and practice over time, this self-talk will become easier and seem less forced. Eventually, it no longer requires conscious effort, and becomes automatic.

With CBT-guided changes in mental responses, the problem frequently improves. The hypercritical, self-deprecating person may start to see him- or herself in a more positive light, and previously limiting depression may lift.

Unlike traditional psychoanalytic therapy, CBT is not usually performed long term. Most CBT is targeted on specific behaviors, and can usually be accomplished within a few months to a year.

How does cognitive behavioral therapy help people with sleep problems?

Mental habits can also lead to sleep disorders. As discussed elsewhere in this book, poor sleep hygiene such as irregular bedtimes and watching TV in bed may interfere with preparing for sleep. Many people ruminate about their problems while lying in bed, which can lead to anxiety and difficulty falling asleep. Others may become upset when they do not fall asleep quickly, and become anxious or frustrated, which prevents them from sleeping. Some people have very fixed ideas about how, when, and how long a person should sleep. Failing to meet their expectations can cause insomnia.

A therapist performing CBT for sleep problems will ask many questions about the patient's bedtimes, wake times, routines before bed, and what happens when they attempt to fall asleep. Often, the therapist will ask the participant to keep written logs of their sleep, night by night. The therapist will identify elements that are interfering with good sleep and discuss them with the patient, aiming to build understanding of why they are counterproductive.

The therapist may recommend specific rules or schedules to follow. For example, they may advise that no activities other than sleep or sex may be done in bed. Other common measures include keeping regular sleep and wake times, and not laying awake in bed for more than fifteen minutes at a time. Initially restricting the number of hours slept is also sometimes useful.

In addition to specific behaviors and sleep hygiene, a CBT therapist will explore the patient's thoughts and beliefs regarding sleep. The therapist will also assess for anxiety and mood disorders, which frequently impact upon sleep, and may address these issues as well.

Relaxation techniques are frequently utilized in CBT for sleep disorders. Many people with insomnia have difficulty relaxing sufficiently for good sleep. Deep breathing, progressive muscle relaxation, and use of positive mental imagery can help in achieving a state more conducive to falling asleep. Some therapists will provide audio recordings for the participant to listen to when trying to fall asleep, which coach and reinforce these techniques. With practice, the CBT participant learns to incorporate relaxation into their bedtime, and better sleep usually results.

Which sleep disorders can be treated with cognitive behavioral therapy?

Generally, any sleep disorder where psychophysiologic insomnia or a mood disorder is felt to be a factor is a candidate for treatment with CBT.

Psychophysiologic insomnia is a broad term that encompasses sleep problems related to poor sleep behaviors and conditioned emotional responses. Examples include the night shift worker who tries to remain awake during the day, or the anxious individual who lays awake for hours, frustrated by his or her inability to fall asleep. These types of sleep disorders frequently respond well to CBT, and typically have better outcomes than treatment with sleeping medications.

It is quite common for more than one sleep disorder to exist in the same individual. Psychophysiologic insomnia often accompanies other "medical" sleep disorders such as sleep apnea, restless leg syndrome, and pain due to arthritis or other conditions. Therefore, the range of patients who may benefit from CBT for sleep disorders is quite broad.

How do I find a CBT therapist?

Some CBT therapists treat sleep disorders as part of a broader mental health practice. However, many therapists who treat sleep disorders with CBT are specialized and limit their practices to these disorders. Most sleep disorder clinics either have CBT practitioners on staff, or have close working relationships with therapists in the area. Therefore, inquiring at a sleep disorders clinic is often the best way to find an appropriate practitioner.

The National Association of Cognitive Behavioral Therapists issues certifications in the technique, and maintains a national database of practitioners certified by the organization. You can search for therapists on their website, www.nacbt.org. The Association For Behavioral and Cognitive Therapies also provides certifications, and has a searchable directory at www.abct.org.

Note

The author acknowledges the assistance of Rochelle L. Cooke, MSW, in the preparation of this article.

Chapter 42

Devices and Appliances for the Treatment of Sleep Disorders

Chapter Contents

Section 42.1

Continuous Positive Airway Pressure (CPAP)

"CPAP," National Heart Lung and Blood Institute, National
Institutes of Health, March 2009.

What Is CPAP?

CPAP, or continuous positive airway pressure, is a treatment that
uses mild air pressure to keep your airways open while you sleep.
CPAP is used for people who have breathing problems, such as sleep
apnea.

This treatment is done using a CPAP machine. CPAP machines
have three main parts:

- A mask or other device that fits over your nose or your nose and
  mouth. Straps keep the mask in place while you're wearing it.

- A tube that connects the mask to the machine's motor.

- A motor that blows air into the tube.

Some CPAP machines have other features as well, such as heated
humidifiers. CPAP machines are small, lightweight, and fairly quiet.
The noise that they make is soft and rhythmic.

Overview

CPAP is the most effective treatment for obstructive sleep apnea.
Sleep apnea is a common disorder in which you have pauses in breathing or shallow breaths while you sleep. When this happens, not enough
air reaches your lungs.

In obstructive sleep apnea, your airways collapse or are blocked
during sleep. The blockage may cause shallow breathing or breathing pauses. When you try to breathe, any air that squeezes past the
blockage can cause loud snoring. Your snoring may wake other people
in the house.

The mild pressure from CPAP can prevent your airway from collapsing or becoming blocked.

If your doctor prescribes CPAP, you will work with someone from a home equipment provider (sometimes called durable medical equipment, or DME) to select a CPAP machine.

Your doctor will work with you to make sure the settings that he or she prescribes for your CPAP machine are correct. He or she may recommend an overnight sleep study to find the correct settings for you. Your doctor will want to make sure the air pressure from the machine is just enough to keep your airways open while you sleep.

There are many different kinds of CPAP machines and masks. Be sure to tell your doctor if you're not happy with the type you're using. He or she may suggest switching to a different kind that may work better for you.

Outlook

CPAP has many benefits. It can do the following things:

• Keep your airways open while you sleep

• Correct snoring so others in your household can sleep

• Improve the quality of your sleep

• Relieve symptoms of sleep apnea, such as excessive daytime sleepiness

• Decrease or prevent high blood pressure

Many people who use CPAP report feeling better once they begin treatment. They feel more attentive and better able to work during the day. They also report fewer complaints from bed partners about snoring and sleep disruption.

Who Needs CPAP?

You may need CPAP if you have obstructive sleep apnea. CPAP is often the best treatment for adults who have this condition.

Children also can have obstructive sleep apnea. The most common treatment for children is surgery to remove the tonsils and adenoids. If symptoms don't improve after surgery, or if the condition is severe, CPAP may be an option.

If you have sleep apnea symptoms, your doctor may recommend an overnight sleep study. A sleep study measures how much and how well you sleep. It also can show whether you have sleep problems and how severe they are.

Your doctor will likely refer you to a sleep specialist for the sleep study. Sleep specialists are doctors who diagnose and treat people who have sleep problems.

A special type of CPAP device is used to treat breathing disorders that are similar to sleep apnea, such as chronic hypoventilation or central sleep apnea. In these conditions, the airways aren't blocked. However, the brain may not send the signals needed for breathing to occur properly. This causes breaths that are too shallow or slow to meet your body's needs.

In central sleep apnea, you may stop breathing for brief periods. This disorder can occur alone or with obstructive sleep apnea. Only a sleep study can find out what type of sleep apnea you have and how severe it is.

In addition to CPAP, there are other positive airway pressure devices. If you don't feel that CPAP is working for you, talk to your sleep specialist about other possible options.

What to Expect Before Using CPAP

Before your sleep specialist prescribes CPAP, you'll likely have a sleep study called a polysomnogram, or PSG.

A PSG usually is done while you stay overnight at a sleep center. This study records brain activity, eye movements, heart rate, blood pressure, and other important data while you sleep.

What to Expect During a Polysomnogram

Your sleep specialist may suggest a split-night sleep study. During the first half of the night, your sleep will be checked without a CPAP machine. This will show whether you have sleep apnea and how severe it is.

If the PSG shows that you have sleep apnea, you may use a CPAP machine during the second half of the split-night study. A technician will help you select a CPAP mask that fits and is comfortable.

While you sleep, the technician checks the amount of oxygen in your blood and whether your airways stay open. He or she adjusts the flow of air through the mask to find the setting that's right for you. This process is called CPAP titration.

In some cases, this isn't done all in the same night. Some people need to go back to the sleep center for the CPAP titration study. Your sleep specialist will decide which type of study is best for you and leave instructions with the technician.

What to Expect After a Polysomnogram

Your sleep specialist will review the results from your sleep study. If CPAP will benefit you, he or she will prescribe the type of CPAP machine and the correct settings for you.

Most health insurance companies now cover CPAP treatment. You may want to contact your health insurance provider to learn more about this coverage.

Your sleep specialist may be able to refer you to a local home equipment provider. The home equipment provider will use your prescription to set up your CPAP machine. Ask your sleep specialist to recommend a home equipment provider that has a lot of experience with CPAP.

It's important to continue to work with your sleep specialist as you adjust to CPAP treatment. Talk to him or her about how to handle follow-up questions. Your sleep specialist can answer some questions, but your home equipment provider may need to address others.

Selecting a CPAP Machine and Mask

CPAP units come with many features designed to improve fit and comfort. Your home equipment provider will help you select a machine based on your prescription and the features that meet your needs.

You may be able to use the CPAP unit for a trial period to make sure you're happy with your choice.

There are many types of CPAP masks. The fit of your mask is important, not only for comfort, but also to keep air from leaking out. A mask that fits will help maintain proper air pressure and keep your airways open.

CPAP masks come in different shapes, sizes, and materials. Some fit over your nose and mouth; others cover only your nose. Some masks can be worn with eyeglasses. If you need oxygen, masks are available that have room for an oxygen tube.

Nasal pillows may be used instead of a mask. Nasal pillows are small, flexible, mushroom-shaped cones that fit into each nostril.

Let your home equipment provider know whether your sleep on your back, side, or stomach. Different types of plastic tubing connect the mask to the CPAP machine. Some types may make it easier for you to sleep on your side or stomach.

What to Expect While Using CPAP

CPAP is a long-term treatment. Many people have questions when they first start using CPAP.

Talk to your sleep specialist about how to handle follow-up questions. He or she can answer some questions, but your home equipment provider may need to address others. Ask your sleep specialist to recommend a home equipment provider that has a lot of experience with CPAP.

To achieve the full benefits of CPAP, use it every time you sleep—during naps and at night. Most people should use CPAP for at least 7.5 hours each night for the best results.

The CPAP Machine

It can take time to adjust to using CPAP. It may feel strange wearing a mask on your face at night or feeling the flow of air. Some people feel confined by the mask. If you feel this way, it may help to adjust to the mask slowly.

First, hold the mask up to your face for short periods during the day. Next, try wearing it with the straps for short periods. Then, add the hose.

Breathing with a machine doesn't feel natural. If your machine has a "ramp" feature, you can use it to slowly "ramp up" from a lower air pressure to the pressure that's needed to keep your airways open during sleep. Once you're comfortable using CPAP during the day, try using it at night while you sleep.

Relaxation exercises, such as progressive muscle relaxation, help some people adjust to using CPAP. Talk to your doctor about whether relaxation exercises may help you.

If you're having trouble adjusting to the mask or the CPAP machine, contact your home equipment provider. Your provider may have staff who can help you adjust. You may want to try a different mask that has fewer straps or less contact with your skin.

Follow-Up Care

Your sleep specialist may ask you to schedule a follow-up visit about a month after you begin using CPAP. He or she will want to see how well you're adjusting to treatment. After that, you may have follow-up care every six or twelve months.

Your sleep specialist may need to adjust the air pressure setting of your CPAP machine if any of the following are true:

- You gain or lose a lot of weight

- Your symptoms, such as daytime sleepiness, persist or recur

- You have another treatment for sleep apnea, such as upper airway surgery or a mouthpiece

Benefits of CPAP

CPAP has many benefits. It can do the following:

- Keep your airways open while you sleep

- Correct snoring so others in your household can sleep

- Improve the quality of your sleep

- Relieve symptoms of sleep apnea, such as excessive daytime sleepiness

- Decrease or prevent high blood pressure

With CPAP, you may fall asleep faster and wake fewer times during the night. The pauses in breathing that are typical with sleep apnea won't interrupt your sleep.

Studies also show that treatment with CPAP is linked to a decrease in reported car accidents and near accidents. Some studies have shown that CPAP improves reaction times, concentration, and memory in people who use the treatment.

Many people who use CPAP report feeling better once they begin treatment. They feel more attentive and better able to work during the day. They also report fewer complaints from bed partners about snoring and sleep disruption.

You may feel better after the first night you use CPAP. You may wake feeling refreshed, alert, and in a better mood. You also may feel less tired during the day.

However, it may take a week to a month to adjust to CPAP. Some people have trouble falling asleep when they first start using CPAP. This problem usually is short term and goes away as you adjust to the treatment.

Even if you don't notice a change right away, stick with the treatment. The benefits are worth it. Once you adjust to using CPAP, you'll sleep better.

What Are the Risks of CPAP?

CPAP is a safe, painless treatment. Side effects and other problems usually are minor and can be treated or fixed. Talk to your doctor if you're having problems using CPAP. He or she can suggest ways to handle or treat these problems.

Although these problems can be frustrating, stick with the treatment. The benefits of CPAP are worthwhile.

Side Effects

Mask allergies and skin irritation: CPAP masks may cause skin allergies or skin irritation. If this happens, try a different type of mask.

CPAP masks come in different shapes, sizes, and materials. Some have fewer straps and less contact with your face. Certain masks may irritate your skin less than others.

If you have trouble finding a mask that works for you, talk to your sleep specialist about nasal pillows. These are small, flexible, mushroom-shaped cones that fit into each nostril.

Dry mouth: Dry mouth may be due to the CPAP itself or from breathing through your mouth at night. A CPAP machine that has a heated humidifier may help relieve this side effect.

If dry mouth persists, your sleep specialist may recommend a chin strap to keep your mouth closed or a different type of mask.

Talk to your sleep specialist if dry mouth continues. It may mean that your mask is leaking air. The air may be going into your open mouth and causing dry mouth.

Congestion, runny nose, sneezing, sinusitis, and nosebleeds: Congestion, runny nose, sneezing, sinusitis, and nosebleeds can occur while using CPAP. A CPAP machine that uses a heated humidifier can help relieve these side effects. Also, make sure that your mask fits properly.

Some people find that using a saline nasal spray at bedtime prevents these side effects. If these steps don't work, talk to your sleep specialist. He or she may prescribe a steroid nasal spray.

Stomach bloating and discomfort: Stomach bloating and discomfort may be due to a problem with the air pressure setting of your CPAP machine. If you have stomach bloating and discomfort, talk to your sleep specialist. He or she may adjust the settings of your machine to relieve these side effects.

Problems with the CPAP Equipment

Mask leaks: A number of different things can cause a CPAP mask to leak. To avoid a leak, follow the instructions that come with the mask. Try washing the mask daily. Also, wash your face and use a moisturizer so your skin is moist before you put on the mask.

It may help to adjust the mask's straps. When straps are too loose or too tight, a leak may happen. You may need to select a different size or type of mask.

When a CPAP mask leaks air, you don't get the proper amount of air pressure. Also, leaks can lead to skin or eye irritation.

Very small leaks don't stop the machine from producing the correct amount of air pressure. But small leaks can cause a shrill sound that disturbs the sleep of others in the house.

Don't use tape or grease on a mask to prevent leaks unless your home equipment provider or sleep specialist advises you to.

Air pressure problems: The air pressure from CPAP makes some people feel like it's hard to exhale or like they're choking or suffocating. Some people swallow air, which may cause burping.

If you have problems with the air pressure from CPAP, it may help to use the "ramp" feature on your CPAP machine. The feature allows the machine to slowly "ramp up" from a lower air pressure to the pressure that's needed to keep your airways open during sleep.

If your machine doesn't have this feature or if it doesn't help, talk to your sleep specialist. He or she may suggest a different CPAP machine. If that doesn't work, your sleep specialist may suggest another type of positive airway pressure.

Mask removal: To get the full benefit of CPAP, you should use it every time you sleep. Some people remove the CPAP mask while they're asleep. If this happens, you may be able to solve the problem by doing the following:

- Finding a mask that fits better

- Using a CPAP machine that has a humidifier, which might make the treatment more comfortable and stop you from removing the mask

- Using a chin strap to hold the mask in place

Some CPAP machines come with an alarm that sounds if the mask comes off.

Noise: Most new CPAP machines are fairly quiet. The noise that they make is soft and rhythmic. If there's still a noise that bothers you, check the air filter to make sure the machine is working right. Your sleep specialist or home equipment provider also can check the machine for you.

If the CPAP machine is working right, but the noise still bothers you, try using earplugs or a white-noise sound machine.

Living with CPAP

CPAP is a long-term treatment. To achieve the full benefits of CPAP, use it every time you sleep—during naps and at night. Most people should use CPAP for at least 7.5 hours each night for the best results.

CPAP machines are small, lightweight, and fairly quiet. It's possible to take your machine with you when you travel.

Knowing how to maintain your CPAP machine is important. You also should see your sleep specialist for ongoing care as he or she advises.

Maintaining the CPAP Machine

It's important to properly maintain your CPAP machine. Refer to the user manual or ask your home equipment provider how to take care of the machine.

Parts of the machine need daily or routine care and cleaning. For example, if your machine has a humidifier, you will likely need to clean it daily. You also may need to replace parts of the machine after a certain amount of time.

Your home equipment provider should be able to provide replacement filters, masks, and hoses for your machine.

If you suspect a problem with your CPAP machine, call your home equipment provider. Don't try to fix it yourself. There's a small hole in most machines that lets the air that you exhale out and keeps the air supply fresh. This isn't a defect in the machine, and you shouldn't try to cover it.

Getting Ongoing Care

Many people have questions when they first start using CPAP. Talk to your sleep specialist about how to handle follow-up questions. He or she can answer some questions, but your home equipment provider may need to address others.

It's important to continue to work with your sleep specialist as you adjust to CPAP. Ask your sleep specialist to recommend a home equipment provider that has a lot of experience with CPAP.

Your sleep specialist may ask you to schedule a follow-up visit about a month after you begin using CPAP. He or she will want to see how well you're adjusting to treatment. After that, you may have follow-up care every six or twelve months.

Most CPAP machines record the amount of time you use them on a computer card. Your sleep specialist may ask you to bring the card in to see how well you're doing.

During follow-up visits, your sleep specialist may need to adjust the air pressure setting of your CPAP machine if any of the following happen:

• You gain or lose a lot of weight

- Your symptoms, such as daytime sleepiness, persist or recur

- You have another treatment for sleep apnea, such as upper airway surgery or a mouthpiece

During follow-up visits, be sure to tell your sleep specialist if you're not happy with your CPAP machine. He or she may suggest switching to a different machine that may work better for you.

Key Points

- CPAP, or continuous positive airway pressure, is a treatment that uses mild air pressure to keep your airways open while you sleep. CPAP is used for people who have breathing problems, such as sleep apnea.

- CPAP is the most effective treatment for obstructive sleep apnea. Sleep apnea is a common disorder in which you have pauses in breathing or shallow breaths while you sleep. When this happens, not enough air reaches the lungs.

- CPAP is often the best treatment for adults who have obstructive sleep apnea. Children also can have this condition. The most common treatment for children is surgery to remove the tonsils and adenoids. If symptoms don't improve after surgery, or if the condition is severe, CPAP may be an option.

- If you have sleep apnea symptoms, your doctor may recommend an overnight sleep study. A sleep study measures how much and how well you sleep. It also can show whether you have sleep problems and how severe they are. Your doctor will likely refer you to a sleep specialist for the sleep study.

- Your sleep specialist will review the results from your sleep study. If CPAP will benefit you, your sleep specialist will prescribe the type of CPAP machine and the correct settings for you. Once you have your CPAP prescription, you will work with someone from a home equipment provider to select a CPAP machine that meets your needs.

- CPAP is a long-term treatment. Many people have questions when they first start using it. Talk to your sleep specialist about how to handle follow-up questions. He or she can answer some questions, but your home equipment provider may need to address others.

- To achieve the full benefits of CPAP, use it every time you sleep—during naps and at night. Most people should use CPAP for at least 7.5 hours each night for the best results.

- CPAP has many benefits. It can do the following things:
  - Keep your airways open while you sleep
  - Correct snoring so others in your household can sleep
  - Improve the quality of your sleep
  - Relieve symptoms of sleep apnea, such as excessive daytime sleepiness
  - Decrease or prevent high blood pressure

- With CPAP, you may fall asleep faster and wake fewer times during the night. The pauses in breathing that are typical with sleep apnea won't interrupt your sleep.

- Many people who use CPAP report feeling better once they begin treatment. They feel more attentive and better able to work during the day. They also report fewer complaints from bed partners about snoring and sleep disruption.

Section 42.2

Oral Appliances for Snoring and Obstructive Sleep Apnea

Snoring and Obstructive Sleep Apnea

Snoring is the sound of partially obstructed breathing during sleep. While snoring can be harmless, it can also be the sign of a more serious medical condition known as obstructive sleep apnea (OSA).When obstructive sleep apnea occurs, the tongue and soft palate collapse onto the back of the throat and completely block the airway, which restricts the flow of oxygen. The condition known as upper airway resistance syndrome (UARS), is midway between primary snoring and true obstructive sleep apnea. People with UARS suffer many of the symptoms of OSA but require special sleep testing techniques.

Standards of Care

Oral appliance therapy is indicated for:

- Patients with primary snoring or mild OSA who do not respond to, or are not appropriate candidates for treatment with behavioral measures such as weight loss or sleep-position change.

- Patients with moderate to severe OSA should have an initial trial of nasal CPAP, due to greater effectiveness with the use of oral appliances.

- Patients with moderate to severe OSA who are intolerant of or refuse treatment with nasal CPAP. Oral appliances are also indicated for patients who refuse treatment, or are not candidates for tonsillectomy and adenoidectomy, craniofacial operations, or tracheostomy.

Oral Appliances

Oral appliances that treat snoring and obstructive sleep apnea are small plastic devices that are worn in the mouth, similar to orthodontic retainers or sports mouth guards. These appliances help prevent the collapse of the tongue and soft tissues in the back of the throat, keeping the airway open during sleep and promoting adequate air intake. Currently, there are approximately seventy different oral appliances available. Oral appliances may be used alone or in combination with other means of treating OSA, including general health and weight management, surgery, or CPAP.

Types of Oral Appliances

With so many different oral appliances available, selection of a specific appliance may appear somewhat overwhelming. Nearly all appliances fall into one of two categories. The diverse variety is simply a variation of a few major themes. Oral appliances can be classified by mode of action or design variation.

Tongue Retaining Appliances

Tongue retaining appliances function by holding the tongue in a forward position by means of a suction bulb. When the tongue is in a forward position, it serves to keep the back of the tongue from collapsing during sleep and obstructing the airway in the throat.

Mandibular Repositioning Appliances

Mandibular repositioning appliances function to reposition and maintain the lower jaw (mandible) in a protruded position during sleep. This serves to open the airway by indirectly pulling the tongue forward, stimulating activity of the muscles in the tongue and making it more rigid. It also holds the lower jaw and other structures in a stable position to prevent opening of the mouth.

Oral Appliance Therapy

Oral appliance therapy involves the selection, fitting, and use of a specially designed oral appliance worn during sleep that maintains an opened, unobstructed airway in the throat.

Oral appliances work in several ways:

- Repositioning the lower jaw, tongue, soft palate, and uvula

- Stabilizing the lower jaw and tongue
- Increasing the muscle tone of the tongue

Dentists with training in oral appliance therapy are familiar with the various designs of appliances. They can determine which one is best suited for your specific needs. The dentist will work with your physician as part of the medical team in your diagnosis, treatment, and ongoing care. Determination of effective treatment can only be made by joint consultation of your dentist and physician. The initial evaluation phase of oral appliance therapy can take from several weeks to several months to complete. This includes examination, evaluation to determine the most appropriate oral appliance, fitting, maximizing adaptation of the appliance, and the function.

Other Treatment Options

In addition to lifestyle changes, such as good sleep hygiene, exercise, and weight loss, there are three primary ways to treat snoring and sleep apnea. The most common way is with therapy delivered through a continuous positive air pressure (CPAP) machine. CPAP is usually applied through a tube to a mask that covers the nose. The air pressure that is generated splints the structures in the back of the throat, holding the airway open during sleep. Treatment can also be accomplished with surgery to the soft palate, uvula, and tongue to eliminate the tissue that collapses during sleep. More complex surgery can reposition the anatomic structure of your mouth and facial bones. Many of these procedures can be performed by an American Academy of Dental Sleep Medicine (AADSM) member trained as an oral and maxillofacial surgeon.

Ongoing Care

Ongoing care, including short- and long-term follow-up is an essential step in the treatment of snoring and obstructive sleep apnea with oral appliance therapy. Follow-up care serves to assess the treatment of your sleep disorder, the condition of your appliance, your physical response to your appliance, and to ensure that it is comfortable and effective.

Advantages of Oral Appliance Therapy

Oral appliance therapy has several advantages over other forms of therapy:

437

- Oral appliances are comfortable and easy to wear. Most people find that it only takes a couple of weeks to become acclimated to wearing the appliance.

- Oral appliances are small and convenient, making them easy to carry when traveling.

- Treatment with oral appliances is reversible and non-invasive.

Section 42.3

Bright Light Therapy for Circadian Rhythm Sleep Disorders

"Blue Light Special: Treating Circadian Rhythm Sleep Disorders," *Neuropsychiatry Reviews*, September 2006. © 2006 Quadrant HealthCom Inc. Reprinted with permission.

Treatment for patients with circadian rhythm disorders is being cast in a new light—blue. Researchers believe that blue light therapy, though still in the experimental stage, could help patients with certain types of sleep and mood disorders, improve alertness during shift work, overcome jet lag, and even help resolve circadian disruptions in astronauts during spaceflight.

Traditional treatment of patients with circadian rhythm disorders has been based on the premise that the suprachiasmatic nucleus, or the body's internal clock, will only respond to bright light at a certain time of day. The fact that lower-intensity, short-wavelength blue light has been shown to be more effective than the most visible kinds of light in that regard is evidence that a separate photoreceptor system exists within the human eye, other than what is used for sight. Ultimately, color, intensity, and timing of light are all critical factors for stimulating the body clock, which regulates sleep patterns and other physiologic and behavioral functions.

"The circadian system is ubiquitous," said Leon Lack, PhD, at the Twentieth Anniversary Meeting of the Associated Professional Sleep Societies (APSS). "Virtually every physiologic, biochemical, and hormonal measure you can take for twenty-four hours shows a circadian rhythm. Most of these circadian rhythms are endogenous, and they are timed by the internal body clock." Dr. Lack is a professor of psychology at Flinders University of South Australia in Adelaide.

According to Dr. Lack, a normal sleep phase involves a bedtime of about 11:00 p.m. and wake-up time of about 7:00 a.m., with a core temperature minimum in the latter half of the normal sleep period. However, for people with an advanced sleep phase, the core temperature minimum might be as early as midnight. Likewise, people with a delayed circadian rhythm have a core temperature minimum as late as 7:00 or 8:00 a.m.

"Bright light presented just after [core temperature minimum] will cause phase advances, and bright light just before that time will cause phase delays," said Dr. Lack. "Low-intensity light will cause a small phase delay presented just before that temperature minimum. Moderate-intensity light and high-intensity light will cause a greater phase delay. Likewise, light presented after that point, of low, moderate, or high intensity will cause varying degrees of phase advance."

Looking through Blue-Colored Glasses

Light boxes have been the most common tool used in light therapy, but they are large and bulky, not easily transported, and are relatively costly. So Dr. Lack and colleagues devised hi-tech glasses that deliver the same amount of light into the eyes but reduce the overall amount of light produced. "So we actually have a source that is very close to the eyes, emitting very much less light but still getting exactly the same amount of light to the retina."

Dr. Lack's group used light-emitting diodes (LEDs), which are very efficient in converting electricity into light and have relatively narrow spectrum outputs, to compare a standard light box with two portable light sources in suppressing and phase shifting melatonin. They found that the portable LED source was an effective way of administering light to phase-shift the melatonin rhythm, with the blue-green LED light outperforming white LED light.

The investigators also carried out a phase advance study in which amber and red light, which are both long-wavelength light, were compared with short-wavelengths blue, blue-green, and green light emitted via the glasses, as well as with a no-light condition. Dim light melatonin onset (DLMO) was measured on the first evening and again on the third evening, and the glasses were worn between 6:00 and 8:00 a.m. on two consecutive mornings. Dr. Lack's group found that the no-light control condition was associated with no significant change. "That's sort of interesting in a sense, that they woke up earlier than normal for two mornings in a row under dim illumination levels, and that in itself wasn't able to produce any significant phase advance," he said. "The green, blue-green, and blue all produced significant changes from the control condition and from the amber and red conditions. The blue also had a significantly greater phase advance than the green in this experiment."

Into the Blue

George Brainard, PhD, has focused much of his research on the circadian and neuroendocrine capacities of light and the use of light treatment for winter depression. In a recent study that explored short-wavelength sensitivity for the effects of light on alertness and performance, he teamed with lead investigator Steven Lockley, PhD, of the Brigham and Women's Hospital in Boston. The researchers compared the effects of equal photon density exposure to 460-nm blue or 555-nm white light for 6.5 hours during the night. The researchers measured melatonin onset before the light exposure and then again afterward and found that subjects exposed to blue light had significantly lower subjective sleepiness ratings, decreased auditory reaction time, and fewer attention failures, compared with those exposed to white light.

"What is really astonishing about these data is that it takes 5 lux [of blue light] with this very precisely measured method of delivery of light to produce a phase delay equivalent to 10,000 lux of white light without pupil dilation and, of course, without this rigorous control," said Dr. Brainard. He is a professor of neurology at Thomas Jefferson University in Philadelphia.

"We've got a very interesting picture now," he commented. "We've got the development and discovery of a new sensory system, the work of many laboratories. Of course, the classic visual photoreceptor system mediates vision, and then this newly discovered system mediates biologic and behavioral effects, some of them very fast-acting and acute, some of them longer term."

Blue for SAD

Dr. Brainard and colleagues also studied a cohort with seasonal affective disorder (SAD). According to Dr. Brainard, the current standard of therapy for SAD is 10,000 lux white light therapy in the morning. "As with any clinical intervention, you start with something that works, and then ultimately you try to refine it down and optimize it to its most potent elements, because then you can make it more convenient with fewer side effects."

The researchers sought to determine if blue light would be more potent than the longer-wavelength part of the spectrum. Arrays of blue LEDs were developed specifically for the study. "They are not commercially available," Dr. Brainard noted. "They are a bigger bank of light and very much in the developmental stage."

Nineteen females and five males participated in the study. All had major depression with a seasonal pattern, a score of 20 or greater on the Structured Interview Guide for the Hamilton Depression Rating Scale–SAD (SIGH-SAD), and normal sleeping patterns. They were randomly assigned, in a double-blind fashion, to receive either blue light or red light therapy daily for forty-five minutes upon awakening, between 6:00 and 8:00 a.m., for three weeks. Each light unit measured 20 x 24 centimeters and had 267 LEDs in the array and had been given an independent hazard analysis. After one week of therapy, both groups had a reduction in symptoms, "but there was a more dramatic reduction in the blue light group," noted Dr. Brainard. "That reduction continued to go down across the three weeks in the blue light group. Compared to the red light, blue light produced a significantly stronger therapeutic response."

Dr. Brainard's group also looked at remission rates in the cohort. "When we look at it in terms of remission, the blue light group had a 55 percent remission rate, and the red light group had a 31 percent remission rate, and that was statistically significant as well."

When comparing actual photometric and radiometric parameters, the researchers found that the blue light at less than 400 lux evoked a similar therapeutic response to that observed with the 10,000 lux of white light. The blue light also had a lower photon density and a lower microwatt level. "So much less of everything," pointed out Dr. Brainard, "whether you are counting energy, photons, or illuminance, this device achieved equivalent types of therapy in this phase I trial compared to standard therapy.

"We think that these data are supportive of the idea that blue light might have high efficacy for treating winter depression, but there are limitations to this study, and I want to be very clear about these limitations," Dr. Brainard continued. "It's a phase I trial; it's proof of concept. To confirm a specific wavelength effect, the trial must be done in equal photon densities, and that's not been done yet. The study also did not do a direct comparison to 10,000 lux of white light. That's a historical comparison. Still, we think the data are very provocative."

The (Blue) Sky Is the Limit

It is clear that circadian rhythms, in terms of DLMO measurements in people with delayed sleep-phase syndrome, can be retimed with morning blue light, Dr. Lack commented. "Changes in circadian rhythms alone, however, do not result in a change in sleep-wake habits," he said. "We're dealing with real people, with real contingencies and needs and habits. So it is clear to us that we need to follow the blue light treatment with instructions of about what to do to try and maintain their wake-up time in the post-treatment period. So cognitive behavior therapy or at least further instructions obviously will be necessary."

"Basically, I think the bottom line is this," Dr. Brainard continued. "A brand new sensory system has been discovered. There's a lot of neuroanatomy and neurophysiology to be worked out on it, but it has very many exciting potential applications. Essentially, our field has an open door, an opportunity to begin exploring this in greater depth."

Chapter 43

Oral Surgery for Sleep Disorders

Snoring and Obstructive Sleep Apnea

Snoring is the sound of partially obstructed breathing during sleep. While snoring can be harmless, it can also be the sign of a more serious medical condition known as obstructive sleep apnea (OSA). OSA occurs when the tongue and soft palate collapse onto the back of the throat, which completely blocks the airway and restricts the flow of oxygen. The condition known as upper airway resistance syndrome (UARS) is midway between primary snoring and true obstructive sleep apnea. People with UARS suffer many of the symptoms of OSA, but normal sleep testing may be negative.

Treatment Options

In addition to good sleep hygiene, exercise, and weight loss, there are three primary methods to treat snoring and sleep apnea. The most common method is therapy involving a continuous positive air pressure (CPAP) machine. CPAP is usually applied through a tube to a mask that covers the nose. The air pressure that is generated splints the structures in the back of the throat, holding the airway open during sleep. Treatment may also be accomplished through oral appliance therapy. Oral appliances that treat snoring and obstructive sleep apnea are small plastic devices, worn in the mouth, similar to orthodontic retainers or sports mouth guards. These appliances help prevent the collapse of the tongue and soft tissues in the back of the throat, keeping the airway open during sleep and promoting adequate air intake. Treatment can also be accomplished with surgery to the soft palate, uvula, and tongue to eliminate the tissue that collapses during sleep. More complex surgery can reposition the anatomic structure of your mouth and facial bones. Many of these procedures can be performed by an American Academy of Dental Sleep Medicine (AADSM) member trained as an oral and maxillofacial surgeon. There are many surgical procedures available, some of which are detailed below.

Surgical Treatment Options

In general, surgery is indicated when the other therapies are non-applicable, unsuccessful, or intolerable. Surgery may be an effective treatment for snoring and OSA, but only if performed on the correct portions of the upper airway. Surgery is "site-specific," meaning it requires the identification of specific anatomic areas contributing to airway obstruction. This may vary from patient to patient. A detailed examination of the entire upper airway is necessary before deciding which surgical procedures may be most effective.

Maxillomandibular Advancement (MMA)

Maxillomandibular advancement involves osteotomies (bony cuts performed via intraoral incisions) to advance the upper and lower jaws to pull forward and tighten the soft palate, tongue, and other attached soft tissues. This process enlarges and stabilizes the entire upper airway. MMA is the most effective and acceptable surgical treatment of OSA. MMA has published success rates ranging from 94 to 100 percent. An overnight hospital stay is required, and the jaws may be wired shut for several weeks, which may result in weight loss.

Anterior Inferior Mandibular Osteotomy (AIMO) with Hyoid Suspension

The AIMO involves a chin bone osteotomy for advancement of the genial tubercles to pull forward the attached tongue and hyoid (the U-shaped bone in the anterior neck) muscles to enlarge and stabilize the airway behind the tongue base. Although not as effective as MMA, the jaws do not have to be wired shut and there is no change in bite. AIMO may be performed solely as an outpatient procedure or in combination with MMA and other procedures.

Surgery of the Soft Palate

There are many soft-palatal operations that may be effective for snoring, upper airway resistance syndrome (UARS), and obstructive sleep apnea (OSA). Possible adverse side effects of the soft palatal surgery include throat swelling, and nasal reflux of air during speech and fluid during drinking. Throat swelling usually occurs immediately after surgery. The most commonly performed procedure is an uvulopalatopharyngoplasty (UPPP), which involves trimming of a bulky soft palate, often performed in combination with removal of enlarged tonsils and/or adenoids. A laser-assisted uvuloplasty (LAUP) is a modified UPPP that involves "scarring" cuts to tighten the soft palate and sequential trimming of the uvula over several appointments. While LAUP is less painful and has fewer side effects, it is less effective than UPPP in the treatment of OSA. Radiofrequency volumetric tissue reduction (RFVTR), sometimes called somnoplasty, attempts to shrink the soft palate and tongue base using energy waves, similar to microwaves.

Nasal Surgery

Nasal obstruction may be treated by surgical procedures, including septoplasty, to straighten a deviated septum, and turbinate reduction, to remove or reduce large turbinates and polyps. While these procedures may be performed independently as outpatient procedures, they are often used in combination with other procedures to treat snoring and OSA.

Tongue Reduction Surgery

This procedure involves a wedge-shaped surgical reduction of the tongue base. It is not typically performed to treat OSA and may have many potentially adverse side effects.

Weight Reduction Surgery

Bariatric surgery, such as gastric bypass, may be indicated as a last resort treatment of morbidly obese patients with OSA. Cervicofacial liposuction is a relatively safe procedure that selectively removes excessive fatty tissue below the chin and anterior neck to reduce the weight against underlying soft tissues. It also helps minimize airway collapse behind the tongue base. It is usually used in combination with other surgical procedures.

Tracheostomy

This operation bypasses the entire upper airway by creating an opening in the larynx, or windpipe. Although having the highest therapeutic efficacy for OSA, tracheostomy has many psychosocial problems and is typically reserved as a last resort for the treatment of severe OSA. Tracheostomy is particularly beneficial for patients with complicated medical conditions that prevent other above-listed surgical procedures.

Currently, there is no single universal effective and tolerable treatment for sleep-related breathing disorders. Therefore, sleep medicine requires an interdisciplinary approach partnering physician and dentist for the management of snoring, UARS, and OSA.

Part Six

A Special Look at Pediatric Sleep Issues

Chapter 44

Sleep Overview: From Infancy through the Teen Years

Sleep—or lack of it—is probably the most-discussed aspect of baby care. New parents discover its vital importance those first few weeks and months. The quality and quantity of an infant's sleep affects the well-being of everyone in the household—it's the difference between being cheerful, alert parents and members of the walking dead.

And sleep struggles rarely end with a growing child's move from crib to bed. It simply changes form. Instead of cries, it's pleas or refusals. Instead of a feeding at 3:00 a.m., it's a nightmare or request for water.

So how do you get your child to bed through the cries, screams, avoidance tactics, and pleas? How should you respond when you're awakened in the middle of the night? And how much sleep is enough for your child?

How Much Is Enough?

It all depends on your child's age. Charts that list the hours of sleep likely to be required by an infant or a two-year-old may cause concern when individual differences aren't considered. These numbers are simply averages reported for large groups of children of particular ages.

"All About Sleep," November 2007, reprinted with permission from www.Kids Health.org. Copyright © 2007 The Nemours Foundation. This information was provided by KidsHealth, one of the largest resources online for medically reviewed health information written for parents, kids, and teens. For more articles like this one, visit www.KidsHealth.org, or www.TeensHealth.org.

There's no magical number of hours required by all kids in a certain age group. Two-year-old Sarah might sleep from 8:00 p.m. to 8:00 a.m., whereas two-year-old Johnny is just as alert the next day after sleeping from 10:00 p.m. to 5:00 a.m. Still, sleep is very important to a child's well-being. The link between a child's lack of sleep and his or her behavior isn't always obvious. When adults are tired, they can either be grumpy or have low energy, but kids can become hyper, disagreeable, and have extremes in behavior.

Most kids' sleep requirements fall within a predictable range of hours based on their age, but each child is a unique individual with distinct sleep needs. Here are some approximate numbers based on age, accompanied by age-appropriate pro-sleep tactics.

Babies (Up to Six Months)

There is no sleep formula for newborns because their internal clocks aren't fully developed yet. They generally sleep or drowse for sixteen to twenty hours a day, divided about equally between night and day.

Newborns should be awakened every three to four hours until their weight gain is established, which typically happens within the first couple of weeks. After that, it's OK if a baby sleeps for longer periods of time. But don't get your slumber hopes up just yet—most infants won't snooze for extended periods of time because they get hungry.

Newborns' longest sleep periods are generally four or five hours— this is about how long their small bellies can go between feedings. If newborns do sleep for a while, they will likely be extra hungry during the day and may want to nurse or get the bottle more frequently.

Just when parents feel that sleeping through the night seems like a far-off dream, their baby's sleep time usually begins to shift toward night. At three months, a baby averages five hours of sleep during the day and ten hours at night, usually with an interruption or two. About 90 percent of babies this age sleep through the night, meaning six to eight hours in a row.

But it's important to recognize that babies aren't always awake when they sound like they are; they can cry and make all sorts of other noises during light sleep. Even if they do wake up in the night, they may only be awake for a few minutes before falling asleep again on their own. It's best if babies learn early to get themselves to sleep, so let your baby try.

If a baby under six months old continues to cry for several minutes, it's time to respond. Your baby may be genuinely uncomfortable: hungry, wet, cold, or even sick. But routine nighttime awakenings for changing and feeding should be as quick and quiet as possible. Don't provide any unnecessary stimulation, such as talking, playing, or turning on the lights. Encourage the idea that nighttime is for sleeping. You have to teach this because your baby doesn't care what time it is as long as his or her needs are met.

Ideally, your baby should be placed in the crib before falling asleep. And it's not too early to establish a simple bedtime routine. Any soothing activities, performed consistently and in the same order each night, can make up the routine. Your baby will associate these with sleeping, and they'll help him or her wind down. You want your child to fall asleep independently, and a routine encourages babies to go back to sleep if they should wake up in the middle of the night.

Six to Twelve Months

At six months, an infant may nap about three hours during the day and sleep about eleven hours at night. At this age, you can begin to change your response to an infant who awakens and cries during the night.

You can give babies at this age five minutes to settle down on their own and go back to sleep. If they don't, you can comfort them without picking them up (talk softly, rub their backs), then leave—unless they appear to be sick. Sick babies need to be picked up and comforted. If your baby doesn't seem sick and continues to cry, you can wait a little longer than five minutes, then repeat the short crib-side visit.

After several days, your baby should find it easier to get back to sleep on his or her own. But if your six-month-old continues to wake up five or six times each night, talk to your doctor.

Between six and twelve months, separation anxiety becomes a major issue for some babies and may cause them to start waking up again. But the rules for nighttime awakenings are the same through a baby's first birthday: Don't pick up your baby, turn on the lights, sing, talk, play, or feed your child. All of these activities encourage repeat behavior.

If your baby wakes up crying at night, you can check in to make sure he or she isn't sick or in need of a diaper change. You can pat your child lovingly on the back or belly. Using a pacifier or thumb sucking can also help children of this age learn to calm and reassure themselves. If your baby continues to cry, you can institute the five-minute visit pattern.

Toddlers

From ages one to three, most toddlers sleep about ten to thirteen hours. Separation anxiety, or just the desire to be up with mom and dad (and not miss anything), can motivate a child to stay awake. So can simple toddler-style contrariness.

Note the time of night when your toddler begins to show signs of sleepiness, and try establishing this as his or her regular bedtime. And you don't have to force a two- or three-year-old child to nap during the day unless yours gets cranky and overly tired.

Parents sometimes make the mistake of thinking that keeping a child up will make him or her sleepier for bedtime. In fact, though, kids can have a harder time sleeping if they're overtired.

Establishing a bedtime routine helps kids relax and get ready for sleep. For a toddler, the routine may be from fifteen to thirty minutes long and include calming activities such as reading a story, bathing, and listening to soft music.

Whatever the nightly ritual is, your toddler will probably insist that it be the same every night. Just don't allow rituals to become too long or too complicated. Whenever possible, allow your toddler to make bedtime choices within the routine: which pajamas to wear, which stuffed animal to take to bed, what music to play. This gives your little one a sense of control over the routine.

But even the best sleepers give parents an occasional wake-up call. Teething can awaken a toddler and so can dreams. Active dreaming begins at this age, and for very young children, dreams can be pretty alarming. Nightmares are particularly frightening to a toddler, who can't distinguish imagination from reality. (So carefully select what TV programs, if any, your toddler sees before bedtime.)

Comfort and hold your child at these times. Let your toddler talk about the dream if he or she wants to, and stay until your child is calm. Then encourage your child to go back to sleep as soon as possible.

Preschoolers

Preschoolers sleep about ten to twelve hours per night, but there's no reason to be completely rigid about which ten to twelve hours they are. A five-year-old who gets adequate rest at night no longer needs a daytime nap. Instead, a quiet time may be substituted. Most nursery schools and kindergartens have brief quiet periods when the children lie on mats or just rest.

A five-year-old child may still have nightmares and trouble falling asleep some nights. You can prepare a "nighttime kit" that includes activities to pass the time and relax your child. It might include a flashlight, a book, and a cassette or CD player and story tape or CD. Use the kit together, then put it in a special place in your child's room where he or she can get to it in the middle of the night.

School-Age Children and Preteens

Kids ages six to nine need about ten hours of sleep a night. Bedtime difficulties can arise at this age from a child's need for private time with parents, without siblings around. Try to make a little private time just before bedtime and use it to share confidences and have small discussions, which will also prepare your child for sleep.

Children ages ten to twelve need a little over nine hours of shuteye a night. But it's up to parents to judge the exact amount of rest their children need and see that they're in bed in time for sufficient sleep.

Lack of sleep for kids can cause irritable or hyper types of behavior and can also make a condition like attention deficit hyperactivity disorder (ADHD) worse.

Teens

Adolescents need about eight to nine-and-a-half hours of sleep per night, but many don't get it. And as they progress through puberty, teens actually need more sleep. Because teens often have schedules packed with school and activities, they're typically chronically sleep deprived (or lacking in a healthy amount of sleep).

And sleep deprivation adds up over time, so an hour less per night is like a full night without sleep by the end of the week. Among other things, sleep deprivation can lead to:

- decreased attentiveness;

- decreased short-term memory;

- inconsistent performance;

- delayed response time.

These can cause generally bad tempers, problems in school, stimulant use, and driving accidents (more than half of "asleep-at-the-wheel" car accidents are caused by teens).

Adolescents also experience a change in their sleep patterns—their bodies want to stay up late and wake up later, which often leads to them trying to catch up on sleep during the weekend. This sleep schedule irregularity can actually aggravate the problems and make getting to sleep at a reasonable hour during the week even harder.

Ideally, a teenager should try to go to bed at the same time every night and wake up at the same time every morning, allowing for at least eight to nine hours of sleep.

Establishing a Bedtime Routine

Here's a summary of a few ways that may help your child ease into a good night's sleep:

- Include a winding-down period in the routine.

- Stick to a bedtime, alerting your child both half an hour and ten minutes beforehand.

- Allow your child to choose which pajamas to wear, stuffed animal to take to bed, etc.

- Consider playing soft, soothing music.

- Don't give your baby or toddler a bottle (of breast milk, formula, or any sugar-containing drink) to aid sleep. This can cause a serious dental problem called "baby bottle tooth decay" because the fluids tend to pool in the child's mouth.

- Tuck your child into bed snugly for a feeling of security.

- Encourage your older kid or teen to set and maintain a bedtime that allows for the full hours of sleep needed at this age.

There isn't one sure way to raise a good sleeper, but every parent should be encouraged to know that most kids have the ability to sleep well. The key is to try, from early on, to establish healthy sleep habits.

Chapter 45

Infants and Sleeping-Related Concerns

Chapter Contents

Section 45.1

Providing a Safe Sleeping Environment for Infants

"Baby's Safe Sleep," June 2009, reprinted from www.nchealthystart.org, courtesy of the North Carolina Healthy Start Foundation website and the North Carolina Department of Health and Human Services.

For the first few months, your newborn will spend most of his or her time sleeping. Other than the cost of a crib, creating a safe sleep place does not require special equipment. Bumper pads, sleep position wedges, or special pillows are not needed. The Consumer Product Safety Commission does not recommend their use.

Reducing the risk of sudden infant death syndrome (SIDS) continues after your baby is born. Make sure your baby develops healthy and safe sleep habits from the beginning. Share this list with grandparents, babysitters, or others that will be caring for your baby.

Safe Sleep Habits

- Always place healthy babies on their backs for nighttime sleep and for naps. Letting babies sleep on their backs has other advantages besides lowering their chances of SIDS. Research shows that babies who sleep on their backs have fewer colds, fewer ear infections, and fewer fevers.

- Use a sleep place like a crib, bassinet, or playpen designed for babies—do not sleep with the baby in your bed.

- Never put your sleeping baby on pillows, cushions, sofas, or loose bedding.

- Keep excess bedding, toys, stuffed animals, and pillows out of the crib while baby sleeps.

- Do not cover the crib or your baby's face with blankets.

- Don't allow older siblings to sleep with your baby.

- Prevent overheating. Keep room temperature between 68°F and 72°F and never more than 75°F.

- Make sure your baby breathes air that is smoke free; don't allow anyone to smoke near your baby or in your home or car.

Using a Baby Blanket

When using a blanket, practice the feet-to-foot guideline. Tucking the blanket under the crib mattress helps keep the blanket from becoming loose and covering the baby's head:

- Position the baby so his feet are near the foot of the crib.
- Place a lightweight blanket across the baby's chest just under the armpits.
- Tuck the blanket in securely along the two sides and foot of the crib.

Try These Nursery Makeover Tips

- Liven up a bare-looking crib with colorful, printed fitted sheets.
- Hang a colorful quilt on the wall instead of using it in the crib.
- A bed skirt hanging below the bottom of the crib railing to the floor and secured beneath the mattress is a decorative touch to add a splash of color and hide baby items stored underneath the crib.
- Fasten a mobile to the crib footboard, up and out of baby's reach, or hang it from the ceiling.

Section 45.2

Cosleeping: A Controversial Practice

The image of a baby and parent dozing off together isn't an uncommon one. But the practice of cosleeping, or sharing a bed with your infant, is controversial in the United States. Supporters of cosleeping believe that a parent's bed is just where an infant belongs. But is it safe?

Why Do Some People Choose to Cosleep?

Cosleeping supporters believe—and some studies support their beliefs—that cosleeping:

- encourages breastfeeding by making nighttime breastfeeding more convenient;

- makes it easier for a nursing mother to get her sleep cycle in sync with her baby's;

- helps babies fall asleep more easily, especially during their first few months and when they wake up in the middle of the night;

- helps babies get more nighttime sleep (because they awaken more frequently with shorter duration of feeds, which can add up to a greater amount of sleep throughout the night);

- helps parents who are separated from their babies during the day regain the closeness with their infant that they feel they missed.

But do the risks of cosleeping outweigh the benefits?

Is Cosleeping Safe?

Despite the possible pros, the U.S. Consumer Product Safety Commission (CPSC) warns parents not to place their infants to sleep in adult beds, stating that the practice puts babies at risk of suffocation and strangulation. And the American Academy of Pediatrics (AAP) agrees.

Cosleeping is a widespread practice in many non-Western cultures. However, differences in mattresses, bedding, and other cultural practices may account for the lower risk in these countries as compared with the United States.

According to the CPSC, at least 515 deaths were linked to infants and toddlers under two years of age sleeping in adult beds from January 1990 to December 1997:

- 121 of the deaths were attributed to a parent, caregiver, or sibling rolling on top of or against a baby while sleeping;

- more than 75 percent of the deaths involved infants younger than three months old.

Cosleeping advocates say it isn't inherently dangerous and that the CPSC went too far in recommending that parents never sleep with children under two years of age. According to supporters of cosleeping, parents won't roll over onto a baby because they're conscious of the baby's presence—even during sleep.

Those who should not cosleep with an infant, however, include:

- other children—particularly toddlers—because they might not be aware of the baby's presence;

- parents who are under the influence of alcohol or any drug because that could diminish their awareness of the baby;

- parents who smoke because the risk of sudden infant death syndrome (SIDS) is greater.

But can cosleeping cause SIDS? The connection between cosleeping and SIDS is unclear and research is ongoing. Some cosleeping researchers have suggested that it can reduce the risk of SIDS because cosleeping parents and babies tend to wake up more often throughout the night. However, the AAP reports that some studies suggest that, under certain conditions, cosleeping may increase the risk of SIDS, especially cosleeping environments involving mothers who smoke.

CPSC also reported more than one hundred infant deaths between January 1999 and December 2001 attributable to hidden hazards for babies on adult beds, including:

- suffocation when an infant gets trapped or wedged between a mattress and headboard, wall, or other object;

- suffocation resulting from a baby being face-down on a waterbed, a regular mattress, or on soft bedding such as pillows, blankets, or quilts;

- strangulation in a bed frame that allows part of an infant's body to pass through an area while trapping the baby's head.

In addition to the potential safety risks, sharing a bed with a baby can sometimes prevent parents from getting a good night's sleep. And infants who cosleep can learn to associate sleep with being close to a parent in the parent's bed, which may become a problem at nap time or when the infant needs to go to sleep before the parent is ready.

Making Cosleeping as Safe as Possible

If you do choose to share your bed with your baby, make sure to follow these precautions:

- Always place your baby on his or her back to sleep to reduce the risk of SIDS.

- Always leave your child's head uncovered while sleeping.

- Make sure your bed's headboard and footboard don't have openings or cutouts that could trap your baby's head.

- Make sure your mattress fits snugly in the bed frame so that your baby won't become trapped in between the frame and the mattress.

- Don't place a baby to sleep in an adult bed alone.

- Don't use pillows, comforters, quilts, and other soft or plush items on the bed.

- Don't drink alcohol or use medications or drugs that may keep you from waking and may cause you to roll over onto, and therefore suffocate, your baby.

- Don't place your bed near draperies or blinds where your child could be strangled by cords.

Transitioning Out of the Parent's Bed

Most medical experts say the safest place to put an infant to sleep is in a crib that meets current standards and has no soft bedding. But if you've been cosleeping with your little one and would like to stop, talk to your doctor about making a plan for when your baby will sleep in a crib.

Transitioning to the crib by six months is usually easier—for both parents and baby—before the cosleeping habit is ingrained and other developmental issues (such as separation anxiety) come into play. Eventually, though, the cosleeping routine will likely be broken at some point, either naturally because the child wants to or by the parents' choice.

But there are ways that you can still keep your little one close by, just not in your bed. You could:

- Put a bassinet, play yard, or crib next to your bed. This can help you maintain that desired closeness, which can be especially important if you're breastfeeding. The AAP says that having an infant sleep in a separate crib, bassinet, or play yard in the same room as the mother reduces the risk of SIDS.

- Buy a device that looks like a bassinet or play yard minus one side, which attaches to your bed to allow you to be next to each other while eliminating the possibility of rolling over onto your infant.

Of course, where your child sleeps—whether it's in your bed or a crib—is a personal decision. As you're weighing the pros and cons, talk to your child's doctor about the risks, possible personal benefits, and your family's own sleeping arrangements.

Section 45.3

Positional Plagiocephaly (Flattened Head)

Passage through the birth canal often makes a newborn's head appear pointy or elongated for a short time. It's normal for a baby's skull, which is made up of several separate bones that will eventually fuse together, to be slightly misshapen during the few days or weeks after birth.

But if you've noticed that your baby is developing a persistent flat spot, either in the back or on one side of the head, it could be a sign of positional plagiocephaly. Also known as flattened head syndrome, this can occur when a baby sleeps in the same position repeatedly or because of problems with the neck muscles.

Fortunately, positional plagiocephaly usually is easy to treat, and with appropriate intervention will correct itself by the time a child is one year old.

About Positional Plagiocephaly

Positional plagiocephaly is a disorder in which the back or one side of an infant's head is flattened, often with little hair growing in that area. It's most often the result of babies spending a lot of time lying on their backs or often being in a position where the head is resting against a flat surface (such as in cribs, strollers, swings, and playpens).

Because infants' heads are soft to allow for the incredible brain growth that occurs in the first year of life, they're susceptible to being "molded" into a flat shape.

The number of positional plagiocephaly cases increased sixfold from 1992 to 1994, occurring in approximately 33 out of every 10,000 births. This dramatic increase started when the American Academy of Pediatrics (AAP) began its "Back to Sleep" campaign, which continues to recommend that babies sleep on their backs to reduce the risk of sudden infant death syndrome (SIDS).

Since the AAP's campaign, the incidence of SIDS in the United States has decreased by almost 40 percent while the incidence of flattened head syndrome has risen. Still, the prevention of SIDS is worth the increased risk of a flattened head, especially because positional plagiocephaly will often correct itself with appropriate intervention.

Causes of Positional Plagiocephaly

The most common cause of a flattened head is a baby's sleep position. Because an infant sleeps so many hours on the back of his or her head, the head sometimes assumes a flat shape.

Another thing that can contribute to flattening is torticollis, which means the neck muscles are too tight, have inadequate tone, or are shorter on one side than the other, causing the head to tilt one way while the chin points in the opposite direction.

Premature babies are more prone to positional plagiocephaly—their skulls are softer than those of full-term babies, and they spend a great deal of time on their backs without being moved or picked up because of their medical needs and extreme fragility after birth, which usually requires a stay in the neonatal intensive care unit.

A baby might even start to develop positional plagiocephaly before birth, if pressure is placed on the baby's skull by the mother's pelvis or a twin. In fact, it's not at all unusual to see plagiocephaly in multiple birth infants.

But the differences in head shape seen in children with positional plagiocephaly shouldn't be confused with those caused by craniosynostosis, a more serious condition that occurs when skull bones fuse together too soon, causing an abnormal skull shape and possible brain damage if the condition is not corrected. A child with craniosynostosis may have deformities in the front of the head and a bony ridge over the abnormally fused skull bones. Craniosynostosis is usually corrected with surgery.

Signs and Symptoms

Positional plagiocephaly is usually easy for parents to notice. Typically, the back of the child's head (called the occiput) and the ear on the flattened side may be pushed forward. In severe cases, there may be bulging on the side opposite from the flattening and the forehead may be asymmetrical (or uneven), although this is unusual in full-term infants. If torticollis is the cause, the neck, jaw, and face may be asymmetrical.

Diagnosis

Most often, a doctor can make the diagnosis of positional plagiocephaly simply by examining your child's head, without having to order lab tests or x-rays. The doctor will also note whether regular repositioning of your child's head during sleep successfully reshapes the growing skull over time (craniosynostosis, on the other hand, typically will worsen).

If there's still some doubt, x-rays or a computed tomography (CT) scan of the head will show the doctor if the skull bones are normally separated or if they fused together too soon. If the bones aren't fused, the doctor will probably rule out craniosynostosis and confirm that the child has positional plagiocephaly.

Treatment

Treatment for positional plagiocephaly caused by sleeping position is usually easy and painless, entailing simple repositioning of babies during sleep to encourage them to alternate their head position while sleeping on their backs.

Even though they'll probably move around throughout the night, alternating sides is still beneficial. Wedge pillows are available that keep babies lying on one side or the other, but be sure to check with your doctor before using one to ensure that it's appropriate and safe for your baby. The AAP does not recommend routinely using any devices that might restrict the movement of an infant's head.

In addition, you may want to consider moving your baby's crib to a different area of the room. If there's something in the room (a window or toy, for example) that's catching your baby's attention and causing him or her to hold the head in a similar position day after day, moving the crib will coax your child to look at it from another position.

Always be sure your baby gets plenty of supervised time on the stomach while awake during the day. Not only does "tummy time" promote normal shaping of the back of the head, it also helps in other ways. Looking around from a new perspective encourages your baby's learning and discovery of the world. Plus, it helps babies learn to push up on their arms, which helps develop the muscles needed for crawling and sitting up. It also helps to strengthen the neck muscles.

If torticollis is the cause of your baby's flattened head, a course of physical therapy and a home exercise program will usually do the trick. A physical therapist can teach you exercises to do with your baby involving stretching techniques that are gradual and progressive. Most moves will consist of stretching your child's neck to the side opposite the tilt. Eventually, the neck muscles will be elongated and the neck will straighten itself out. Although they're very simple, the exercises must be performed correctly.

For kids with severe positional plagiocephaly, doctors may prescribe a custom-molded helmet or head band. These work best if started between the ages of four and six months, when a child grows the fastest, and are usually less helpful after ten months of age. They work by applying gentle but constant pressure on a baby's growing skull in an effort to redirect the growth.

But never purchase or use any devices like these without having your child evaluated by a doctor. Only a small percentage of babies wear helmets. The decision to use helmet therapy is made on a case-by-case basis (for example, if the condition is so severe that a baby's face is becoming misshapen or the parents are very upset). Although helmets might not improve the outcome in all children, some kids with severe torticollis can benefit from their use.

Prognosis

The outlook for babies with positional plagiocephaly is excellent. As babies grow, they begin to reposition themselves naturally during sleep much more often than they did as newborns, which allows their heads to be in different positions throughout the night. After babies are able to roll over, the AAP still recommends that parents put them to sleep on their backs, but then allow them to move into the position that most suits them without repositioning them onto their backs.

Most skull-flattening deformities are self-corrected by the time the child is one year old. A persistent, severe, or cosmetically obvious deformity can be corrected with reconstructive surgery between twelve and eighteen months of age, but very few cases require this.

It's important to remember that plagiocephaly itself does not affect your child's brain growth or cause developmental delays or brain damage.

Prevention

Babies should be put down to sleep on their backs to help prevent SIDS, despite the possibility of developing an area of flattening on the back of the head. However, alternating their head position every night while they sleep and providing lots of tummy time and stimulation during the day while they're awake can reduce the risk of positional plagiocephaly.

Section 45.4

Sudden Infant Death Syndrome

"Sudden Infant Death Syndrome (SIDS)," November 2008, reprinted with permission from www.kidshealth.org. Copyright © 2008 The Nemours Foundation. This information was provided by KidsHealth, one of the largest resources online for medically reviewed health information written for parents, kids, and teens. For more articles like this one, visit www.KidsHealth .org or www.TeensHealth.org.

Reducing the Risk

A lack of answers is part of what makes sudden infant death syndrome (SIDS) so frightening. SIDS is the leading cause of death among infants one month to one year old, and claims the lives of about 2,500 each year in the United States. It remains unpredictable despite years of research.

Even so, the risk of SIDS can be greatly reduced. First and foremost, infants younger than one year old should be placed on their backs to sleep—never face-down on their stomachs.

Searching for Answers

As the name implies, SIDS is the sudden and unexplained death of an infant who is younger than one year old. It's a frightening prospect because it can strike without warning, usually in seemingly healthy babies. Most SIDS deaths are associated with sleep (hence the common reference to "crib death") and infants who die of SIDS show no signs of suffering.

While most conditions or diseases usually are diagnosed by the presence of specific symptoms, most SIDS diagnoses come only after all other possible causes of death have been ruled out through a review of the infant's medical history and environment. This review helps distinguish true SIDS deaths from those resulting from accidents, abuse, and previously undiagnosed conditions, such as cardiac or metabolic disorders.

When considering which babies could be most at risk, no single risk factor is likely to be sufficient to cause a SIDS death. Rather, several risk factors combined may contribute to cause an at-risk infant to die of SIDS.

Most deaths due to SIDS occur between two and four months of age, and incidence increases during cold weather. African-American infants are twice as likely and Native American infants are about three times more likely to die of SIDS than Caucasian infants. More boys than girls fall victim to SIDS.

Other potential risk factors include:

- smoking, drinking, or drug use during pregnancy;

- poor prenatal care;

- prematurity or low birth weight;

- mothers younger than twenty;

- tobacco smoke exposure following birth;

- overheating from excessive sleepwear and bedding;

- stomach sleeping.

Stomach Sleeping

Foremost among these risk factors is stomach sleeping. Numerous studies have found a higher incidence of SIDS among babies placed on their stomachs to sleep than among those sleeping on their backs or sides. Some researchers have hypothesized that stomach sleeping puts pressure on a child's jaw, therefore narrowing the airway and hampering breathing.

Another theory is that stomach sleeping can increase an infant's risk of "rebreathing" his or her own exhaled air, particularly if the infant is sleeping on a soft mattress or with bedding, stuffed toys, or a pillow near the face. In that scenario, the soft surface could create a small enclosure around the baby's mouth and trap exhaled air. As the baby breathes exhaled air, the oxygen level in the body drops and carbon dioxide accumulates. Eventually, this lack of oxygen could contribute to SIDS.

Also, infants who succumb to SIDS may have an abnormality in the arcuate nucleus, a part of the brain that may help control breathing and awakening during sleep. If a baby is breathing stale air and not getting enough oxygen, the brain usually triggers the baby to wake up and cry. That movement changes the breathing and heart rate, making up for the lack of oxygen. But a problem with the arcuate nucleus could deprive the baby of this involuntary reaction and put him or her at greater risk for SIDS.

Going "Back to Sleep"

The striking evidence that stomach sleeping might contribute to the incidence of SIDS led the American Academy of Pediatrics (AAP) to recommend in 1992 that all healthy infants younger than one year of age be put to sleep on their backs (also known as the supine position).

Since the AAP's recommendation, the rate of SIDS has dropped by over 50 percent. Still, SIDS remains the leading cause of death in young infants, so it's important to keep reminding parents about the necessity of back sleeping.

Many parents fear that babies put to sleep on their backs could choke on spit-up or vomit. According to the AAP, however, there is no increased risk of choking for healthy infants who sleep on their backs. (For infants with chronic gastroesophageal reflux disease [GERD] or certain upper airway malformations, sleeping on the stomach may be the better option. The AAP urges parents to consult with their child's doctor in these cases to determine the best sleeping position for the baby.)

Placing infants on their sides to sleep is not a good idea, either, the AAP said, as there's a risk that infants will roll over onto their bellies while they sleep.

Some parents also may be concerned about positional plagiocephaly, a condition in which babies develop a flat spot on the back of their heads from spending too much time lying on their backs. Since the Back to Sleep campaign, this condition has become quite common—but it is usually easily treatable by changing your baby's position frequently and allowing for more "tummy time" while he or she is awake.

Of course, once babies can roll over consistently—usually around four to seven months—they may choose not to stay on their backs all night long. At this point, it's fine to let babies pick a sleep position on their own.

Tips for Reducing the Risk of SIDS

In addition to placing healthy infants on their backs to sleep, the AAP suggests these measures to help reduce the risk of SIDS:

- Place your baby on a firm mattress to sleep, never on a pillow, waterbed, sheepskin, couch, chair, or other soft surface. To prevent rebreathing, do not put blankets, comforters, stuffed toys, or pillows near the baby.

- Make sure your baby does not get too warm while sleeping. Keep the room at a temperature that feels comfortable for an adult in a short-sleeve shirt. Some researchers suggest that a baby who gets too warm could go into a deeper sleep, making it more difficult to awaken.

- Do not smoke, drink, or use drugs while pregnant and do not expose your baby to secondhand smoke. Infants of mothers who smoked during pregnancy are three times more likely to die of SIDS than those whose mothers were smoke-free; exposure to secondhand smoke doubles a baby's risk of SIDS. Researchers speculate that smoking might affect the central nervous system, starting prenatally and continuing after birth, which could place the baby at increased risk.

- Receive early and regular prenatal care.

- Make sure your baby has regular well-baby checkups.

- Breastfeed, if possible. There is some evidence that breastfeeding may help decrease the incidence of SIDS. The reason for this is not clear, though researchers think that breast milk may help protect babies from infections that increase the risk of SIDS.

- If your baby has GERD, be sure to follow your doctor's guidelines on feeding and sleep positions.

- Put your baby to sleep with a pacifier during the first year of life. If your baby rejects the pacifier, don't force it. Pacifiers have been linked with lower risk of SIDS. If you're breastfeeding, try to wait until after the baby is one month old so that breastfeeding can be established.

- While infants can be brought into a parent's bed for nursing or comforting, parents should return them to their cribs or bassinets when they're ready to sleep. It's a good idea to keep the cribs and bassinets in the room where parents' sleep. This has been linked with a lower risk of SIDS.

For parents and families who have experienced a SIDS death, many groups, including the Sudden Infant Death Syndrome Alliance, can provide grief counseling, support, and referrals.

And growing public awareness of SIDS and precautions to prevent it should leave fewer parents searching for answers in the future.

Chapter 46

Apnea: When Breathing Stops

Chapter Contents

Section 46.1

Sleep-Related Apnea in Children

Everyone has brief pauses in their breathing pattern called apnea. Usually these brief stops are completely normal.

Sometimes, though, apnea can cause a prolonged pause in breathing, making the breathing pattern irregular. Someone with apnea might actually stop breathing for short amounts of time, decreasing oxygen levels in the body and disrupting sleep.

Types of Apnea

The word apnea comes from the Greek word meaning "without wind." Although it's perfectly normal for everyone to experience occasional pauses in breathing, apnea can be a problem when breathing stops for twenty seconds or longer.

There are three types of apnea:

1. obstructive
2. central
3. mixed

Obstructive Apnea

A common type of apnea in children, obstructive apnea is caused by an obstruction of the airway (such as enlarged tonsils and adenoids). This is most likely to happen during sleep because that's when the soft tissue at back of the throat is most relaxed. As many as 1 to 3 percent of otherwise healthy preschool-age kids have obstructive apnea.

Symptoms include:

- snoring (the most common) followed by pauses or gasping;
- labored breathing while sleeping;

- very restless sleep and sleeping in unusual positions;
- changes in color.

Because obstructive sleep apnea may disturb sleep patterns, these children may also show continued sleepiness after awakening in the morning and tiredness and attention problems throughout the day. Sometimes apnea can affect school performance. One recent study suggests that some kids diagnosed with attention deficit hyperactivity disorder (ADHD) actually have attention problems in school because of disrupted sleep patterns caused by obstructive sleep apnea.

Treatment for obstructive apnea involves keeping the throat open to aid air flow, such as with adenotonsillectomy (surgical removal of the tonsils and adenoids) or continuous positive airway pressure (CPAP), which is delivered by having the child wear a nose mask while sleeping.

Central Apnea

Central apnea occurs when the part of the brain that controls breathing doesn't start or properly maintain the breathing process. In very premature infants, it's seen fairly commonly because the respiratory center in the brain is immature. Other than being seen in premature infants, central apnea is the least common form of apnea and often has a neurological cause.

Mixed Apnea

Mixed apnea is a combination of central and obstructive apnea and is seen particularly in infants or young children who have abnormal control of breathing. Mixed apnea may occur when a child is awake or asleep.

Conditions Associated with Apnea

Apnea can be seen in connection with:

Apparent life-threatening events (ALTEs): An ALTE itself is not a sleep disorder—it's a serious event with a combination of apnea and change in color, change in muscle tone, choking, or gagging. Call 911 immediately if your child shows the signs of an ALTE.

ALTEs, especially in young infants, are often associated with medical conditions that require treatment. Examples of these medical conditions include gastroesophageal reflux (GERD), infections, or neurological disorders. ALTEs are scary to observe, but can be uncomplicated and may not happen again. However, any child who has an ALTE should be seen and evaluated immediately.

Apnea of prematurity (AOP): AOP can occur in infants who are born prematurely (before thirty-four weeks of pregnancy). Because the brain or respiratory system may be immature or underdeveloped, the baby may not be able to regulate his or her own breathing normally. AOP can be obstructive, central, or mixed.

Treatment for AOP can involve the following:

- Keeping the infant's head and neck straight (premature babies should always be placed on their backs to sleep to help keep the airways clear)

- Medications to stimulate the respiratory system

- Continuous positive airway pressure (CPAP)—to keep the airway open with the help of forced air through a nose mask

- Oxygen

Premature infants with AOP are followed closely in the hospital. If AOP doesn't resolve before discharge from the hospital, an infant may be sent home on an apnea monitor and parents and other caregivers will be taught cardiopulmonary resuscitation (CPR). The family will work closely with the child's doctor to have a treatment plan in place.

Apnea of infancy (AOI): Apnea of infancy occurs in children who are younger than one year old and who were born after a full-term pregnancy. Following a complete medical evaluation, if a cause of apnea isn't found, it's often called apnea of infancy. AOI usually goes away on its own, but if it doesn't cause any significant problems (such as low blood oxygen), it may be considered part of the child's normal breathing pattern.

Infants with AOI can be observed at home with the help of a special monitor prescribed by a sleep specialist. This monitor records chest movements and heart rate and can relay the readings to a hospital apnea program or save them for future examination by a doctor. Parents and caregivers will be taught CPR before the child is sent home.

If You Think Your Child Has Apnea

If you suspect that your child has apnea, call your doctor. If you suspect that your child is experiencing an ALTE, call 911 immediately.

Although prolonged pauses in breathing can be serious, after a doctor does a complete evaluation and makes a diagnosis, most cases of apnea can be treated or managed with surgery, medications, monitoring devices, or sleep centers. And many cases of apnea go away on their own.

Section 46.2

Having Your Child Evaluated for Obstructive Sleep Apnea

If you suspect that your child has obstructive sleep apnea (OSA), you may want to consult first with your child's primary care provider (usually a pediatrician or family physician) and share your concerns. You may also choose to consult with an otolaryngologist (ear, nose, and throat specialist or ENT) or a pulmonologist (a specialist in lung problems) who deals with children. Sometimes, because of the hyperactivity, inattentiveness, aggressive behavior, irritability, and mood swings associated with pediatric OSA, a mental health provider, such as a child psychiatrist or psychologist, or a neurologist may be the first to recognize the problem. However, before seeing any specialist for an evaluation, you should check with your insurance company as you may need a referral or have to go to a specific provider.

Doctors who specialize in sleep medicine may also practice in your area. They have usually trained under other sleep specialists and/or studied sleep medicine through a residency program, continuing medical education (CME) courses, and scientific meetings. Physicians certified by the American Board of Sleep Medicine have passed standardized tests on both pediatric and adult sleep disorders. You should ask any doctor or health-care provider about his or her credentials and experience, especially in dealing with children. You should be satisfied with the explanations and how it will be diagnosed and treated in your child's particular case.

In most cases, the initial evaluation for children with suspected OSA includes a complete medical history (symptoms; previous and current medical problems; operations, especially removal of the tonsils and/or adenoids; medications; and allergies), a review of any behavioral or developmental problems, a sleep history, and a physical exam (including weight and height). Blood tests, x-rays, and other specialized tests may be needed in some cases.

Based on the initial evaluation, your healthcare provider may suggest an overnight sleep study. A sleep study or polysomnogram can help to make a diagnosis of OSA in children and can help to judge the severity of the problem.

The recording devices used during a sleep study are similar in adults and children. These generally include an electroencephalogram (EEG) to measure brain waves and an electrooculogram (EOG) to measure eye and chin movement, both to monitor the different stages of sleep; an electrocardiogram (EKG) to measure heart rate and rhythm; chest bands to measure breathing movements; and additional monitors to sense oxygen and carbon dioxide levels in the blood as well as monitors to record leg movement. None of the devices is painful and there are no needles involved, and sometimes the technician can attach the monitoring devices after the child has fallen asleep in the lab. Still the process may be a little frightening for a young child. Most sleep labs accommodate a parent's stay with the child overnight.

There are currently only a few clinics around the country that specialize specifically in pediatric sleep problems. However, many sleep study facilities (usually called sleep labs or sleep centers) perform studies on children as well as adults. Check first to make sure that the facility you use is equipped to handle children and that the sleep lab technicians are comfortable working with them. You should also ask if the doctor who will interpret the sleep study is familiar with reading pediatric sleep studies, as they differ some from those of adults.

If you are not given a list of doctors and sleep testing facilities, you can find a referral from a few different sources. There is no one complete list of all such facilities, and as a nonprofit organization, the American Sleep Apnea Association (ASAA) does not endorse or recommend any company, product, or healthcare provider. However, there is a list of sleep centers and laboratories accredited by the American Academy of Sleep Medicine (AASM) that pay their AASM membership dues. (The AASM, formerly known as the American Sleep Disorders Association or ASDA, is the professional society in the field of sleep medicine that accredits such facilities; accreditation implies adherence to a certain set of standards). The most up-to-date list of accredited member sleep centers and laboratories appears on the AASM's website: www.aasmnet.org. You can request a list from the ASAA as well. Remember that other centers are in the process of being accredited, have chosen not to be accredited, or do not qualify for accreditation. You can also check with local hospitals and healthcare professionals to find a testing facility. It is technically possible to have a sleep study in the home, but home sleep studies have yet to be validated for children.

A different type of portable monitoring system has been approved by the Food and Drug Administration specifically for use in children aged five to seventeen. It can be used at home as well as in a sleep center but it does not gather some of the information that is obtained in a sleep center study. It is recommended that you check with your insurance carrier to see if they will pay for this type of study or pay for treatment based on a portable study.

OSA in children is a serious disorder that, untreated, may result in health problems as well as behavior and academic problems. Although common, OSA often goes unrecognized, but it can usually be easily treated if detected. Symptoms of pediatric OSA should not be ignored.

This section is written for children age one or older who have not yet entered puberty and does not encompass infantile apnea or apnea of prematurity. As children begin to enter puberty, their symptoms—and hence the diagnosis and treatment of the disorder—become more like those of adults.

Some insurance policies specifically exclude the diagnosis and/or treatment of sleep disorders and some do not cover durable medical equipment (however, relatively few children are treated with durable medical equipment or DME; surgery is more common). Such coverage is worth considering when examining your policy and whenever thinking about changing your policy (such as during your employer's open season).

Chapter 47

Getting Children to Bed: Bedtime Guidelines

If these are common concerns:

- You are spending "too much" time helping your child fall asleep at night

- Your child is waking up frequently throughout the night

- You are losing sleep (and patience) because of your child's sleep problems

- Your relationship with your child is starting to suffer because of lack of sleep

Your child may have a sleep disorder.

It is important to better understand your child's sleep difficulties and take steps to help her sleep better. The most common childhood sleep disorders can be remedied quickly once they have been properly identified and treated.

Three of the most common sleep problems for young children include:

- **Sleep-onset association disorder:** Sleep-onset association disorder occurs when your child associates or closely connects his ability to fall asleep with "something in the environment" (such as being held by his parent; being rocked to sleep; nursing, drinking, or eating at bedtime; watching television; or even sleeping in a parent's or sibling's bed). When this "something in the environment" is absent, your child cannot fall asleep. All of us wake up briefly a number of times each night, but we are usually not aware that we wake up because we fall back asleep very quickly. For the child with sleep-onset association disorder, when they awaken during the night, they are not able to fall back asleep if their "something in the environment" is not present. If your child is only able to nap or fall asleep at night in the car (or in one bed but not another), he likely has a sleep onset association problem.

- **Nighttime eating/drinking disorder:** Nighttime eating/drinking disorder is more common among infants and toddlers and involves "excessive" nighttime feeding (often nursing or bottle-feeding) that is required in order for the child to fall asleep or return to sleep. For infants, feeding during the night is a normal part of development. However, by the age of five or six months most children are not drinking more than eight ounces of fluid during the night (or nursing more than once or twice).

- **Limit-setting sleep disorder:** Limit-setting sleep disorder is more common for children who are fully ambulatory (i.e., able to walk/run) and have developed receptive and expressive language skills (typically after age two). Limit-setting problems are characterized by a child refusing or stalling bedtime (e.g., "I need to go to the bathroom, get a drink of water, one more hug, tell you something really, really important," etc.) and making it hard for the parent to leave the child's room without them getting up out of bed. Attempts to have the child return to bed may result in behavioral outbursts (e.g., crying; screaming; destruction of property or aggression).

How should we treat our child's bedtime problem?

A consistent sleep routine is helpful for treating and/or preventing the most common childhood sleep disorders. Routines that integrate relaxing pre-sleep activities and an environment free of overstimulating or distracting activities are best for your child.

Spending time with your child before bed each night is a critical part of the bedtime ritual. Do not substitute television or videos for personal time with your child each night. Positive parent-child interactions before bed help your child to calm and feel comfortable with the transition to bed.

For children with a sleep-onset association problem a bedtime routine that promotes the child's ability to fall asleep by herself is important. Teach your child to fall asleep independently at all sleep intervals (including naps):

- Set up an environment (sleep associations) at bedtime that does not require a response from you. For example, play music, put on a night light, provide comfort items.

- Avoid having your child fall asleep in your arms or while you are rocking her. Place her in her bed before she falls asleep.

- For the young child (that is still napping) it may be easiest to start the relearning process at night.

- Your child is expected to cry at first during this process.

- You are not abandoning your child by intentionally ignoring her mild distress for set periods of time. When you allow her to experience increasingly longer periods by herself followed by brief encouragement and reassurance, she can learn to fall asleep without your presence.

- Place your awake or drowsy child in his bed after you have completed a calming and quiet bedtime routine.

- Say goodnight and leave the room. You may keep the door open to allow some dim light into the room or use a night light.

- If your child begins to cry and is still crying after a few minutes, return to the room and provide brief reassurance with words or light physical touch (placing hand on back or belly). Do not pick up your child, turn on the lights, or respond to requests (e.g., another bedtime story). Do not stay in the room longer than one or two minutes. Repeat this process, extending the time that you give your child to fall asleep independently (e.g., two minutes; then five minutes; then ten minutes; then fifteen minutes). Increase the time that you are out of the room in increments of five minutes to help your child gradually become more comfortable being alone in her bed.

- On subsequent nights increase the intervals of time that you allow your child to self-sooth. For example on the second night start at five minutes and on the third night start at ten minutes.

- The first few nights are going to be the most difficult for you and your child as you learn this new routine. The time that you

481

spend away from your child when he is upset can be very difficult for you. However, it is important to keep in mind that you are teaching him to learn a very important developmental skill (falling asleep independently).

If you are able to use this approach consistently on consecutive nights, you are likely to see results in five to ten days.

If your child becomes sick or there is some other event that interferes with this process, you will likely have to start the process again.

If you feel you have been consistent with this approach for a two-week period and you are not seeing results, you should consider having your child evaluated for another underlying sleep disorder.

For a child with nighttime feeding problems it is important to gradually wean your child from this habit by reducing access to food/drink. This can be accomplished by reducing the frequency of nighttime feedings (i.e., increase the interval of time between feedings). It may help to set defined time intervals to offer your child her bottle (e.g., every two hours) and slowly increase the interval periodically until you are no longer offering the bottle at night. If your child wakes up and signals hunger before the time you have set for access to food/drink, provide brief reassurance and give her an opportunity to fall back asleep without access to food (see above for guidelines on helping your child to self-soothe and fall asleep independently).

For a child with limit-setting problems at bedtime it is important to have a consistent bedtime routine as well as very clearly defined behavioral limits for bedtime. Parents should focus on having a relaxing pre-sleep ritual each night, however, the transition to bed may require a more "matter of fact" approach. A firm and consistent response to your child's delay at bedtime will prevent you from inadvertently reinforcing your child's "delay behaviors." Limit-setting during the day and night are important. It may be helpful to establish a behavioral reinforcement system that provides behavioral incentives for your child's cooperation with bedtime and staying in bed through the night.

Chapter 48

Bedwetting

Why does my child wet the bed?

Many children wet the bed until they are five years old, or even older. In most cases, the cause is physical and not the child's fault. The child's bladder might be too small. Or the amount of urine produced overnight is too much for the bladder to hold. As a result, the bladder fills up before the night is over. Some children sleep too deeply or take longer to learn bladder control. Children don't wet the bed on purpose. Bedwetting is a medical problem, not a behavior problem. Scolding and punishment will not help a child stay dry.

Bedwetting may run in the family. If both parents wet the bed as children, their child is likely to have the same problem. If only one parent has a history of bedwetting, the child has about a fifty-fifty chance of having the problem. Some children wet the bed even if neither parent ever did.

Bedwetting may be caused by an infection or a nerve disease. Children with nerve disease often also have daytime wetting.

A child who has been dry for several months or even years may return to wetting the bed. The cause might be emotional stress, such as loss of a loved one, problems at school, a new sibling, or even training too early.

"What I Need to Know about My Child's Bedwetting," National Institute of Diabetes and Digestive and Kidney Diseases, National Institutes of Health, NIH Publication No. 06-5631, April 2006.

How can I help my child stay dry?

The answer is rarely easy. Try skipping drinks before bedtime. Avoid drinks with caffeine, like colas or tea. These drinks speed up urine production. Give your child one drink with dinner. Explain that it will be the last drink before going to bed. Make sure your child uses the bathroom just before bed. Many children will still wet the bed, but these steps are a place to start.

Your child may feel bad about wetting the bed. Let your child know he isn't to blame. Let her help take off the wet sheets and put them in the washer, but don't make this a punishment. Be supportive. Praise your child for dry nights.

Be patient. Most children grow out of bedwetting. Some children just take more time than others.

Should I take my child to the doctor?

If your child is younger than five, don't worry about bedwetting. Many children do not stay dry at night until age seven. Most children outgrow wetting the bed. A single episode of bedwetting should not cause alarm, even in an older child.

If your child is seven years old or older and wets the bed more than two or three times in a week, a doctor may be able to help. If both day and night wetting occur after age five, your child should see a doctor before age seven.

The doctor will ask questions about your child's health and the wetting problem. Your child will likely be asked for a urine sample. The doctor uses the sample to look for signs of infection. By testing the reflexes in the child's legs and feet, the doctor can check for nerve damage. Sometimes bedwetting is a sign of diabetes, a condition that can cause frequent urination.

If your child has an infection, the doctor can prescribe medicine. In most cases, the doctor finds that the child is normal and healthy. If your child is basically healthy, a variety of ways are available to help your child stop wetting the bed.

What treatments can help my child stay dry?

Talk with your doctor about ways to help your child. Many choices exist. Let your child help decide which ones to try.

Bladder training: Bladder training can help your child hold urine longer. Write down what times your child urinates during the day. Then figure out the times between trips to the bathroom. After a day or two, have your child try to wait an extra fifteen minutes before using the bathroom. If the child usually goes to the bathroom at 3:30 p.m., have him wait until 3:45. Slowly make the times longer and longer. This method is designed for children with small bladders. It helps stretch the bladder to hold more urine. Be patient. Bladder training can take several weeks, or even months.

Moisture alarm: A small moisture alarm can be put in the child's bed or underwear. The alarm triggers a bell or buzzer with the first drops of urine. The sound wakes the child. Your child can then stop the flow of urine, get up, and use the bathroom. Waking also teaches the child how a full bladder feels.

Medicine: Two kinds of medicine are available for treating bedwetting. One medicine slows down how fast your body makes urine. The other medicine helps the bladder relax so it can hold more urine. These medicines often work well. Remember wetting may return when the child stops taking the medicine. If this occurs, keeping the child on medicine for a longer time helps.

Points to Remember

- Normal, healthy children may wet the bed.

- Bedwetting may be a sign of infection or other problems.

- Many children are dry at night by the time they are five years old. Others take longer to stay dry.

- Scolding and punishment do not help a child stop bedwetting.

- If your child is seven or older and wets the bed more than two or three times a week, a doctor may be able to help.

- Treatments include bladder training, alarms, and medicines.

- Most children grow out of bedwetting naturally.

Chapter 49

Bruxism (Teeth Grinding)

When you look in on your sleeping child, you want to hear the sounds of sweet dreams: easy breathing and perhaps an occasional sigh. But some parents hear the harsher sounds of gnashing and grinding teeth, called bruxism, which is common in kids.

About Bruxism

Bruxism is the medical term for the grinding of teeth or the clenching of jaws. Bruxism often occurs during deep sleep or while under stress. Two to three out of every ten kids will grind or clench, experts say, but most outgrow it.

Causes of Bruxism

Though studies have been done, no one knows why bruxism happens. But in some cases, kids may grind because the top and bottom teeth aren't aligned properly. Others do it as a response to pain, such as an earache or teething. Kids might grind their teeth as a way to ease the pain, just as they might rub a sore muscle. Many kids outgrow these fairly common causes for grinding.

Stress—usually nervous tension or anger—is another cause. For instance, a child might worry about a test at school or a change in routine (a new sibling or a new teacher). Even arguing with parents and siblings can cause enough stress to prompt teeth grinding or jaw clenching.

Some kids who are hyperactive also experience bruxism. And sometimes kids with other medical conditions (such as cerebral palsy) or on certain medications can develop bruxism.

Effects of Bruxism

Many cases of bruxism go undetected with no adverse effects, while others cause headaches or earaches. Usually, though, it's more bothersome to other family members because of the grinding sound.

In some circumstances, nighttime grinding and clenching can wear down tooth enamel, chip teeth, increase temperature sensitivity, and cause severe facial pain and jaw problems, such as temporomandibular joint disease (TMJ). Most kids who grind, however, do not have TMJ problems unless their grinding and clenching is chronic.

Diagnosing Bruxism

Lots of kids who grind their teeth aren't even aware of it, so it's often siblings or parents who identify the problem.

Some signs to watch for:

• Grinding noises when your child is sleeping

• Complaints of a sore jaw or face in the morning

• Pain with chewing

If you think your child is grinding his or her teeth, visit the dentist, who will examine the teeth for chipped enamel and unusual wear and tear, and spray air and water on the teeth to check for unusual sensitivity.

If damage is detected, the dentist may ask your child a few questions, such as:

• How do you feel before bed?

• Are you worried about anything at home or school?

• Are you angry with someone?

• What do you do before bed?

The exam will help the dentist determine whether the grinding is caused by anatomical (misaligned teeth) or psychological (stress) factors and come up with an effective treatment plan.

Treating Bruxism

Most kids outgrow bruxism, but a combination of parental observation and dental visits can help keep the problem in check until they do.

In cases where the grinding and clenching make a child's face and jaw sore or damage the teeth, dentists may prescribe a special night guard. Molded to a child's teeth, the night guard is similar to the protective mouthpieces worn by football players. Though a mouthpiece may take some getting used to, positive results happen quickly.

Helping Kids with Bruxism

Whether the cause is physical or psychological, kids might be able to control bruxism by relaxing before bedtime—for example, by taking a warm bath or shower, listening to a few minutes of soothing music, or reading a book.

For bruxism that's caused by stress, ask about what's upsetting your child and find a way to help. For example, a kid who is worried about being away from home for a first camping trip might need reassurance that mom or dad will be nearby if anything happens.

If the issue is more complicated, such as moving to a new town, discuss your child's concerns and try to ease any fears. If you're concerned, talk to your doctor.

In rare cases, basic stress relievers aren't enough to stop bruxism. If your child has trouble sleeping or is acting differently than usual, your dentist or doctor may suggest further evaluation. This can help determine the cause of the stress and an appropriate course of treatment.

How Long Does Bruxism Last?

Childhood bruxism is usually outgrown by adolescence. Most kids stop grinding when they lose their baby teeth. However, a few kids do continue to grind into adolescence. And if the bruxism is caused by stress, it will continue until the stress is relieved.

Preventing Bruxism

Because some bruxism is a child's natural reaction to growth and development, most cases can't be prevented. Stress-induced bruxism can be avoided, however, by talking with kids regularly about their feelings and helping them deal with stress. Take your child for routine dental visits to find and, if needed, treat bruxism.

Chapter 50

Pediatric Movement Disorders in Sleep

Head Banging and Body Rocking

What is head banging and body rocking?

Head banging and body rocking—also called rhythmic movement disorder—usually involve some type of repetitive stereotypical rocking, rolling, or head banging behaviors. These behaviors are usually seen in children around nap time and bedtime and may recur after awakenings throughout the night.

Typical movements:

- Head banging typically occurs with the child lying face down—banging the head down into a pillow or mattress. In the upright position, the head is banged against the wall or headboard repeatedly.

- Body rocking is typically done with the entire body while on the hands and knees. In the upright position, the upper body can be rocked.

Body rocking and head banging may occur at the same time. Other less common types of rhythmic movement disorders include body rolling, leg banging, and leg rolling.

"Head Banging and Body Rocking" and "Restless Legs Syndrome in Children and Adolescents," © 2009 The Cleveland Clinic Foundation, 9500 Euclid Avenue, Cleveland, OH 44195, http://my.clevelandclinic.org. Additional information is available from the Cleveland Clinic Health Information Center, 216-444-3771, toll-free 800-223-2273 extension 43771, or at http://my.clevelandclinic.org/health.

One or two movements can occur every second or two and "episodes" often last up to fifteen minutes. Sometimes this may be accompanied by humming or other vocalizations. The movements usually stop if the child is distracted or after sleep is established. Usually, there is no recall (amnesia) upon awakening.

As a parent, should I be concerned about my child's head banging and body rocking behaviors?

If your child is normal and healthy and only shows these behaviors during the night or at nap time, you should not be concerned—these are common ways for children to fall asleep. They are seen in many healthy infants and children beginning at an average of six to nine months of age. These behaviors typically subside by age two or three and by age five are only still seen in 5 percent of normal, healthy children. These movements tend to occur at the same rate in both girls and boys and may run in families with a history of these movement disorders.

Note: Head banging and body rocking behaviors should only be considered a disorder if they markedly interfere with sleep or result in bodily injury.

Parents of certain children with other health issues—including developmental delay, neurological or psychological problems, autism spectrum disorder, or those who are blind—will need to be watchful of these behaviors, as they can (though rarely) lead to injury. Of note, rhythmic behaviors in children with health problems may occur both during the day and night.

What response or protective action should a parent take?

Simply keep in mind that head banging and body rocking are normal activities that some children engage in to fall asleep. There is not much you need to do and most children will grow out of this behavior by school age. There is no real need to put extra pillows or bumpers in the crib—they usually don't work. Also, don't forget that by visiting your child while they are doing these activities, you may be reinforcing what may be an attention-seeking behavior. So, make sure you are giving your child plenty of attention during the day, and ignore this behavior at night.

As far as your child's safety is concerned, do make sure the bed or crib they are in is secure—that all the bolts and screws are checked and tightened on a regular basis. If your child is in a bed, put a guardrail up, so he or she does not roll out of bed. You may want to move the bed/crib away from the wall to reduce the noise factor at night.

When should I consult a doctor?

You may wish to discuss this with your doctor if:

- there is injury associated or you fear there is potential for harm;

- there is a lot of disruption to the home environment due to noisy head banging;

- you feel there may be other sleep disorders such as snoring and sleep apnea involved;

- you are concerned about the development of your child;

- you worry your child may be having seizures.

Restless Legs Syndrome in Children and Adolescents

What is restless legs syndrome?

Restless legs syndrome (RLS) is a movement disorder in which the child or adolescent reports an uncomfortable and irresistible urge to move his or her legs. This urge usually happens at bedtime but can occur at other times when the legs have been inactive, such as when sitting still for a long period of time (e.g., during long car rides or while watching a movie). To relieve the discomfort, the child or adolescent moves his or her legs, stretches his or her legs, tosses and turns, or gets up and walks or runs around. The relief experienced is usually immediate.

What causes restless legs syndrome?

The exact cause of this disorder is not known. RLS can be related to a low iron level or sometimes associated with diabetes, kidney, or some neurological diseases. RLS sometimes runs in families and there is thought to be a genetic link in these cases. Many types of drugs used in the treatment of other disorders may cause RLS as a side effect.

What are the signs and symptoms of restless legs syndrome?

Symptoms of restless legs syndrome include:

- **Leg discomfort or "heebie-jeebies":** Uncomfortable leg sensations described as creeping, itching, pulling, crawling, cramping, tugging, tingling, burning, gnawing, or pain. Feeling of "Coca Cola in the veins" has been described. These sensations usually occur at bedtime but can occur at other times of leg inactivity.

- **Urge to move legs:** To relieve leg discomfort, children and adolescents have an uncontrollable urge to move their legs.

- **Sleep disruption:** Additional time is often needed to fall asleep because of the urge to move the legs to relieve the discomfort. Sometimes staying asleep may also be difficult.

- **Bedtime behavior problems:** Because children have a hard time falling asleep, they may not always stay in bed and sometimes need to get out of bed to stretch their legs to relieve discomfort.

- **Daytime sleepiness:** Problems with falling asleep and staying asleep may result in problems with daytime sleepiness.

- **Behavior and school performance problems:** Again, due to sleep disruption, problems may emerge in the child's academic performance or in daytime behavior (irritability, moodiness, difficulty concentrating, hyperactivity, etc.)

How is restless legs syndrome diagnosed?

Unfortunately, there is no specific test for restless legs syndrome. Diagnosis is made based on symptoms. A medical history and complete physical exam are conducted to rule out any other possible health problems. An overnight sleep study may be recommended to evaluate for other sleep disorders, especially periodic limb movement disorder (a movement disorder in which legs kick or twitch during sleep but the child is usually not aware of the symptoms).

According to the Restless Legs Syndrome Foundation, to be officially diagnosed with restless legs syndrome, the following criteria must be met in a child older than twelve years old:

- The individual must have nearly an irresistible urge to move his or her legs. The urge is often accompanied by uncomfortable sensations described above.

- The symptoms start or become worse at rest. The longer the rest period, the greater the chance that symptoms will occur and the more severe they are likely to be.

- Symptoms are temporarily relieved when legs are moved. Relief can be complete or partial but only persists as long as legs continue to be moved.

- The restless legs symptoms are worse in the evening and especially when lying down.

Modified criteria are in place for children younger than twelve years where the diagnosis may be more uncertain. Your sleep doctor will be able to discuss this further with you and may even suggest a sleep study to help with the diagnosis.

How is restless legs syndrome treated?

Treatment options for RLS can include any of the following:

- **Adopt appropriate bedtime habits:** The child or adolescent is only to get into bed and lay in bed when it is time to go to bed. Do not get into bed and spend time reading, watching television, or playing any games.

- **Say "no" to caffeine:** Caffeine can make RLS worse, so avoid caffeinated products (e.g., coffees, teas, colas, chocolates, and some medications).

- **Use local comfort aids for legs:** Apply a heating pad, cold compress, or consider rubbing your legs to provide temporary relief to the discomfort in your legs. Also consider massage, acupressure, walking, stretching, or other relaxation techniques.

- **Supplement micronutrients:** Have your physician check your child's iron stores and if necessary, folic acid levels. Low levels of these substances can contribute to restless legs syndrome symptoms.

- **Consider medication options:** Your child's doctor may discuss several different types of drugs as options. The simplest is iron or folate supplementation as mentioned above. Other categories of drugs include dopaminergic agents (e.g., carbidopa-levodopa), dopamine agonists (e.g., ropinirole, pramipexole), benzodiazepines (e.g., clonazepam), anticonvulsants (e.g., gabapentin), and others, including clonidine.

- **Eliminate unnecessary medications:** Talk with your doctor about other medications (both prescription and over-the-counter) and herbal products your child may be taking. They may be making RLS worse. Some of the types of products to discuss with your doctor include drugs to treat nausea, colds, allergies, and depression.

- **Conduct a dietary review:** Make sure your child is eating a healthy and well-balanced diet. You may wish to review this with the doctor.

Chapter 51

Sleepwalking in Children

About Sleepwalking

Hours after bedtime, do you find your little one wandering the hall looking dazed and confused? If you have a sleepwalking child, you're not alone. It can be unnerving to see, but sleepwalking is very common in kids and most sleepwalkers only do so occasionally and outgrow it by the teen years. Still, some simple steps can keep your young sleepwalker safe while traipsing about.

Despite its name, sleepwalking (also called somnambulism) actually involves more than just walking. Sleepwalking behaviors can range from harmless (sitting up), to potentially dangerous (wandering outside), to just inappropriate (kids may even open a closet door and urinate inside). No matter what kids do during sleepwalking episodes, though, it's unlikely that they'll remember ever having done it!

As we sleep, our brains pass through five stages of sleep—stages 1, 2, 3, 4, and REM (rapid eye movement) sleep. Together, these stages make up a sleep cycle. One complete sleep cycle lasts about ninety to one hundred minutes. So a person experiences about four or five sleep cycles during an average night's sleep.

"Sleepwalking," May 2009, reprinted with permission from www.KidsHealth .org. Copyright © 2009 The Nemours Foundation. This information was provided by KidsHealth, one of the largest resources online for medically reviewed health information written for parents, kids, and teens. For more articles like this one, visit www.KidsHealth.org, or www.TeensHealth.org.

Sleepwalking most often occurs during the deeper sleep of stages 3 and 4. During these stages, it's more difficult to wake someone up, and when awakened, a person may feel groggy and disoriented for a few minutes.

Kids tend to sleepwalk within an hour or two of falling asleep and may walk around for anywhere from a few seconds to thirty minutes.

Causes of Sleepwalking

Sleepwalking is far more common in kids than in adults, as most sleepwalkers outgrow it by the early teen years. It may run in families, so if you or your partner are or were sleepwalkers, your child may be too.

Other factors that may bring on a sleepwalking episode include:

- lack of sleep or fatigue;
- irregular sleep schedules;
- illness or fever;
- certain medications;
- stress (sleepwalking is rarely caused by an underlying medical, emotional, or psychological problem).

Behaviors during Sleepwalking

Of course, getting out of bed and walking around while still sleeping is the most obvious sleepwalking symptom. But young sleepwalkers may also:

- sleep talk;
- be hard to wake up;
- seem dazed;
- be clumsy;
- not respond when spoken to;
- sit up in bed and go through repeated motions, such as rubbing their eyes or fussing with their pajamas.

Also, sleepwalkers' eyes are open, but they don't see the same way they do when they're awake and they often think they're in different rooms of the house or different places altogether.

Sometimes, these other conditions may accompany sleepwalking:

- sleep apnea (brief pauses in breathing while sleeping);

- bedwetting (enuresis);

- night terrors.

Is Sleepwalking Harmful?

Sleepwalking itself is not harmful. However, sleepwalking episodes can be hazardous since sleepwalking kids aren't awake and may not realize what they're doing, such as walking down stairs or opening windows.

Sleepwalking is not usually a sign that something is emotionally or psychologically wrong with a child. And it doesn't cause any emotional harm. Sleepwalkers probably won't even remember the nighttime stroll.

How to Keep a Sleepwalker Safe

Although sleepwalking isn't dangerous by itself, it's important to take precautions so that your sleepwalking child is less likely to fall down, run into something, walk out the front door, or drive (if your teen is a sleepwalker).

To help keep your sleepwalker out of harm's way:

- Try not to wake a sleepwalker because this might scare your child. Instead, gently guide him or her back to bed.

- Lock the windows and doors, not just in your child's bedroom but throughout your home, in case your young sleepwalker decides to wander. You may consider extra locks or child safety locks on doors. Keys should be kept out of reach for kids who are old enough to drive.

- To prevent falls, don't let your sleepwalker sleep in a bunk bed.

- Remove sharp or breakable things from around your child's bed.

- Keep dangerous objects out of reach.

- Remove obstacles from your child's room and throughout your home to prevent a stumble. Especially eliminate clutter on the floor (i.e., in your child's bedroom or playroom).

- Install safety gates outside your child's room and/or at the top of any stairs.

Other Ways to Help a Sleepwalker

Unless the episodes are very regular, cause your child to be sleepy during the day, or your child is engaging in dangerous sleepwalking behaviors, there's usually no need to treat sleepwalking. But if the sleepwalking is frequent, causing problems, or your child hasn't out-grown it by the early teen years, talk to your doctor. Also talk to your doctor if you're concerned that something else could be going on, like reflux or trouble breathing.

For kids who sleepwalk often, doctors may recommend a treatment called scheduled awakening. This disrupts the sleep cycle enough to help stop sleepwalking. In rare cases, a doctor may prescribe medication to help a child sleep.

Other ways to help minimize sleepwalking episodes:

- Have your child relax at bedtime by listening to soft music or re-laxation tapes.

- Establish a regular sleep and nap schedule and stick to it—both nighttime and wake-up time.

- Make your child's bedtime earlier. This can improve excessive sleepiness.

- Don't let kids drink a lot in the evening and be sure they go to the bathroom before going to bed. (A full bladder can contribute to sleepwalking.)

- Avoid caffeine near bedtime.

- Make sure your child's bedroom is quiet, cozy, and conducive to sleeping. Keep noise to a minimum while kids are trying to sleep (at bedtime and nap time).

The next time you encounter your nighttime wanderer, don't panic. Simply steer your child back to the safety and comfort of his or her bed.

Chapter 52

Sleep Concerns among Teens

Chapter Contents

Section 52.1

School Start Time: Should It Be Pushed Back?

"Sleep Loss Affects High Schoolers," by Elizabeth Crown, June 7, 2005, Northwestern University News Center. © 2005 Northwestern University. Reprinted with permission. Reviewed by David A. Cooke, MD, FACP, August 2010.

Current high school start times deprive adolescents of sleep and force students to perform academically in the early morning, a time of day when they are at their worst, according to a study in the June 2005 issue of the journal *Pediatrics*.

Results from high school senior sleep/wake diaries kept for the study also showed that adolescents lost as much as two hours of sleep per night during the school week, but weekend sleep times during the school year were similar to those in summer.

The study was a collaborative project involving researchers at the Feinberg School of Medicine and the Center for Sleep and Circadian Biology at Northwestern University and faculty, students, and parents from Evanston Township High School, Evanston, Illinois. The students were advanced placement biology students who helped conduct the study and analyze the collected data.

Martha Hansen, advanced placement biology teacher and current science department chair at Evanston Township High School, headed the project in collaboration with Margarita L. Dubocovich, professor of molecular pharmacology and biological chemistry and of psychiatry and behavioral sciences, Feinberg; and Phyllis C. Zee, M.D., professor of neurology, Feinberg.

The study assessed the impact of sleep loss after the start of school on cognitive performance and mood and examined the relationship of weekday to weekend sleep in adolescents.

The study also showed that exposure to bright light in the morning did not modify students' sleep-wake cycle or improve daytime performance during weekdays, probably because of their strict school schedule. All students performed better in the afternoon than in the morning. Students in early morning classes reported being wearier, less alert, and having to expend greater effort.

Potential solutions to this problem could be solved by changing school start times and by giving standardized tests later in the day, the authors suggested.

For example, classes at Evanston Township High School start at 8:05 a.m. and run until 3:35 p.m.—one of the longest school days in Illinois. Many high schools in the country have start times of 7:15 or 7:30 a.m. In addition, almost all standardized tests in high school begin at 8 a.m.

Since this is when adolescents show their poorest performance levels, a change is clearly needed and would be relatively easy to negotiate, the researchers suggest.

While the authors emphasized that more research on adolescent circadian rhythms is needed, they also believe that all groups dealing with adolescents—pediatricians, parents, teachers, and teenagers themselves—need to be aware of adolescents' lifestyle patterns and the unusual weekday/weekend sleep phenomena.

"Knowledge of adolescent circadian rhythms could promote better family relationships if parents understood that sleeping late on weekends is part of their children's in-born cycle and not 'lazy' or antisocial behavior," the researchers said.

Finally, this sleep study forged collaboration between high school students and faculty where everyone learned and benefited from the experience.

"Students were able to learn about the process of collecting and analyzing data and to discover more about the fascinating topic of themselves," the authors said.

Other researchers on the study were Imke Janssen, statistician and Evanston Township High School parent; and Adam Schiff, a former Evanston Township High School student, currently in medical school.

Section 52.2

Sleepy Teens: Problems at School and Behind the Wheel

Reprinted from "Sleepy Teens at School and Behind the Wheel," Substance Abuse and Mental Health Services Administration, U.S. Department of Health and Human Services, March 31, 2004. Reviewed by David A. Cooke, MD, FACP, April 2010.

"Kids have so much energy!" is not true for many American teens, who actually require more sleep than they did as children. A poll by the National Sleep Foundation (NSF) shows that most teens are not getting the 9.25 hours of sleep they need each night.[1] One reason is that a teen's biological clock changes during puberty and disrupts his or her normal sleep-wake cycle. Many teens find it is hard to fall asleep until late at night; then they want to sleep later in the morning. However, many demands on teens, such as early school times, conflict with their new sleeping pattern. As a result, teens often do not get the sleep they need. They are sleepy when they most need to be alert. Teens can have trouble paying attention and learning in school, especially in the morning. In the NSF poll, 15 percent of teens said they fell asleep at school sometime during the year.[2]

Teens who drive while sleepy are a danger to themselves and others. Driving drowsy can be like driving under the influence of drugs or alcohol. Sleepy teens are more likely to have breaks in attention, impaired memory and judgment, and slower reactions at critical times.[3] Police report that drowsiness or fatigue causes at least 100,000 traffic crashes each year. These crashes kill more than 1,500 people and injure another 71,000. Drivers aged twenty-five and younger are involved in more than half of the crashes in which the driver has fallen asleep.[4]

Parents need to find ways to help their teens be well rested, ready to face the school day and the road. The tips below may help.

Sleep-Smart Tips for Parents and Teens

Set a bedtime routine: A regular bedtime helps the body get used to a sleep schedule. Your teen's bedtime routine should include at least fifteen to thirty minutes of low-key activities such as reading or taking a warm bath. He or she should avoid exercise, telephone use, and playing video games during this time. For a few hours before bedtime, your teen also should avoid caffeine, which is found in many beverages, in chocolate, and in other products.

Make sleep an important activity: Help your teen set priorities for activities. Make sure that downtime and sleep are high on the list. Many teens lose sleep because they have too many demands on their time. Too many activities can lead to stress, poor health, and sleep problems.

Look for signs of lack of sleep: Your teen may not be getting enough sleep if he or she finds it hard to wake up in the morning or falls asleep during quiet times of the day. Another sign is that your teen sleeps for extra long periods whenever he or she can. A teen who isn't getting enough sleep also may be cranky in the afternoon or may seem depressed.

Follow the light: Use bright light and sunshine to help your teen wake up in the morning. Low light at night will help a teen's body get ready for sleep.

Be a good role model: Create a home life that supports healthy sleep habits for the whole family. Set an example by making sure that you get enough sleep. You also need to be able to deal well with the challenges of your day, including being a good parent.

Sources

1. National Sleep Foundation. Too Many Teens May Be Sleepy Behind Their Desks—and Behind the Wheel: Back to School Means Adjusting Sleep Habits of Teens, last referenced 3/3/04.

2. Ibid.

3. National Institutes of Health. Sustained Reduced Sleep Can Have Serious Consequences, last referenced 3/4/04.

4. National Sleep Foundation. Adolescent Sleep Needs and Patterns: Research Report and Resource Guide, last referenced 3/3/04.

Section 52.3

Caffeine and Teens' Sleep

Reprinted from "Caffeine and Teens' Sleep: An Eye-Opening Study," Substance Abuse and Mental Health Services Administration, U.S. Department of Health and Human Services, March 29, 2004. Reviewed by David A. Cooke, MD, FACP, April 2010.

You may have spotted your teen staying up later than he or she used to. Activities that could be filling his or her late hours might include computer games, TV shows, phone calls, or music. Have you ever thought about caffeine intake as one of the reasons your teen is a night owl?

According to a recent study, eating foods, drinking beverages, or taking medications that have caffeine may lead to daytime sleepiness and breaks in sleep at night. Almost two hundred high school students took part in this fourteen-day study. They reported on the time they went to bed and woke up, any caffeine intake, and any naps they took. At the end of the study, the researchers found that teens with higher caffeine intake slept fewer hours at night and took more naps during the day than those who had less caffeine.[1]

What Does This Mean?

Broken sleep patterns can have many effects on a child. These include the following[2]:

- Academic trouble
- Anxiety
- Decrease in cognitive development
- Depression (more common among females)
- Decreased immunity to illness
- Moodiness
- Reduced motivation

Caffeine can be found in many sodas, coffee, tea, and chocolate. It is also one of the most commonly used drugs in some pain medications and over-the-counter drugs. Caffeine stimulates the central nervous system and raises the heart rate, which can lead to nervous system disorders and heart problems.

Like many drugs, caffeine can be addictive. Once the body becomes used to the caffeine intake, it needs more to feel the same effect. This often causes a continued increase in caffeine intake.

What to Do?

Now that you know some of the problems linked to loss of sleep and caffeine intake, you might be wondering how you can help your teen. Here are some tips:

- Avoid caffeinated drinks and products in the evening. Offer juice, milk, and water instead of soft drinks or tea and coffee.

- Adjust plans to allow plenty of time for homework, studying, and writing reports and don't allow all-nighters. This will cut down on the desire to take coffee or drugs with caffeine.

- Talk with your teen and agree on a bedtime. Help your teen plan how to get enough sleep. Some activities may need to be cut out or cut down to keep with the bedtime.

- Urge your teen to stick to the plan as much as possible over the weekend.

These ideas can help reduce sleep deprivation. How do you help your teen kick the caffeine habit? Stopping caffeine intake cold turkey can cause withdrawal symptoms, including headaches, short-term depression or moodiness, and muscle aches. To avoid withdrawal, suggest slowly cutting back on caffeine.[3] Cutting back may be hard at first, but after a few days your teen most likely will feel better rested and no longer suffer the effects of losing sleep.

References

1. Pollak, Charles, and David Bright. January 2003 Caffeine Consumption and Weekly Sleep Patterns in U.S. Seventh-, Eighth, and Ninth-Grader. *Pediatrics*. Vol. 111, No. 1, 42–46.

2. Sleep Foundation. Adolescent Sleep Needs and Patterns, last referenced, 3/3/04.

3. University of California at Berkeley. Exploring the Link Between Caffeine Withdrawal Symptoms and the Neurochemical

Changes Caused by Regular Caffeine Consumption, last referenced 3/3/04.

4. Johns Hopkins Bayview Medical Center. Information About Caffeine Dependence, last referenced 3/3/04.

Section 52.4

Sleep May Reduce Depression in Teens

Researchers at Columbia University Medical Center have found new evidence that inadequate sleep can lead to depression and suicidal thoughts in adolescents.

The study of nearly sixteen thousand teenagers in grades seven to twelve found that adolescents with bedtimes set at midnight or later were 24 percent more likely to suffer from depression than those with bedtimes of 10 p.m. or earlier. Teenagers with later bedtimes also were 20 percent more likely to have suicidal thoughts.

The study was published in the January 2010 issue of the journal *Sleep*.

Depression and poor sleep often go hand in hand, but sleep difficulties are usually seen as a symptom of depression, not a cause, says James Gangwisch, Ph.D., assistant professor in the Department of Psychiatry and lead investigator of the new study.

To see if sleep deprivation can lead to depression, researchers would have to alter teenagers' sleep schedules and record the results. Such an experiment would be unethical, given other known detriments of sleep deprivation, and too expensive with large numbers of teenagers.

Instead, Dr. Gangwisch did the next best thing. He gathered data from a "natural experiment": what happened when teenagers had their bedtimes imposed by their parents. These data on bedtime and depression came from a previous survey, the National Longitudinal Study of Adolescent Health, conducted between 1994 and 1996.

"Depression in adolescents can affect their choice of bedtime, but it's less likely to affect their parents' choice," Dr. Gangwisch says, "By using data from the survey, we got some of the benefits of a large experimental study without the drawbacks.

"Together with smaller studies that have shown sleep deprivation alters mood in teenagers, our finding is strong evidence that inadequate sleep plays a role in causing depression."

The reasons why sleep deprivation may lead to depression, though, are still unclear. Dr. Gangwisch says moodiness from a lack of sleep may interfere with a teenager's ability to cope with daily stress or impair relationships with friends and family. Suicidal thoughts may increase due to the effects of insufficient sleep on judgment, aggression, and impulse control.

Of course, telling teenagers to go to bed at 10 p.m. does not mean they will actually go to sleep. But nearly 70 percent of the teenagers in the study reported going to bed at or before bedtimes set by their parents.

"The biggest question I get from parents is how to get their teenagers to bed earlier," Dr. Gangwisch says. "I think it's a matter of motivating teenagers to see the benefits. I'd encourage teenagers to try a few nights of eight or nine hours of sleep and see if they feel better during the day.

"In our society we think we can cut back on sleep to be more productive during the day, but the loss of concentration, energy, motivation, and now mood changes resulting from insufficient sleep can make us less productive during the day, making the extra time devoted to sleep well worth it."

Section 52.5

Lack of Sleep May Lead to High Blood Pressure in Teens

"Catch Your ZZZZZs!" *Medline Plus Magazine*, Fall 2008 (3, no. 4): 27.

Nodding off in school may not be the only outcome for otherwise healthy teens who don't get enough sleep. A recent study links poor sleep in teens (ages thirteen to sixteen years old) to higher blood pressure. Researchers found that teens who got less than 6.5 hours sleep were two and a half times more likely to have elevated blood pressure than teens who slept longer. Also, teens who had trouble falling asleep or staying asleep were three and a half times more likely to have high blood pressure or pre–high blood pressure than teens who slept well. These results are similar to findings from other studies in adults. High blood pressure, if left untreated, can increase the risk of stroke and heart diseases later in life.

The research study funded by the National Heart, Lung, and Blood Institute was conducted by a team at Case Western Reserve University in Cleveland, Ohio.

Sleep Facts

- School-aged children and teens need at least nine hours of sleep a night.

- Adults need seven to eight hours of sleep a night.

Sleep Tips

- Set a sleep schedule; going to bed and waking up the same times each day.

- Keep room temperature on the cool side.

- A TV or computer in the bedroom can be a distraction.

Part Seven

Additional Help and Information

Chapter 53

Glossary of Terms Related to Sleep and Sleep Disorders

advanced sleep phase syndrome (ASPS): A circadian rhythm disorder in which sleep onset occurs in early evening and as a consequence, wakefulness occurs in early morning. This disorder is more common in the elderly.

alpha waves: Electroencephalogram (EEG, or brain) wave activity that occurs during quiet wakefulness, such as when the eyes are closed. The frequency of alpha waves is between 8 to 12 hertz (cycles per second). It is indicative of the wakeful state in humans.

alternative medicine: Any of the various practices or healing methods for treating illness that are not taught in a traditional curricula of a U.S. or U.K. medical school. Some of these include homeopathy, herbal remedies, acupuncture, meditation, chiropractic medicine, and faith healing.

anticonvulsant: A class of drugs that work to suppress sensory disturbances; they are often used to treat epileptic seizures.

antidepressant: A type of drug traditionally used to relieve or prevent psychiatric disorders associated with depression, anxiety, and obsessive-compulsive disorder but also used in the treatment of cataplexy, hypnagogic hallucinations, and sleep paralysis.

"Sleep Dictionary," © 2000 Talk About Sleep (www.talkaboutsleep.com). Revised by David A. Cooke, M.D., F.A.C.P., May 2010. All rights reserved. Reprinted with permission.

antihistamine: A drug that inhibits histamine, a compound that mediates inflammation and produces allergic reactions; antihistamines are a common ingredient in over-the-counter sleeping pills because of their sedative effect.

anxiolytics: A drug that relieves anxiety.

apnea: Derived from Greek translated as "want of breath"; episodes of nonrespiration during sleep that last at least ten seconds. See central or mixed sleep apnea.

arousal: "Partial" arousal is an abrupt change from a "deep" stage of non–rapid eye movement (NREM) sleep (stage 3–4) to a "lighter" one (stage 2 or 1). "Full" arousal means awakening. During an arousal, your muscle tone increases, your heart may beat faster, and you may move.

augmentation: A result of prolonged use of dopaminergic agents in which symptoms (of restless legs syndrome) are chased into the daytime, sometimes necessitating daytime dosing.

automatic behavior: Performing activities or tasks with little or no recollection of the event.

awakening: "Spontaneous" awakenings most often start while you are in REM sleep, although you may awaken from NREM sleep, as well. When you are awake, your brain waves are of the alpha or beta pattern (see brain wave rhythms), your muscle tone is high, and you can move voluntarily.

bedtime: Defined as the time when one attempts to fall asleep (as distinguished from the time one gets into bed).

beta waves: EEG (brain) wave activity with a frequency of 13 to 35 hertz (cycles per second) that is typically seen in active wakefulness and also associated with taking psychotropic drugs, in which the eyes blink repeatedly.

benzodiazepine: A class of central nervous system depressants; examples include Valium® (diazepam), Klonopin® (clonazepam), Restoril® (temazepam), and Halcion® (triazolam); useful for managing insomnia, restless legs syndrome, periodic limb movement disorder, sleepwalking, and rapid eye movement (REM) behavior disorder. Ambien® (zolpidem), Sonata® (Zaleplon), and Lunesta® (eszopiclone) have very similar effects but are not technically considered benzodiazepines.

bilevel positive airway pressure (BiPAP): An air compressor that blows a higher pressure for inhaling and a lower pressure for exhaling. BiPAP is generally used for apnea patients who cannot tolerate high constant air pressure with continuous positive airway pressure (CPAP).

bimaxillary advancement: A surgical procedure in which the upper and lower jawbones and teeth are moved forward and held in place with titanium plates and screws so that soft tissue structures are pulled forward, creating more space for the tongue.

"biological clock": The term used to describe an internal timing mechanism that exists in most living systems and is thought to be located in the suprachiasmatic nucleus. It is the current explanation by which various cyclical behaviors and physiological processes are regulated and synchronized with environmental events.

biological rhythm: A regular pattern or cycle of change in an organism related to a physical variable, such as heart rate, body temperature, sleep-wake cycle, and so on.

BiPAP: An acronym for bilevel positive airway pressure; an alternative therapy to continuous positive airway pressure (CPAP) for the treatment of obstructive sleep apnea that allows for choosing a separate respiratory and expiratory pressure.

brain-wave rhythms: Patterns of electrical activity of the brain. They include: alpha rhythms (most consistent and predominant during relaxed wakefulness, particularly when your eyes are closed or you are in the dark, they cycle eighteen times per second); beta rhythms (usually associated with alert wakefulness, they are faster than alpha waves, cycling about thirteen to thirty-five times per second); delta rhythms (occurring chiefly in deep sleep stages 3 to 4, also known as slow sleep, they cycle less than four times per second); and theta rhythms (associated with the light sleep stages 1 and 2, these cycle four to eight times per second).

bright light therapy: A treatment used to treat circadian rhythm disturbances; also used to treat seasonal affective disorder (SAD).

bruxism: also called teeth grinding; a parasomnia characterized by the grinding or clenching of teeth during sleep.

cataplexy: A temporary decrease or complete loss of muscle control triggered by an emotional response that is often seen in narcoleptics. Also, a sudden, dramatic drop in muscle tone and loss of deep reflexes, which leads to muscle weakness or paralysis (an attack may cause a person to collapse). It is usually triggered by an emotional stimulus such as laughing or being startled, or by some sudden physical exertion. Cataplexy is a symptom of narcolepsy, a neurologic disorder that causes excessive sleepiness.

central nervous system (CNS): The part of the nervous system that consists of the brain and the spinal cord, which are responsible for the coordination of all motor and mental activities.

central sleep apnea: Episodes of nonrespiration during sleep for ten seconds or longer that are caused by the brain failing to signal the respiratory muscles to breathe.

chronic insomnia: Regular sleeplessness that lasts for more than three weeks and is persistent without treatment.

chronobiology: The scientific study of biological rhythms and timing mechanisms, sleep-wake cycles, heart rate, hibernation cycles, and body temperature.

circadian: A cycle that lasts about twenty-four hours.

circadian rhythms: The process of biological variations over twenty-four hours, coordinated by the suprachiasmatic nuclei in the brain, which regulate body temperature, hormone secretions, and other physiological functions.

cognitive-behavioral therapy: Psychological therapy which focuses on changing attitudes and beliefs related to sleep and insomnia.

complementary medicine: The science of combining one or more conventional treatments with one or more alternative treatments to aid in the healing process. For example, treatment for insomnia might include a medication in combination with relaxation therapy.

compulsive hyperphagia: A disorder of excessive and compulsive overeating; it is often accompanied by other disorders, such as hypersexuality and hypersomnia, and is also associated with Kleine-Levin syndrome.

continuous positive airway pressure: Also known as CPAP; A type of therapy used to effectively treat obstructive sleep apnea in which an air compressor forces air through the nose and into the airway by way of a light mask worn over the nose during sleep.

cortisol: (The same as hydrocortisone) a steroid hormone produced in the adrenal gland that influences the metabolism of various cell types.

CPAP: An acronym for continuous positive airway pressure; an effective therapy used to treat obstructive sleep apnea.

delayed sleep phase syndrome: Also known as DSPS; A circadian rhythm sleep disorder characterized by difficulty achieving sleep onset in the evening and difficulty waking up at a desired time in the morning. It involves a desired sleep time out of sync with physiologic sleep time.

delta waves: EEG activity with a frequency of less than 4 hertz (cycles per second) that is most often seen in stage 3 and 4 of non-REM sleep.

delta sleep: Also called slow wave sleep; a term used to describe the stages of sleep characterized by delta waves. It is regarded as the most restorative time of sleep.

dopaminergic agents: A class of drugs synthesized with the neurotransmitter dopamine and most often used to treat Parkinson patients; often helpful in managing restless legs syndrome and periodic limb movement disorder. Examples include Parlodel® (bromocriptine), Requip® (ropinirole), and Mirapex® (pramipexole).

dreams: Periods of intense vivid imagery during sleep, often associated with rapid eye movements.

electroencephalogram: Also called an EEG; the measurement and recording of brain wave activity. Frequency measurement in hertz ranges from below 3.5 per second (delta), 4 to 7.5 per second (theta), 8 to 12 per second (alpha), and above 13 per second (beta). Electrodes are typically placed at C3 and C4 positions on the scalp.

electromyogram: Also called an EMG; the measurement and recording of muscle activity, particularly under the chin, along the jaw, and on the legs.

electrooculogram: Also called an EOG; the detection and recording of eye movements, essential for determining the different sleep stages.

endogenous circadian pacemaker: An internal mechanism in the brain, thought to be at the site of the suprachiasmatic nucleus, that drives periodic processes, such as the sleep-wake cycle, body temperature, and cortisol release, in the human circadian timing system.

enuresis: Also called bedwetting or sleep enuresis; uncontrolled urination during sleep. This disorder is more common in children and often related to maturation; however, repeated nocturnal bedwetting can indicate other physical or emotional problems.

excessive daytime sleepiness: Sometimes called excessive sleepiness, the inability to stay awake during the normal wake period of a sleep-wake cycle or may involve involuntary sleep. Common causes include: insufficient sleep, sleep apnea, narcolepsy, and insomnia.

"Factor S": A substance in the cerebrospinal fluid that has sleep-inducing properties.

fragmentation: The interruption of any stage of sleep due to appearance of another stage or waking. Sleep fragmentation connotes repetitive interruptions of sleep by arousals and awakenings.

genioglossus muscle: A muscle that attaches from the back of the tongue to a region on the back of the chin and serves to advance, retract, and depress the tongue.

genioglossus advancement: A surgical operation that detaches the genioglossus muscle from its insertion point and reattaches it in a more advanced position in order to pull the back of the tongue forward, enlarging the air space behind the tongue.

glossectomy: The surgical reduction or removal of the tongue, used to open the lower airway or to remove cancerous tissue.

Hertz (Hz): The unit of measurement for cycles per second; used to measure EEGs.

homeostatic: (homeostasis, n.) The balanced state of the living body (i.e., temperature, chemistry, blood pressure, sleep and wakefulness, and so on), despite variations in the environment.

hyoid advancement: A surgical operation in which the hyoid bone is moved forward and either attached to the Adam's apple or to the jawbone, enlarging the air space behind the tongue.

hyoid bone: A C-shaped bone in the upper neck positioned above the Adam's apple with muscle attachments to the back of the tongue, as well as the sides of the lower throat.

hypersomnia: Also called excessive (daytime) sleepiness or somnolence; the inability to remain awake during an individual's normal wake period.

hypnagogic hallucinations: Vivid, often frightening, dreamlike images and sounds experienced at REM sleep onset, usually accompanied by fear and anxiety; a characteristic feature of narcolepsy.

hypnic jerk: Also called sleep starts; the sensation of falling and then a physical jerk into wakefulness, usually during stage 1 sleep.

hypnotic: Also called a sleeping pill, sedative, or a sedative-hypnotic medication; a medication that causes drowsiness, induces sleep onset, and/or maintains sleep.

"hypnotoxin": Also called sleep-promoting substance (SPS); the term coined by Henri Pieron in 1907 that described a sleep-inducing substance thought to be in the cerebrospinal fluid.

hypopnea: An episode of abnormally slow or shallow respiration during sleep that lasts longer than ten seconds. Hypopnea differs from apnea in that some airflow is present.

hypothalamus: The region at the base of the brain involved in autonomic processes such as temperature regulation, food intake, and emotional activity, and thought to be important in the role of sleep and wakefulness.

idiopathic: Occurring spontaneously and without known cause.

idiopathic hypersomnia: A disorder of excessive sleepiness in which the affected individual sleeps longer than normal (greater than ten hours), is excessively sleepy, falls asleep at inappropriate times, and frequently takes naps. Its exact cause is unknown.

insomnia: The inability to sleep applied to the general complaint of having trouble falling or staying asleep; insomnia is a symptom usually caused by underlying problems. See also transient, short-term, chronic, and sleep onset insomnia.

jet lag: A condition that occurs following air travel through multiple time zones (usually three or more zones) and is characterized by various psychological and physiological effects, such as fatigue, gastrointestinal disturbances, and irritability, caused by a disruption in circadian rhythms.

K-complex: High-voltage EEG activity that consists of a sharp upward component followed by a slower downward component and lasts more than 0.5 seconds; required for definition of stage 2 non-REM sleep.

Kleine-Levin syndrome: A disorder distinguished by recurrent hypersomnia, compulsive overeating, and hypersexuality and first described by Willi Kleine in 1925 and then by Max Levin in 1929.

lark: Also called a morning person or morning lark; a person who prefers go to bed early in the evening and rise early in the morning. This tendency becomes more common in the elderly.

laser-assisted uvulopalatoplasty (LAUP): A surgical procedure for the treatment of habitual loud snoring or obstructive sleep apnea that involves removal of the back edge of the palate, the uvula, and if present, the tonsils.

latency period: An interval. Sleep latency is the interval from "lights out" until sleep begins. REM latency is the period from the beginning of sleep to the first appearance of rapid eye movement (REM) sleep.

L-Dopa: A drug which is converted into dopamine within the central nervous system, most often used to treat Parkinson patients. It is also often helpful in managing restless legs syndrome and periodic limb movement disorder. It is usually prescribed as a combination tablet with a peripheral dopa decarboxylase inhibitor to prevent overly rapid breakdown. Commonly used combinations include Sinemet® and Sta-levo®.

"leucomaines": The name for the poisonous substances that supposedly accumulated during the day and passed from the blood to the brain. Leo Errera proposed that these substances in the 1880s were the cause of sleep.

light box: A commercially available, electrically powered instrument that provides artificial light; a treatment option for patients with seasonal affective disorder, advanced phase sleep disorder, or delayed phase sleep disorder.

light therapy: A treatment for various disorders including seasonal affective disorder, depression, hypersomnia, and delayed phase sleep disorder. It involves properly timed exposure to bright light to promote a normal sleep-wake cycle and decrease sleep disturbances.

lingualplasty: A surgical procedure that involves a resection of the tongue with additional removal of side wedges in order to reduce the back of the tongue and open the lower airway.

lingual tonsils: Tonsil-like tissue on the back part of the tongue.

lux: A measure of light intensity; the unit used by light box manufacturers to describe light output.

maintenance of wakefulness test: also called MWT; a test that consists of four twenty-minute trials conducted every two hours and used to determine a patient's ability to stay awake during the day. Contrary to a multiple sleep latency test (MSLT), the MWT is scored on the patient's ability to remain awake during the trials.

melatonin: In nature, a hormone that is secreted by the pineal gland in the brain in response to darkness, and has been linked to regulation of circadian rhythms; a derivative of melatonin marketed as a health food supplement is commercially available.

mental imagery: The process of creating images in the mind.

microsleep: A lapse from wakefulness into sleep that lasts just a few seconds.

mixed sleep apnea: The combination of central and obstructive sleep apnea.

montage: The term applied to the testing variables and their order on polysomnogram paper or a computer monitor, such EEG, EOG, heart rate, and so on.

MSLT: The acronym for multiple sleep latency test; a test used to study and document excessive daytime sleepiness by way of a series of naps at two-hour intervals.

multiple sleep latency test: A test used to study and document excessive daytime sleepiness by way of a series of naps at two-hour intervals.

MWT: An acronym for the maintenance of wakefulness test, in which four twenty-minute trials are conducted every two hours and the patient is encouraged to stay awake.

myoclonus: See nocturnal myoclonus.

narcolepsy: A physical condition characterized by episodes of inappropriate and often involuntary sleep in the form of naps that may last a few minutes to hours; usually accompanied by cataplexy, sleep paralysis, and hypnagogic hallucinations.

National Sleep Foundation (NSF): Established in 1990 as an "independent nonprofit organization dedicated to improving public health and safety by achieving public understanding of sleep and sleep disorders."

negative sleep conditioning: A psychological state perpetuated by self-induced stress and anxiety of needing to attain sleep; specifically, it refers to an inability to sleep at night in one's own bed.

neuron: A type of nerve cell (or brain cell) that has a central cell body (axon) and long endings (dendrites) specialized to receive, conduct, and transmit signals in the nervous system.

nightmare: A sleep-disrupting dream that is often recalled in detail. An anxiety-filled dream that often wakes the sleeper from REM sleep. It is distinguished from "sleep terror," which is sudden, partial arousal from NREM sleep that may cause the sleeper to cry out in fright but that seldom includes vivid images.

night owl: Also called a night person or evening person; a name applied to someone who prefers to stay up into the night or early morning and arise in late morning.

nocturia: Also called nycturia; frequent urination at night that results in arousal of sleep and rising frequently to go to the bathroom. It can be caused by urological problems, infection, a tumor, or medication and has been associated with the development of obstructive sleep apnea.

nocturnal: Of the night or night-related; the opposite of diurnal.

nocturnal myoclonus: A brief rapid twitch that occurs at night as a result of a sudden contraction of one or more muscle groups; former name of periodic limb movement disorder.

non-REM sleep: A state of sleep characterized by four stages that range from light dozing to deep sleep; 75 percent of sleep is spent in non-REM sleep. In stages 3 and 4 of NREM sleep, there is a decrease in blood pressure, muscle activity, and respiratory rate as the sleeper relaxes.

normal hypersomnia: A disorder in which the affected individual requires more sleep than normal, that is, more than ten hours of sleep per day, and which may be the result of a genetic predisposition. Normal hypersomniacs are also called "naturally long sleepers."

obstructive sleep apnea (syndrome): Also called OSA; a common form of apnea, in which the airway is blocked, resulting in a lack of respiration and a momentary interruption of sleep; usually caused by physical abnormality.

opiate: A class of controlled narcotics, such as Tylenol #3, Percocet® (oxycodone), Darvon® (propoxyphene), and methadone; used to manage severe cases of restless legs syndrome and periodic limb movement disorder.

OTCs: An acronym for over-the-counter medications, those that are available for purchase without a prescription.

OSA: An acronym for obstructive sleep apnea; a common form of apnea.

otolaryngology: The medical study of the ears, nose, and throat (ENT).

over-the-counter medications: Drugs that are available to the general public without a prescription.

paradoxical therapy: An effective therapeutic approach to conquering insomnia that asks the insomniac to do the exact opposite of trying to fall asleep.

parasomnia: A term used to describe uncommon disruptive sleep-related disorders, such as sleepwalking, sleep talking, and nightmares.

pavor nocturnus: A term derived from Latin *pavor,* terror, and *nocturnus,* at night. See also sleep terrors.

periodic limb movement disorder: Also called PLMD, periodic limb movement syndrome, or PLMS; a condition in which the legs or arms twitch or move involuntarily and periodically during sleep.

periodic limb movement index: The record of the number of leg or arm movements during each hour of sleep, measured by sensors placed on the legs and arms.

Pickwickian syndrome: The first term applied to obstructive sleep apnea, originally described by Charles Dickens in 1836. It referred to people who were excessively sleepy, loud snorers, and overweight.

PLMD: An acronym for periodic limb movement disorder; a condition in which the legs or arms twitch or move involuntarily and periodically during sleep.

polyp: A projecting growth or mass, usually benign, that forms in a mucous membrane and in the nasal passages, causes obstructed airflow.

polysomnogram: Also called a PSG, sleep study, or sleep test; a noninvasive test that records vital signs and physiology during a night of sleep. It includes measurements from an EEG, EMG, and EOG, as well as respiratory airflow, blood oxygen saturation, pulse rate, heart rate, body position, and respiratory effort.

postprandial dip: A slight drowsiness caused by a natural drop in body temperature, particularly in early afternoon and after a meal.

post-traumatic hypersomnia: A disorder of excessive sleepiness that appears within eighteen months of a traumatic event involving a central nervous system-related accident.

primary snoring: Snoring not associated with apnea.

process C: The natural behavior and tendency, regulated by human circadian rhythms, to sleep during the "sleepy phase" of the body, usually between 11:00 p.m. and 7:00 a.m.

process S: Also known as the homeostatic process, it is the disposition of a normal person who is sleep-deprived to become sleepy when awake, and sleep deeper and longer when sleep is achieved.

pupillometry: The measurement of pupil diameter and activity as related to alertness or sleepiness. This test is used more for research rather than a diagnostic assessment.

radio-frequency tissue ablation: A technique that uses radio-frequency waves via a needle electrode placed under the surface of the tissue, resulting in contraction and subsequent shrinkage of excessive tissues that cause snoring.

recurrent hypersomnia: A disorder of excessive sleepiness that occurs weeks or months apart, often accompanied by other disorders such as hypersexuality or compulsive eating.

relaxation therapy: Also termed relaxation imagery; various methods or techniques for the alleviation of insomnia that help to relax the mind and the body and which can facilitate sleep onset.

REM latency: The period of time in the sleep period from sleep onset to the first appearance of REM sleep.

REM onset: The designation for commencement of a REM period.

REM percent: The proportion of total sleep time constituted by the REM stage of sleep.

REM rebound or recovery: An increased amount of REM sleep for a few nights after a period of REM deprivation. REM rebound may occur after several days without sleep, or upon withdrawal from certain drugs, including some sleeping pills, that suppress REM sleep. Increased amounts of REM sleep may be reflected by disturbing dreams.

REM sleep: Also known as "paradoxical" sleep, this state of sleep is characterized by rapid eye movement (REM), muscle paralysis, and irregular breathing, heart rate, and blood pressure. Dreaming takes place during REM sleep.

respiratory disturbance index (RDI): A record of the number and duration of apnea episodes, both obstructive and central, during each hour of sleep. An RDI of greater than 5 is regarded as abnormal.

restless legs syndrome: Also called RLS; a neurological disorder of unknown cause that causes irrepressible twitching and creeping sensations in the legs while sitting or lying down.

RLS: An acronym for restless legs syndrome; a disorder that causes irrepressible and uncontrollable tingling sensations in the legs.

SAD: An acronym for seasonal affective disorder; a disorder with depression-like symptoms that occurs in the late fall because of less light exposure and diminishes with the onset of spring.

SCN: An acronym for suprachiasmatic nuclei and sometimes called the endogenous circadian pacemaker; small structures in the brain, sensitive to the presence or absence of light, that coordinate circadian rhythms.

seasonal affective disorder: A disorder characterized by depression, sleeping too much, overeating, diminished sex drive, working less productively, and other depression-related symptoms that occurs in the mid-to-late fall due to less light exposure. Symptoms usually diminish with the onset of spring.

sedative: Also called a sleeping pill or hypnotic; a medication that causes drowsiness, induces sleep onset, and/or maintains sleep.

selective serotonin reuptake inhibitors: a class of antidepressants that assist nerve impulses along pathways using the neurotransmitter serotonin; effective in treating narcolepsy symptoms. Examples include: Zoloft®, Prozac®, Celexa®, Lexapro®, and Paxil®.

septoplasty: A surgery sometimes used to treat obstructive sleep apnea in which a small incision is made inside a nostril, and the cartilage and bone of the septum is straightened.

septum: The divider between the two nasal passages; if deviated (crooked), the septum can obstruct the nasal passages.

serotonin: A neurotransmitter found in brain stem cells and other parts of the central nervous system; in animal studies, the inhibition of the formation of serotonin led to severe insomnia.

short-term insomnia: Temporary sleeplessness that arises because of ongoing stress, a temporary illness, or a traumatic experience.

sleep: A physical and mental resting state in which a person becomes relatively inactive and unaware of his or her environment.

sleep apnea: Episodes of nonrespiration during sleep that last at least ten seconds and occur five times per hour of sleep; see central, or mixed sleep apnea.

sleep architecture: The structure of the sleep cycle and wakefulness as it occurs over a period of sleep.

"sleep center": A localized area in the brain believed to regulate sleep.

sleep cycle: The cycle in which non-REM and REM sleep alternate in 90- to 110- minute phases. A normal sleep pattern has four to five sleep cycles.

sleep debt: The deficiency of sleep created when personal sleep requirements are not met.

sleep deprivation: A mental and physical state that arises when sleep has not been attained or has been inhibited. In some cases, it can cause an inability to concentrate, loss of memory, and rarely, hallucinations and erratic behavior.

sleep disorders: Physical and psychological conditions or disturbances of sleep and wakefulness, usually caused by abnormalities that occur during sleep or by abnormalities of specific sleep mechanisms.

sleep efficiency: The proportion of sleep in the period potentially filled by sleep; that is, the ratio of total sleep time in bed.

sleep hygiene: The practice of achieving and maintaining proper habits to promote good sleep.

sleep latency: The period of time measured from "lights out," or bedtime, to the commencement of sleep.

sleep maintenance insomnia: One or more episodes of wakefulness that occur later in the night and may be due to medical illness, primary sleep disorders, or depression.

sleep medicine: The science of the study of sleep and its processes; also refers to the clinical practice of assessing and treating sleep disorders.

sleep mentation: The imagery and thinking (and emotion) experienced during sleep.

sleep onset: The transition from the awake to the sleep state, normally into NREM stage 1 (but in certain conditions, such as infancy and narcolepsy, into REM.) Most polysomnographers accept EEG slowing, reduction and eventual disappearance of alpha activity, presence of EEG vertex spikes, and slow rolling eye movements (the components of NREM stage 1) as sufficient for sleep onset; others require appearance of stage 2 wave forms. See sleep latency.

sleep onset insomnia: Insomnia characterized by a delay in falling asleep, lasting thirty minutes or longer, at the time when one goes to bed; it is most commonly caused by anxiety.

sleep paralysis: A brief loss of muscle control that occurs at the onset of sleep or upon awakening; a condition usually associated with narcolepsy. May last from a few seconds to a few minutes. Occurs in one in twenty healthy people but is more common in those with narcolepsy.

sleep restriction therapy: A behavioral treatment developed by Dr. Arthur Spielman and colleagues that follows a simple principle: Restrict time in bed to only the number of hours asleep, then increase time in bed as sleep efficiency increases.

sleep spindles: A pattern of EEG waves that consist of a burst of 11 to 15 hertz waves that last for 0.5 to 1.5 seconds; an identifying feature of stage 2 sleep.

sleep talking: Also called somniloquy; a parasomnia characterized by talking during sleep.

sleep terrors: Also called pavor nocturnus or night terrors; a parasomnia characterized by episodes of screaming or shouting and occasionally, sleepwalking. Sleep terrors are usually associated with fear and anxiety.

sleep-wake cycle: The repeated pattern over twenty-four hours that consists of periods of sleep alternating with periods of wakefulness.

sleepwalking: Also called somnambulism; a parasomnia characterized by walking or performing other complicated activities while asleep.

slow wave sleep (SWS): Synonymous with sleep stages 3 and 4.

snoring: The noise produced by a sleeping individual in which the soft palate and the uvula vibrate during respiration.

somnambulism: See also sleepwalking; a parasomnia characterized by walking or performing other complicated activities while asleep.

somniloquy (somniloquism): See also sleep talking; a parasomnia characterized by talking during sleep.

somnolence: Also called excessive sleepiness or excessive daytime sleepiness; the inability to stay awake during the normal wake period of a sleep-wake cycle. It can be measured by a multiple sleep latency test (MSLT).

somnologist: A specialist in the study of sleep and in the diagnosis and treatment of sleep disorders.

somnoplasty: A noninvasive procedure that uses radio frequency to reduce structures in the mouth in the treatment of snoring and obstructive sleep apnea.

stage 1 sleep: The brief, dozing stage of non-REM sleep in which a person transitions to very light sleep and can be awakened easily, characterized by low voltage EEG and slow rolling eye movements; 5 percent of non-REM sleep is spent in stage 1.

stage 2 sleep: The stage of consolidated sleep in non-REM sleep characterized by sleep spindles and K-complexes; 45 percent of non-REM sleep is spent in stage 2.

stage 3 sleep: The stage of deeper sleep in non-REM sleep characterized by delta waves interspersed with smaller, faster waves; 12 percent of non-REM sleep is spent in stage 3.

stage 4 sleep: The stage of very deep sleep in non-REM sleep almost exclusively composed of delta waves and the stage in which sleep terrors or sleepwalking may occur; 13 percent of non-REM sleep is spent in stage 4.

stimulant: A type of drug, such as Cylert®, Ritalin®, and Dexedrine®, that stimulates the central nervous system; often used to treat excessive daytime sleepiness. Provigil® and Nuvigil® are two newer stimulants of a somewhat different type.

stimulus control: An effective insomnia technique developed by Dr. Richard Bootzin and colleagues which proposes that an individual has ten minutes to fall asleep. If sleep is not achieved, the person must get up, go into another room, and return to bed only when sleepy. Also called the ten-minute rule.

suprachiasmatic nuclei: Also called the SCN or the endogenous circadian pacemaker; small structures in the brain, sensitive to the presence or absence of light, that coordinate circadian rhythms.

teeth grinding: Also called bruxism; a parasomnia characterized by the grinding or clenching of teeth during sleep.

The Ten-Minute Rule: A relaxation and sleeping technique that suggests that an individual who has laid awake in bed for an estimated ten minutes get up, go into another room, relax by doing something boring, and then return to bed when sleepy.

tonsils: Masses of lymphoid tissue at the back of both sides of the mouth whose primary function is fighting infection.

tonsillectomy: Surgical removal of the tonsils.

total sleep period: The period of time measured from sleep onset to final wakening. In addition to total sleep time, it is comprised of the time taken up by arousals and movement time until wake-up.

total sleep time: The amount of actual sleep time in a sleep period; equal to total sleep period less movements and awake time. Total sleep time is the total of all REM and NREM sleep in a sleep period.

tracheostomy: Also known as a tracheotomy; a surgical procedure that creates an opening in the windpipe via the neck in order to insert a tube that facilitates breathing. This procedure is reserved for patients with severe sleep apnea.

transient insomnia: Sometimes called adjustment sleep disorder or situational insomnia, it is sleeplessness that lasts a few consecutive nights and is often triggered by stress or excitement.

turbinate: Also called the nasal concha; any of three bones (lowest, middle, and upper) within the nose that are surrounded by soft tissue and form the sides of the nasal cavity.

turbinate reduction: A surgical procedure used to reduce the size of an enlarged turbinate, which can improve the size of the nasal airway, thereby relieving obstructive sleep apnea.

UPPP: An acronym for uvulopalatopharyngoplasty; the surgical procedure for the removal of the uvula and tightening of loose tissue in the back of the throat.

"urotoxins": Coined by Abel Bouchard in 1886, a term he used to describe toxic agents excreted in the urine during sleep.

uvula: The tissue that hangs down in the back of the throat.

uvulopalatopharyngoplasty: Also called UPPP; the surgical procedure for the removal of the uvula and tightening of loose tissue in the back of the throat.

vigilance testing: The process of assessing the level of alertness during wakefulness in a clinical or research setting. It may include a series of tests such as the Epworth sleepiness scale, pupillometry, reaction time tests, a MSLT, or MWT.

wakefulness: A brain state that occurs when a healthy individual is not asleep.

Chapter 54

Directory of
Sleep-Related Resources

General

American Academy of Dental Sleep Medicine
2510 N. Frontage Road
Darien, IL 60561
Phone: 630-737-9705
Fax: 630-737-9790
Website: http://www.aadsm.org
E-mail: info@aadsm.org

American Academy of Sleep Medicine
2510 N. Frontage Road
Darien, IL 60561
Phone: 630-737-9700
Fax: 630-737-9790
Website: http://www.aasmnet.org

American Sleep Association
Website: http://www.
sleepassociation.org

Better Sleep Council
501 Wythe Street
Alexandria, VA 22314-1917
Phone: 703-683-8371
Website: http://www.bettersleep
.org

Cleveland Clinic
9500 Euclid Avenue
Cleveland, Ohio 44195
Phone: 866.594.2091
TTY: 216-444-0261
Website: http://
my.clevelandclinic.org

The information in this chapter was compiled from various sources deemed accurate. All contact information was verified and updated in November 2009. Inclusion does not imply endorsement. This list is intended to serve as a starting point for information gathering; it is not comprehensive.

KidsHealth
Website: http://www.KidsHealth
.org

National Center on Sleep Disorders Research
Two Rockledge Centre
Suite 10038
U.S. National Heart, Lung, and Blood Institute
6701 Rockledge Drive, MSC 7920
Bethesda, MD 20892-7920
Phone: 301-435-0199
Website: www.nhlbi.nih.gov/
about/ncsdr/

National Heart, Lung, and Blood Institute Health Information Center
P.O. Box 30105
Bethesda, MD 20824-0105
Toll-Free: 800-575-WELL (9355)
Phone: 301-592-8573
Website: http://www.nhlbi.nih
.gov
E-mail: NHLBIinfo@nhlbi.nih
.gov

National Institute of Neurological Disorders and Stroke
NIH Neurological Institute
P.O. Box 5801
Bethesda, MD 20824
Toll-Free: 800-352-9424
Phone: 301-496-5751
TTY: 301-468-5981
Website: http://www.ninds.nih
.gov

National Sleep Foundation
1522 K Street NW, Suite 500
Washington, DC 20005
Phone: 202-347-3471
Fax: 202-347-3472
Website: http://www
.sleepfoundation.org
E-mail: nsf@sleepfoundation.org

Ohio Sleep Medicine Institute
4975 Bradenton Avenue
Dublin, OH 43017
Phone: 614-766-0773
Fax: 614-766-2599
Website: http://www.sleepohio.com

Scottsdale Sleep Center
9767 North 91st Street, Suite 104
Scottsdale, AZ 85258
Phone: 480-767-8811
Fax: 480-657-0737
Website: http://www
.scottsdalesleepcenter.com

Talk About Sleep, Inc.
P.O. Box 146
Chaska, MN 55318
Phone: 866-657-5337
Website: http://www
.talkaboutsleep.com
E-mail: info@talkaboutsleep.com

Washington University Sleep Medicine Center
Department of Neurology
212 North Kings Highway
Suite 237
St. Louis, Missouri 63108
Phone: 314-362-4342
Fax: 314-747-3813
Website: http://sleep.wustl.edu

Insomnia

American Insomnia Association
Phone: 708-492-0930
Website: http://www
.americaninsomniaassociation
.org/

Narcolepsy

Narcolepsy Network, Inc.
110 Ripple Lane
North Kingstown, RI 02852
Toll-free: 888-292-6522
Phone: 401-667-2523
Fax: 401-633-6567
Website: http://www
.narcolepsynetwork.org
E-mail: narnet
@narcolepsynetwork.org

Other Disorders Affecting Sleep

Alzheimer's Association
225 N. Michigan Ave., Fl. 17
Chicago, IL 60601-7633
Toll-Free: 800-272-3900
(24/7 Helpline)
Phone: 312-335-8700
(National Office)
Fax: 866-699-1246
TDD: 866-403-3073
Website: http://www.alz.org
E-mail: info@alz.org

American Gastroenterological Association
4930 Del Ray Avenue
Bethesda, MD 20814
Phone: 301-654-2055
Fax: 301-654-5920
Website: http://www.gastro.org
E-mail: member@gastro.org

American Parkinson Disease Association
135 Parkinson Avenue
Staten Island, NY 10305
Toll-Free: 800-223-2732
Phone: 718-981-8001
Fax: 718-981-4399
Website: http://www
.apdaparkinson.org
E-mail: apda@apdaparkinson
.org

Anxiety Disorders Association of America
8730 Georgia Ave.
Silver Spring, MD 20910
Phone: 240-485-1001
Website: http://www.adaa.org

National Center for Posttraumatic Stress Disorder
Website: http://www.ptsd.va.gov

National Institute of Mental Health
Science Writing, Press, and Dissemination Branch
6001 Executive Boulevard
Room 8184, MSC 9663
Bethesda, MD 20892-9663
Toll-Free: 866-615-6464
Phone: 301-443-4513
Fax: 301-443-4279
TTY: 866-415-8051
Website: http://www.nimh.nih.gov
E-mail: nimhinfo@nih.gov

National Multiple Sclerosis Society
733 Third Avenue, 3rd Floor
New York, NY 10017
Toll-Free: 800-344-4867
Website: http://www.nationalmssociety.org

Restless Legs Syndrome

Restless Legs Syndrome Foundation
1610 14th St. NW, Suite 300
Rochester, MN 55901
Phone: 507-287-6465
Fax: 507-287-6312
Website: http://www.rls.org
E-mail: rlsfoundation@rls.org

WE MOVE (Worldwide Education & Awareness for Movement Disorders)
204 West 84th Street
New York, NY 10024
Phone: 212-875-8312
Fax: 212-875-8389
Website: http://www.wemove.org
E-mail: wemove@wemove.org

Sleep Apnea

American Sleep Apnea Association
6856 Eastern Avenue, NW
Suite 203
Washington, DC 20012
Phone: 202-293-3650
Fax: 202-293-3656
Website: http://www.sleepapnea.org
E-mail: asaa@sleepapnea.org

Infant & Children Sleep Apnea Awareness Foundation, Inc.
P.O. Box 2328
New Smyrna Beach, FL 32170
Phone: 386-423-5430
Fax: 386-428-2001
Website: http://www.infantsleepapnea.org

Index

Index

Page numbers followed by 'n' indicate a footnote. Page numbers in *italics* indicate a table or illustration.

bilevel positive airway pressure
(BiPAP), defined 515
Bils, Pete 98–99
bimaxillary advancement,
defined 515
biological clock
defined 515
described 7
biological rhythm, defined 515
BiPAP *see* bilevel positive airway
pressure
bladder training, bedwetting 484–85
blindness, circadian rhythms 8
"Blue Light Special: Treating
Circadian Rhythm Sleep Disorders"
(Quadrant HealthCom Inc.) 438n
body clock *see* circadian rhythms
body rocking, described 491–93
Bonine (meclizine) 319
BPH *see* benign prostatic hyperplasia
"Brain, Heal Thyself" (American
Psychological Association) 104n
brain activity, sleep 102–7, 114–18
Brainard, George 440–42
"Brain Basics: Understanding Sleep"
(NINDS) 7n, 22n
brain development, sleep 6
brain injuries, narcolepsy 201
brain-wave rhythms, defined 515
Brawn, Timothy 114
breathing devices, sleep apnea 148–49
see also continuous positive airway
pressure
bright light therapy
defined 515
overview 438–42
sleep deprivation 77
bromocriptine, described 517
bruxism
defined 515
described 216, 528
overview 487–89
"Bruxism (Teeth Grinding
or Clenching)" (Nemours
Foundation) 487n
BSCS, publications
sleep information 4n
sleep physical characteristics 9n
bumetanide 263

bupropion
depression 251
sleep disorders 319
butisol sodium 385

C

caffeine
adolescents 506–8
drowsy driving 137
insomnia 181
overview 313–17
periodic limb movement
disorder 187
pregnancy 46
shift work 336
sleep deprivation 77
sleep disorders 320
sleep hygiene 41, 294, 297
"Caffeine and Teens' Sleep:
An Eye-Opening Study"
(SAMHSA) 506n
Caffo, B.S. 54n
Cai, Denise 110–11
calcium carbonate 242
CAM *see* complementary and
alternative medicine
cancer
melatonin 393
sleep disorders 235–38
"Can Exercise Help Me Sleep
Better?" (Nieman) 349n
Carbitol (pentobarbital;
carbromal) 386
cardiopulmonary resuscitation
(CPR), children 474
Caruso, Lauren 256–57
cataplexy
defined 515–16
described 72, 199
narcolepsy 202
"Catch Your ZZZZs!" (*Medline Plus
Magazine*) 510n
CBT *see* cognitive-behavioral therapy
CDC *see* Centers for Disease Control
and Prevention
Celexa (citalopram)
described 525
sleep disorders 318

Health Reference Series
Complete Catalog
List price $93 per volume. School and library price $84 per volume.

Adolescent Health Sourcebook, 3rd Edition

Basic Consumer Health Information about Adolescent Growth and Development, Puberty, Sexuality, Reproductive Health, and Physical, Emotional, Social, and Mental Health Concerns of Teens and Their Parents, Including Facts about Nutrition, Physical Activity, Weight Management, Acne, Allergies, Cancer, Diabetes, Growth Disorders, Juvenile Arthritis, Infections, Substance Abuse, and More

Along with Information about Adolescent Safety Concerns, Youth Violence, a Glossary of Related Terms, and a Directory of Resources

Edited by Amy L. Sutton. 600 pages. 2010. 978-0-7808-1140-9.

Adult Health Concerns Sourcebook

Basic Consumer Health Information about Medical and Mental Concerns of Adults, Including Facts about Choosing Healthcare Providers, Navigating Insurance Options, Maintaining Wellness, Preventing Cancer, Heart Disease, Stroke, Diabetes, and Osteoporosis, and Understanding Aging-Related Health Concerns, Including Menopause, Cognitive Changes, and Changes in the Coronary and Vascular Systems

Along with Tips on Caring for Aging Parents and Dealing with Health-Related Work and Travel Issues, a Glossary, and a Directory of Resources for Additional Help and Information

Edited by Sandra J. Judd. 648 pages. 2008. 978-0-7808-0999-4.

"Provides a thorough list of topics that are important to adult health and for caregivers."
—*CHOICE, Nov '08*

"Written in easy-to-understand language... the content is well-organized and is intended to aid adults in making health care-related decisions."
—*AORN Journal, Dec '08*

AIDS Sourcebook, 4th Edition

Basic Consumer Health Information about Human Immunodeficiency Virus (HIV) and Acquired Immunodeficiency Syndrome (AIDS), Featuring Updated Statistics and Facts about Risks, Prevention, Screening, Diagnosis, Treatments, Side Effects, and Complications, and Including a Section about the Impact of HIV/AIDS on the Health of Women, Children, and Adolescents

Along with Tips on Managing Life with AIDS, Reports on Current Research Initiatives and Clinical Trials, a Glossary of Related Terms, and Resource Directories for Further Help and Information

Edited by Ivy L. Alexander. 680 pages. 2008. 978-0-7808-0997-0.

SEE ALSO *Contagious Diseases Sourcebook, 2nd Edition*

Alcoholism Sourcebook, 3rd Edition

Basic Consumer Health Information about Alcohol Use, Abuse, and Dependence, Featuring Facts about the Physical, Mental, and Social Health Effects of Alcohol Addiction, Including Alcoholic Liver Disease, Pancreatic Disease, Cardiovascular Disease, Neurological Disorders, and the Effects of Drinking during Pregnancy

Along with Information about Alcohol Treatment, Medications, and Recovery Programs, in Addition to Tips for Reducing the Prevalence of Underage Drinking, Statistics about Alcohol Use, a Glossary of Related Terms, and Directories of Resources for More Help and Information

Edited by Joyce Brennfleck Shannon. 600 pages. 2010. 978-0-7808-1141-6.

SEE ALSO *Drug Abuse Sourcebook, 3rd Edition*

Allergies Sourcebook, 3rd Edition

Basic Consumer Health Information about Allergic Disorders, Such as Anaphylaxis, Hives,

Eczema, Rhinitis, Sinusitis, and Conjunctivitis, and Their Triggers, Including Pollen, Mold, Dust Mites, Animal Dander, Insects, Chemicals, Food, Food Additives, and Medications

Along with Advice about the Diagnosis and Treatment of Allergy Symptoms, a Glossary of Related Terms, a Directory of Resources for Help and Information, and Suggestions for Additional Reading

Edited by Amy L. Sutton. 588 pages. 2007. 978-0-7808-0950-5.

SEE ALSO Asthma Sourcebook, 2nd Edition

Alzheimer Disease Sourcebook, 4th Edition

Basic Consumer Health Information about Alzheimer Disease, Other Dementias, and Related Disorders, Including Multi-Infarct Dementia, Dementia with Lewy Bodies, Frontotemporal Dementia (Pick Disease), Wernicke-Korsakoff Syndrome (Alcohol-Related Dementia), AIDS Dementia Complex, Huntington Disease, Creutzfeldt-Jacob Disease, and Delirium

Along with Information about Coping with Memory Loss and Forgetfulness, Maintaining Skills, and Long-Term Planning for People with Dementia, and Suggestions Addressing Common Caregiver Concerns, Updated Information about Current Research Efforts, a Glossary of Related Terms, and Directories of Sources for Additional Help and Information

Edited by Karen Bellenir. 603 pages. 2008. 978-0-7808-1001-3.

"An invaluable resource for persons who have received a diagnosis, for caregivers, and for family members dealing with this insidious disease. It is recommended for public, community college, and ready-reference sections in academic libraries."
—American Reference Books Annual, 2009

SEE ALSO Brain Disorders Sourcebook, 3rd Edition

Arthritis Sourcebook, 3rd Edition

Basic Consumer Health Information about the Risk Factors, Symptoms, Diagnosis, and Treatment of Osteoarthritis, Rheumatoid Arthritis, Juvenile Arthritis, Gout, Infectious Arthritis, and Autoimmune Disorders Associated with Arthritis

Along with Facts about Medications, Surgeries, and Self-Care Techniques to Manage Pain and Disability, Tips on Living with Arthritis, a Glossary of Related Terms, and Resources for Additional Help and Information

Edited by Amy L. Sutton. 600 pages. 2010. 978-0-7808-1077-8.

Asthma Sourcebook, 2nd Edition

Basic Consumer Health Information about the Causes, Symptoms, Diagnosis, and Treatment of Asthma in Infants, Children, Teenagers, and Adults, Including Facts about Different Types of Asthma, Common Co-Occurring Conditions, Asthma Management Plans, Triggers, Medications, and Medication Delivery Devices

Along with Asthma Statistics, Research Updates, a Glossary, a Directory of Asthma-Related Resources, and More

Edited by Karen Bellenir. 581 pages. 2006. 978-0-7808-0866-9.

SEE ALSO Lung Disorders Sourcebook; Respiratory Disorders Sourcebook, 2nd Edition

Attention Deficit Disorder Sourcebook

Basic Consumer Health Information about Attention Deficit/Hyperactivity Disorder in Children and Adults, Including Facts about Causes, Symptoms, Diagnostic Criteria, and Treatment Options Such as Medications, Behavior Therapy, Coaching, and Homeopathy

Along with Reports on Current Research Initiatives, Legal Issues, and Government Regulations, and Featuring a Glossary of Related Terms, Internet Resources, and a List of Additional Reading Material

Edited by Dawn D. Matthews. 447 pages. 2002. 978-0-7808-0624-5.

"Recommended reference source."
—Booklist, Jan '03

SEE ALSO Learning Disabilities Sourcebook, 3rd Edition

Autism and Pervasive Developmental Disorders Sourcebook

Basic Consumer Health Information about Autism Spectrum and Pervasive Developmental Disorders, Such as Classical Autism, Asperger Syndrome, Rett Syndrome, and Childhood Disintegrative Disorder, Including Information about Related Genetic Disorders and Medical Problems and Facts about Causes, Screening Methods, Diagnostic Criteria, Treatments and Interventions, and Family and Education Issues

Along with a Glossary of Related Terms, Tips for Evaluating the Validity of Health Claims, and a Directory of Resources for Additional Help and Information

Edited by Sandra J. Judd. 603 pages. 2007. 978-0-7808-0953-6.

"This book provides a current overview of disorders on the autism spectrum and information about various therapies, educational resources, and help for families with practical issues such as workplace adjustments, living arrangements, and estate planning. It is a useful resource for public and consumer health libraries."
—American Reference Books Annual, 2009

SEE ALSO Learning Disabilities Sourcebook, 3rd Edition

Back and Neck Disorders Sourcebook, 2nd Edition

Basic Consumer Health Information about Spinal Pain, Spinal Cord Injuries, and Related Disorders, Such as Degenerative Disk Disease, Osteoarthritis, Scoliosis, Sciatica, Spina Bifida, and Spinal Stenosis, and Featuring Facts about Maintaining Spinal Health, Self-Care, Pain Management, Rehabilitative Care, Chiropractic Care, Spinal Surgeries, and Complementary Therapies

Along with Suggestions for Preventing Back and Neck Pain, a Glossary of Related Terms, and a Directory of Resources

Edited by Amy L. Sutton. 607 pages. 2004. 978-0-7808-0738-9.

"Recommended... An easy to use, comprehensive medical reference book."
—E-Streams, Sep '05

"For anyone who has back or neck problems, this book is ideal. Its easy-to-understand language and variety of topics makes this sourcebook a worthwhile read. The price... is reasonable for the amount of information contained in the book"
—Occupational Therapy in Health Care, 2007

Blood & Circulatory Disorders Sourcebook, 3rd Edition

Basic Consumer Health Information about Blood and Circulatory System Disorders, Such as Anemia, Leukemia, Lymphoma, Rh Disease, Hemophilia, Thrombophilia, Other Bleeding and Clotting Deficiencies, and Artery, Vascular, and Venous Diseases, Including Facts about Blood Types, Blood Donation, Bone Marrow and Stem Cell Transplants, Tests and Medications, and Tips for Maintaining Circulatory Health

Along with a Glossary of Related Terms and a List of Resources for Additional Help and Information

Edited by Sandra J. Judd. 600 pages. 2010. 978-0-7808-1081-5.

SEE ALSO Leukemia Sourcebook

Brain Disorders Sourcebook, 3rd Edition

Basic Consumer Health Information about Acquired and Traumatic Brain Injuries, Brain Tumors, Cerebral Palsy and Other Genetic and Congenital Brain Disorders, Infections of the Brain, Epilepsy, and Degenerative Neurological Disorders Such as Dementia, Huntington Disease, and Amyotrophic Lateral Sclerosis (ALS)

Along with Information on Brain Structure and Function, Treatment and Rehabilitation Options, a Glossary of Terms Related to Brain Disorders, and a Directory of Resources for More Information

Edited by Joyce Brennfleck Shannon. 600 pages. 2010. 978-0-7808-1083-9.

SEE ALSO Alzheimer Disease Sourcebook, 4th Edition

Breast Cancer Sourcebook, 3rd Edition

Basic Consumer Health Information about Breast Health and Breast Cancer, Including Facts about Environmental, Genetic, and Other Risk Factors, Prevention Efforts, Screening and Diagnostic Methods, Surgical Treatment Options and Other Care Choices, Complementary and Alternative Therapies, and Post-Treatment Concerns

Along with Statistical Data, News about Research Advances, a Glossary of Related Terms, and Directories of Resources for Additional Information and Support

Edited by Karen Bellenir. 606 pages. 2009. 978-0-7808-1030-3.

"A very useful reference for people wanting to learn more about breast cancer and how to negotiate their care or the care of a loved one. The third edition is necessary as information/treatment options continue to evolve."
—*Doody's Review Service, 2009*

SEE ALSO *Cancer Sourcebook for Women, 3rd Edition, Women's Health Concerns Sourcebook, 3rd Edition*

Breastfeeding Sourcebook

Basic Consumer Health Information about the Benefits of Breastmilk, Preparing to Breastfeed, Breastfeeding as a Baby Grows, Nutrition, and More, Including Information on Special Situations and Concerns Such as Mastitis, Illness, Medications, Allergies, Multiple Births, Prematurity, Special Needs, and Adoption

Along with a Glossary and Resources for Additional Help and Information

Edited by Jenni Lynn Colson. 367 pages. 2002. 978-0-7808-0332-9.

SEE ALSO *Pregnancy and Birth Sourcebook, 3rd Edition*

Burns Sourcebook

Basic Consumer Health Information about Various Types of Burns and Scalds, Including Flame, Heat, Cold, Electrical, Chemical, and Sun Burns

Along with Information on Short-Term and Long-Term Treatments, Tissue Reconstruction, Plastic Surgery, Prevention Suggestions, and First Aid

Edited by Allan R. Cook. 604 pages. 1999. 978-0-7808-0204-9.

"This is an exceptional addition to the series and is highly recommended for all consumer health collections, hospital libraries, and academic medical centers."
—*E-Streams, Mar '00*

"This key reference guide is an invaluable addition to all health care and public libraries in confronting this ongoing health issue."
—*American Reference Books Annual, 2000*

SEE ALSO *Dermatological Disorders Sourcebook, 2nd Edition*

Cancer Sourcebook, 5th Edition

Basic Consumer Health Information about Major Forms and Stages of Cancer, Featuring Facts about Head and Neck Cancers, Lung Cancers, Gastrointestinal Cancers, Genitourinary Cancers, Lymphomas, Blood Cell Cancers, Endocrine Cancers, Skin Cancers, Bone Cancers, Metastatic Cancers, and More

Along with Facts about Cancer Treatments, Cancer Risks and Prevention, a Glossary of Related Terms, Statistical Data, and a Directory of Resources for Additional Information

Edited by Karen Bellenir. 1105 pages. 2007. 978-0-7808-0947-5.

"The 5th, updated edition of Cancer Sourcebook should be in every public and health lending library collection... An unparalleled discussion essential for any health collections considering an all-in-one basic general reference."
—*California Bookwatch, Aug '07*

SEE ALSO *Breast Cancer Sourcebook, 3rd Edition, Cancer Survivorship Sourcebook, Leukemia Sourcebook*

Cancer Sourcebook for Women, 4th Edition

Basic Consumer Health Information about Gynecologic Cancers and Other Cancers of Special Concern to Women, Including Cancers of the Breast, Cervix, Colon, Lung, Ovaries, Thyroid, and Uterus

Along with Facts about Benign Conditions of the Female Reproductive System, Cancer Risk

Factors, Diagnostic and Treatment Procedures, Side Effects of Cancer and Cancer Treatments, Women's Issues in Cancer Survivorship, a Glossary of Related Terms, and a Directory of Resources for Additional Help and Information

Edited by Karen Bellenir. 600 pages. 2010. 978-0-7808-1139-3.

SEE ALSO Breast Cancer Sourcebook, 3rd Edition, Women's Health Concerns Sourcebook, 3rd Edition

Cancer Survivorship Sourcebook

Basic Consumer Health Information about the Physical, Educational, Emotional, Social, and Financial Needs of Cancer Patients from Diagnosis, through Cancer Treatment, and Beyond, Including Facts about Researching Specific Types of Cancer and Learning about Clinical Trials and Treatment Options, and Featuring Tips for Coping with the Side Effects of Cancer Treatments and Adjusting to Life after Cancer Treatment Concludes

Along with Suggestions for Caregivers, Friends, and Family Members of Cancer Patients, a Glossary of Cancer Care Terms, and Directories of Related Resources

Edited by Karen Bellenir. 633 pages. 2007. 978-0-7808-0985-7.

"Well organized and comprehensive in coverage, the book speaks to issues encountered both during and after cancer treatment. Recommended for consumer health and public libraries."
—*Library Journal, Aug 1 '07*

"Cancer Survivorship Sourcebook will be useful to anyone who has a friend or loved one with a cancer diagnosis."
—*American Reference Books Annual, 2008*

SEE ALSO *Cancer Sourcebook, 5th Edition, Disease Management Sourcebook*

Cardiovascular Disorders Sourcebook, 4th Edition

Basic Consumer Health Information about Heart and Blood Vessel Diseases and Disorders, Such as Angina, Heart Attack, Heart Failure, Cardiomyopathy, Arrhythmias, Valve Disease, Atherosclerosis, Aneurysms, and

Congenital Heart Defects, Including Information about Cardiovascular Disease in Women, Men, Children, Adolescents, and Minorities

Along with Facts about Diagnosing, Managing, and Preventing Cardiovascular Disease, a Glossary of Related Medical Terms, and a Directory of Resources for Additional Information

Edited by Amy L. Sutton. 600 pages. 2010. 978-0-7808-1080-8.

Caregiving Sourcebook

Basic Consumer Health Information for Caregivers, Including a Profile of Caregivers, Caregiving Responsibilities and Concerns, Tips for Specific Conditions, Care Environments, and the Effects of Caregiving

Along with Facts about Legal Issues, Financial Information, and Future Planning, a Glossary, and a Listing of Additional Resources

Edited by Joyce Brennfleck Shannon. 583 pages. 2001. 978-0-7808-0331-2.

"Essential for most collections."
—*Library Journal, Apr 1 '02*

"An ideal addition to the reference collection of any public library. Health sciences information professionals may also want to acquire the Caregiving Sourcebook for their hospital or academic library for use as a ready reference tool by health care workers interested in aging and caregiving."
—*E-Streams, Jan '02*

Child Abuse Sourcebook, 2nd Edition

Basic Consumer Health Information about the Physical, Sexual, and Emotional Abuse of Children, Neglect, Münchhausen Syndrome by Proxy (MSBP), and Shaken Baby Syndrome, and Featuring Facts about Withholding Medical Care, Corporal Punishment, Child Maltreatment in Youth Sports, and Parental Substance Abuse

Along with Information about Child Protective Services, Foster Care, Adoption, Parenting Challenges, Abuse Prevention Programs, and Intervention, Treatment, and Recovery Guidelines, a Glossary of Related Terms, and Resources for Additional Help and Information

Edited by Joyce Brennfleck Shannon. 600 pages. 2009. 978-0-7808-1037-2.

SEE ALSO Domestic Violence Sourcebook, 3rd Edition

Childhood Diseases and Disorders Sourcebook, 2nd Edition

Basic Consumer Health Information about the Physical, Mental, and Developmental Health of Pre-Adolescent Children, Including Facts about Infectious Diseases, Asthma, Allergies, Diabetes, and Other Acute and Chronic Conditions Affecting the Gastrointestinal Tract, Ears, Nose, Throat, Liver, Kidneys, Heart, Blood, Brain, Muscles, Bones, and Skin

Along with Reports on Recommended Childhood Vaccinations, Wellness Guidelines, a Glossary of Related Medical Terms, and a List of Resources for Parents

Edited by Sandra J. Judd. 694 pages. 2009. 978-0-7808-1031-0.

"The strength of this source is the wide range of information given about childhood health issues... It is most appropriate for public libraries and academic libraries that field medical questions."
—American Reference Books Annual, 2009

SEE ALSO Healthy Children Sourcebook

Colds, Flu and Other Common Ailments Sourcebook

Basic Consumer Health Information about Common Ailments and Injuries, Including Colds, Coughs, the Flu, Sinus Problems, Headaches, Fever, Nausea and Vomiting, Menstrual Cramps, Diarrhea, Constipation, Hemorrhoids, Back Pain, Dandruff, Dry and Itchy Skin, Cuts, Scrapes, Sprains, Bruises, and More

Along with Information about Prevention, Self-Care, Choosing a Doctor, Over-the-Counter Medications, Folk Remedies, and Alternative Therapies, and Including a Glossary of Important Terms and a Directory of Resources for Further Help and Information

Edited by Chad T. Kimball. 622 pages. 2001. 978-0-7808-0435-7.

"A good starting point for research on common illnesses. It will be a useful addition to public and consumer health library collections."
—American Reference Books Annual, 2002

"Will prove valuable to any library seeking to maintain a current, comprehensive reference collection of health resources... Excellent reference."
—The Bookwatch, Aug '01

SEE ALSO Contagious Diseases Sourcebook, 2nd Edition

Communication Disorders Sourcebook

Basic Information about Deafness and Hearing Loss, Speech and Language Disorders, Voice Disorders, Balance and Vestibular Disorders, and Disorders of Smell, Taste, and Touch

Edited by Linda M. Ross. 533 pages. 1996. 978-0-7808-0077-9.

"This is skillfully edited and is a welcome resource for the layperson. It should be found in every public and medical library."
—Booklist Health Sciences Supplement, Oct '97

Complementary & Alternative Medicine Sourcebook, 4th Edition

Basic Consumer Health Information about Ayurveda, Acupuncture, Aromatherapy, Chiropractic Care, Diet-Based Therapies, Guided Imagery, Herbal and Vitamin Supplements, Homeopathy, Hypnosis, Massage, Meditation, Naturopathy, Pilates, Reflexology, Reiki, Shiatsu, Tai Chi, Traditional Chinese Medicine, Yoga, and Other Complementary and Alternative Medical Therapies

Along with Statistics, Tips for Selecting a Practitioner, Treatments for Specific Health Conditions, a Glossary of Related Terms, and a Directory of Resources for Additional Help and Information

Edited by Amy L. Sutton. 600 pages. 2010. 978-0-7808-1082-2.

Congenital Disorders Sourcebook, 2nd Edition

Basic Consumer Health Information about Nonhereditary Birth Defects and Disorders

Related to Prematurity, Gestational Injuries, Congenital Infections, and Birth Complications, Including Heart Defects, Hydrocephalus, Spina Bifida, Cleft Lip and Palate, Cerebral Palsy, and More

Along with Facts about the Prevention of Birth Defects, Fetal Surgery and Other Treatment Options, Research Initiatives, a Glossary of Related Terms, and Resources for Additional Information and Support

Edited by Sandra J. Judd. 619 pages. 2007. 978-0-7808-0945-1.

"Congenital Disorders Sourcebook provides an excellent, non-technical overview of many aspects of pregnancy with the focus on congenital disorders."
—*American Reference Books Annual, 2008*

"An excellent readable reference aimed at the lay public for difficult to understand medical problems. An excellent starting point for the interested parent or family member who may then be motivated to seek more information."
—*Doody's Review Service, 2007*

SEE ALSO *Pregnancy and Birth Sourcebook, 3rd Edition*

■

Contagious Diseases Sourcebook, 2nd Edition

Basic Consumer Health Information about Diseases Spread from Person to Person through Direct Physical Contact, Airborne Transmissions, Sexual Contact, or Contact with Blood or Other Body Fluids, Including Pneumococcal, Staphylococcal, and Streptococcal Diseases, Colds, Influenza, Lice, Measles, Mumps, Tuberculosis, and Others

Along with Facts about Self-Care and Over-the-Counter Medications, Antibiotics and Drug Resistance, Disease Prevention, Vaccines, and Bioterrorism, a Glossary, and a Directory of Resources for More Information

Edited by Joyce Brennfleck Shannon. 600 pages. 2010. 978-0-7808-1075-4.

SEE ALSO *AIDS Sourcebook, 4th Edition, Hepatitis Sourcebook*

■

Cosmetic and Reconstructive Surgery Sourcebook, 2nd Edition

Basic Consumer Information about Plastic Surgery and Non-Surgical Appearance-Enhancing Procedures, Including Facts about Botulinum Toxin, Collagen Replacement, Dermabrasion, Chemical Peels, Eyelid Surgery, Nose Reshaping, Lip Augmentation, Liposuction, Breast Enlargement and Reduction, Tummy Tucking, and Other Skin, Hair, Facial, and Body Shaping Procedures

Along with Information about Reconstructive Procedures for Congenital Disorders, Disfiguring Diseases, Burns, and Traumatic Injuries, a Glossary of Related Terms, and a Directory of Additional Resources

Edited by Karen Bellenir. 483 pages. 2007. 978-0-7808-0951-2.

"A comprehensive source for people considering cosmetic surgery... also recommended for medical students who will perform these procedures later in their careers; and public librarians and academic medical librarians who may assist patrons interested in this information."
—*Medical Reference Services Quarterly, Fall '08*

"A practical guide for health care consumers and health care workers... This easy-to-read reference guide would be useful for novice and veteran health care consumers, surgical technology students, nursing students, and perioperative nurses new to plastic and reconstructive surgery. It also may be helpful for medical-surgical nurses as a guide for patient teaching in their practices."
—*AORN Journal, Aug '08*

SEE ALSO *Surgery Sourcebook, 2nd Edition*

■

Death and Dying Sourcebook, 2nd Edition

Basic Consumer Health Information about End-of-Life Care and Related Perspectives and Ethical Issues, Including End-of-Life Symptoms and Treatments, Pain Management, Quality-of-Life Concerns, the Use of Life Support, Patients' Rights and Privacy Issues, Advance Directives, Physician-Assisted Suicide, Caregiving, Organ and Tissue Donation, Autopsies, Funeral Arrangements, and Grief

Along with Statistical Data, Information about the Leading Causes of Death, a Glossary, and Directories of Support Groups and Other Resources

Edited by Joyce Brennfleck Shannon. 626 pages. 2006. 978-0-7808-0871-3.

Dental Care and Oral Health Sourcebook, 3rd Edition

Basic Consumer Health Information about Dental Care and Oral Health Throughout the Lifespan, Including Facts about Cavities, Bad Breath, Cold and Canker Sores, Dry Mouth, Toothaches, Gum Disease, Malocclusion, Temporomandibular Joint and Muscle Disorders, Oral Cancers, and Dental Emergencies

Along with Information about Mouth Hygiene, Crowns, Bridges, Implants, and Fillings, Surgical, Orthodontic, and Cosmetic Dental Procedures, Pain Management, Health Conditions that Impact Oral Care, a Glossary of Related Terms, and a Directory of Additional Resources

Edited by Amy L. Sutton. 619 pages. 2008. 978-0-7808-1032-7.

"Could serve as turning point in the battle to educate consumers in issues concerning oral health. Tightly written in terms the average person can understand, yet comprehensive in scope and authoritative in tone, it is another excellent sourcebook in the Health Reference Series... Should be in the reference department of all public libraries, and in academic libraries that have a public constituency."
—*American Reference Books Annual, 2009*

Depression Sourcebook, 2nd Edition

Basic Consumer Health Information about Unipolar Depression, Bipolar Disorder, Dysthymia, Seasonal Affective Disorder, Postpartum Depression, and Other Depressive Disorders, Including Facts about Populations at Special Risk, Coexisting Medical Conditions, Symptoms, Treatment Options, and Suicide Prevention

Along with Statistical Data, a Glossary of Related Terms, and a Directory of Resources for Additional Help and Information

Edited by Sandra J. Judd. 646 pages. 2008. 978-0-7808-1003-7.

"Recommended for public libraries."
—*American Reference Books Annual, 2009*

SEE ALSO Mental Health Disorders Sourcebook, 4th Edition

Dermatological Disorders Sourcebook, 2nd Edition

Basic Consumer Health Information about Conditions and Disorders Affecting the Skin, Hair, and Nails, Such as Acne, Rosacea, Rashes, Dermatitis, Pigmentation Disorders, Birthmarks, Skin Cancer, Skin Injuries, Psoriasis, Scleroderma, and Hair Loss, Including Facts about Medications and Treatments for Dermatological Disorders and Tips for Maintaining Healthy Skin, Hair, and Nails

Along with Information about How Aging Affects the Skin, a Glossary of Related Terms, and a Directory of Resources for Additional Help and Information

Edited by Amy L. Sutton. 617 pages. 2006. 978-0-7808-0795-2.

"Well organized... presents a plethora of information in a manner that is appropriate in style and readability for the intended audience."
—*Physical Therapy, Nov '06*

"Helpfully brings together... sources in one convenient place, saving the user hours of research time."
—*American Reference Books Annual, 2006*

SEE ALSO Burns Sourcebook

Diabetes Sourcebook, 4th Edition

Basic Consumer Health Information about Type 1 and Type 2 Diabetes Mellitus, Gestational Diabetes, Monogenic Forms of Diabetes, and Insulin Resistance, with Guidelines for Lifestyle Modifications and the Medical Management of Diabetes, Including Facts about Insulin, Insulin Delivery Devices, Oral Diabetes Medications, Self-Monitoring of Blood Glucose, Meal Planning, Physical Activity Recommendations, Foot Care, and Treatment Options for People with Kidney Failure

Along with a Section about Diabetes Complications and Co-Occurring Conditions, a Glossary

of Related Terms, and Directories of Resources for Additional Help and Information

Edited by Karen Bellenir. 627 pages. 2008. 978-0-7808-1005-1.

"Completely and comprehensively covering almost everything a student or physician would need to know... well worth the investment."

—*Internet Bookwatch, Dec '08*

SEE ALSO *Endocrine and Metabolic Disorders Sourcebook, 2nd Edition*

Diet and Nutrition Sourcebook, 3rd Edition

Basic Consumer Health Information about Dietary Guidelines and the Food Guidance System, Recommended Daily Nutrient Intakes, Serving Proportions, Weight Control, Vitamins and Supplements, Nutrition Issues for Different Life Stages and Lifestyles, and the Needs of People with Specific Medical Concerns, Including Cancer, Celiac Disease, Diabetes, Eating Disorders, Food Allergies, and Cardiovascular Disease

Along with Facts about Federal Nutrition Support Programs, a Glossary of Nutrition and Dietary Terms, and Directories of Additional Resources for More Information about Nutrition

Edited by Joyce Brennfleck Shannon. 605 pages. 2006. 978-0-7808-0800-3.

"A valuable resource tool for any individual."

—*Journal of Dental Hygiene, Apr '07*

"From different recommended eating habits to reduce disease and common ailments to nutrition advice for those with specific conditions, Diet and Nutrition Sourcebook is especially important because so much is changing in this area, and so rapidly."

—*California Bookwatch, Jun '06*

SEE ALSO *Eating Disorders Sourcebook, 2nd Edition, Vegetarian Sourcebook*

Digestive Diseases and Disorders Sourcebook

Basic Consumer Health Information about Diseases and Disorders that Impact the Upper and Lower Digestive System, Including Celiac Disease, Constipation, Crohn's Disease, Cyclic Vomiting Syndrome, Diarrhea, Diverticulosis and Diverticulitis, Gallstones, Heartburn, Hemorrhoids, Hernias, Indigestion (Dyspepsia), Irritable Bowel Syndrome, Lactose Intolerance, Ulcers, and More

Along with Information about Medications and Other Treatments, Tips for Maintaining a Healthy Digestive Tract, a Glossary, and Directory of Digestive Diseases Organizations

Edited by Karen Bellenir. 323 pages. 2000. 978-0-7808-0327-5.

"An excellent addition to all public or patient-research libraries."

—*American Reference Books Annual, 2001*

"Recommended reference source."

—*Booklist, May '00*

SEE ALSO *Gastrointestinal Diseases and Disorders Sourcebook, 2nd Edition*

Disabilities Sourcebook

Basic Consumer Health Information about Physical and Psychiatric Disabilities, Including Descriptions of Major Causes of Disability, Assistive and Adaptive Aids, Workplace Issues, and Accessibility Concerns

Along with Information about the Americans with Disabilities Act, a Glossary, and Resources for Additional Help and Information

Edited by Dawn D. Matthews. 602 pages. 2000. 978-0-7808-0389-3.

"A must for libraries with a consumer health section."

—*American Reference Books Annual, 2002*

"A much needed addition to the Omnigraphics Health Reference Series. A current reference work to provide people with disabilities, their families, caregivers or those who work with them, a broad range of information in one volume, has not been available until now... It is recommended for all public and academic library reference collections."

—*E-Streams, May '01*

"An excellent source book in easy-to-read format covering many current topics; highly recommended for all libraries."

—*CHOICE, Jan '01*

Disease Management Sourcebook

Basic Consumer Health Information about Coping with Chronic and Serious Illnesses, Navigating the Health Care System, Communicating with Health Care Providers, Assessing Health Care Quality, and Making Informed Health Care Decisions, Including Facts about Second Opinions, Hospitalization, Surgery, and Medications

Along with a Section about Children with Chronic Conditions, Information about Legal, Financial, and Insurance Issues, a Glossary of Related Terms, and Directories of Additional Resources

Edited by Joyce Brennfleck Shannon. 621 pages. 2008. 978-0-7808-1002-0.

"Consumers need to know how to manage their health care the same way they manage anything else in their lives. The text is very readable and is written for the layperson and consumer. The cost is not prohibitive. This book should be in all collections of health care libraries and public libraries."
— *American Reference Books Annual, 2009*

"The information is very current, and the selection of font and layout make the book easy to read. A hardback that will stand up to much usage, this is an excellent resource for consumers... Recommended. General readers."
—*CHOICE, Nov '08*

"Intended for lay readers, this resource clarifies the many confusing and overwhelming details associated with chronic disease care. Meticulous and clearly explained, the book even includes diagrams intended to ease comprehension of over-the-counter medication labels. An essential guide to navigating the health-care rapids."
—*Library Journal, Aug '08*

Domestic Violence Sourcebook, 3rd Edition

Basic Consumer Health Information about Warning Signs, Risk Factors, and Health Consequences of Intimate Partner Violence, Sexual Violence and Rape, Stalking, Human Trafficking, Child Maltreatment, Teen Dating Violence, and Elder Abuse

Along with Facts about Victims and Perpetrators, Strategies for Violence Prevention, and Emergency Interventions, Safety Plans, and Financial and Legal Tips for Victims, a Glossary of Related Terms, and Directories of Resources for Additional Information and Support

Edited by Joyce Brennfleck Shannon. 634 pages. 2009. 978-0-7808-1038-9.

"A recommended pick for any library interested in consumer health and social issues... A 'must' for any serious health collection."
—*California Bookwatch, Jul '09*

SEE ALSO *Child Abuse Sourcebook, 2nd Edition*

Drug Abuse Sourcebook, 3rd Edition

Basic Consumer Health Information about the Abuse of Cocaine, Club Drugs, Hallucinogens, Heroin, Inhalants, Marijuana, and Other Illicit Substances, Prescription Medications, and Over-the-Counter Medicines

Along with Facts about Addiction and Related Health Effects, Drug Abuse Treatment and Recovery, Drug Testing, Prevention Programs, Glossaries of Drug-Related Terms, and Directories of Resources for More Information

Edited by Joyce Brennfleck Shannon. 600 pages. 2010. 978-0-7808-1079-2.

SEE ALSO *Alcoholism Sourcebook, 3rd Edition*

Ear, Nose, and Throat Disorders Sourcebook, 2nd Edition

Basic Consumer Health Information about Disorders of the Ears, Hearing Loss, Vestibular Disorders, Nasal and Sinus Problems, Throat and Vocal Cord Disorders, and Otolaryngologic Cancers, Including Facts about Ear Infections and Injuries, Genetic and Congenital Deafness, Sensorineural Hearing Disorders, Tinnitus, Vertigo, Ménière Disease, Rhinitis, Sinusitis, Snoring, Sore Throats, Hoarseness, and More

Along with Reports on Current Research Initiatives, a Glossary of Related Medical Terms, and a Directory of Sources for Further Help and Information

Edited by Sandra J. Judd. 631 pages. 2007. 978-0-7808-0872-0.

"A resource book for the general public that provides comprehensive coverage of basic up-to-date medical information about the causes, symptoms, diagnosis, and treatment of diseases and disorders that affect the ears, nose, sinuses, throat, and voice... The majority of information is presented in question and answer format, much like questions a patient might ask of a health care provider. An extensive index facilitates the reader's ability to easily access information on any specific topic."
—*Journal of Dental Hygiene*, Oct '07

"A handy compilation of information on common and some not so common ailments of the ears, nose, and throat."
—*Doody's Review Service, 2007*

Eating Disorders Sourcebook, 2nd Edition

Basic Consumer Health Information about Anorexia Nervosa, Bulimia, Binge Eating, Compulsive Exercise, Female Athlete Triad, and Other Eating Disorders, Including Facts about Body Image and Other Cultural and Age-Related Risk Factors, Prevention Efforts, Adverse Health Effects, Treatment Options, and the Recovery Process

Along with Guidelines for Healthy Weight Control, a Glossary, and Directories of Additional Resources

Edited by Joyce Brennfleck Shannon. 557 pages. 2007. 978-0-7808-0948-2.

"Recommended for the reference collection of large public libraries."
—*American Reference Books Annual, 2008*

"A basic health reference any health or general library needs."
—*Internet Bookwatch, Jun '07*

SEE ALSO *Diet and Nutrition Sourcebook, 3rd Edition, Mental Health Disorders Sourcebook, 4th Edition*

Emergency Medical Services Sourcebook

Basic Consumer Health Information about Preventing, Preparing for, and Managing Emergency Situations, When and Who to Call for Help, What to Expect in the Emergency Room, the Emergency Medical Team,

Patient Issues, and Current Topics in Emergency Medicine

Along with Statistical Data, a Glossary, and Sources of Additional Help and Information

Edited by Jenni Lynn Colson. 472 pages. 2002. 978-0-7808-0420-3.

"Handy and convenient for home, public, school, and college libraries. Recommended."
—*CHOICE, Apr '03*

"This reference can provide the consumer with answers to most questions about emergency care in the United States, or it will direct them to a resource where the answer can be found."
—*American Reference Books Annual, 2003*

SEE ALSO *Injury and Trauma Sourcebook*

Endocrine and Metabolic Disorders Sourcebook, 2nd Edition

Basic Consumer Health Information about Hormonal and Metabolic Disorders that Affect the Body's Growth, Development, and Functioning, Including Disorders of the Pancreas, Ovaries and Testes, and Pituitary, Thyroid, Parathyroid, and Adrenal Glands, with Facts about Growth Disorders, Addison Disease, Cushing Syndrome, Conn Syndrome, Diabetic Disorders, Multiple Endocrine Neoplasia, Inborn Errors of Metabolism, and More

Along with Information about Endocrine Functioning, Diagnostic and Screening Tests, a Glossary of Related Terms, and Directories of Additional Resources

Edited by Joyce Brennfleck Shannon. 597 pages. 2007. 978-0-7808-0952-9.

SEE ALSO *Diabetes Sourcebook, 4th Edition*

Environmental Health Sourcebook, 3rd Edition

Basic Consumer Health Information about the Environment and Its Effects on Human Health, Including Facts about Air, Water, and Soil Contamination, Hazardous Chemicals, Foodborne Hazards and Illnesses, Household Hazards Such as Radon, Mold, and Carbon Monoxide, Consumer Hazards from Toxic Products and Imported Goods, and Disorders

Linked to Environmental Causes, Including Chemical Sensitivity, Cancer, Allergies, and Asthma

Along with Information about the Impact of Environmental Hazards on Specific Populations, a Glossary of Related Terms, and Resources for Additional Help and Information.

Edited by Laura Larsen. 600 pages. 2010. 978-0-7808-1078-5

Ethnic Diseases Sourcebook

Basic Consumer Health Information for Ethnic and Racial Minority Groups in the United States, Including General Health Indicators and Behaviors, Ethnic Diseases, Genetic Testing, the Impact of Chronic Diseases, Women's Health, Mental Health Issues, and Preventive Health Care Services

Along with a Glossary and a Listing of Additional Resources

Edited by Joyce Brennfleck Shannon. 648 pages. 2001. 978-0-7808-0336-7.

"Not many books have been written on this topic to date, and the Ethnic Diseases Sourcebook is a strong addition to the list. It will be an important introductory resource for health consumers, students, health care personnel, and social scientists. It is recommended for public, academic, and large hospital libraries."
— American Reference Books Annual, 2002

"Will prove valuable to any library seeking to maintain a current, comprehensive reference collection of health resources... An excellent source of health information about genetic disorders which affect particular ethnic and racial minorities in the U.S."
—The Bookwatch, Aug '01

Eye Care Sourcebook, 3rd Edition

Basic Consumer Health Information about Eye Care and Eye Disorders, Including Facts about the Diagnosis, Prevention, and Treatment of Refractive Disorders, Cataracts, Glaucoma, Macular Degeneration, and Problems Affecting the Cornea, Retina, and Lacrimal Glands

Along with Advice about Preventing Eye Injuries and Tips for Living with Low Vision or

Blindness, a Glossary of Related Terms, and Directories of Resources for More Help and Information

Edited by Amy L. Sutton. 646 pages. 2008. 978-0-7808-1000-6.

"A solid reference tool for eye care and a valuable addition to a collection."
—American Reference Books Annual, 2009

Family Planning Sourcebook

Basic Consumer Health Information about Planning for Pregnancy and Contraception, Including Traditional Methods, Barrier Methods, Hormonal Methods, Permanent Methods, Future Methods, Emergency Contraception, and Birth Control Choices for Women at Each Stage of Life

Along with Statistics, a Glossary, and Sources of Additional Information

Edited by Amy Marcaccio Keyzer. 503 pages. 2001. 978-0-7808-0379-4.

"Recommended for public, health, and undergraduate libraries as part of the circulating collection."
—E-Streams, Mar '02

"Will prove valuable to any library seeking to maintain a current, comprehensive reference collection of health resources... Excellent reference."
—The Bookwatch, Aug '01

SEE ALSO Pregnancy and Birth Sourcebook, 3rd Edition

Fitness and Exercise Sourcebook, 3rd Edition

Basic Consumer Health Information about the Physical and Mental Benefits of Fitness, Including Cardiorespiratory Endurance, Muscular Strength, Muscular Endurance, and Flexibility, with Facts about Sports Nutrition and Exercise-Related Injuries and Tips about Physical Activity and Exercises for People of All Ages and for People with Health Concerns

Along with Advice on Selecting and Using Exercise Equipment, Maintaining Exercise Motivation, a Glossary of Related Terms, and a Directory of Resources for More Help and Information

Edited by Amy L. Sutton. 635 pages. 2007. 978-0-7808-0946-8.

"Updates the consumer information on the physical and mental benefits of physical activity throughout the lifespan offered in earlier editions... Recommended. All readers; all levels."
—CHOICE, Oct '07

"An exceptionally well-rounded coverage perfect for any concerned about developing and understanding a fitness program."
—California Bookwatch, Jun '07

SEE ALSO Sports Injuries Sourcebook, 3rd Edition

Food Safety Sourcebook

Basic Consumer Health Information about the Safe Handling of Meat, Poultry, Seafood, Eggs, Fruit Juices, and Other Food Items, and Facts about Pesticides, Drinking Water, Food Safety Overseas, and the Onset, Duration, and Symptoms of Foodborne Illnesses, Including Types of Pathogenic Bacteria, Parasitic Protozoa, Worms, Viruses, and Natural Toxins

Along with the Role of the Consumer, the Food Handler, and the Government in Food Safety, a Glossary, and Resources for Additional Help and Information

Edited by Dawn D. Matthews. 327 pages. 1999. 978-0-7808-0326-8.

"Recommended reference source."
—Booklist, May '00

"This book takes the complex issues of food safety and foodborne pathogens and presents them in an easily understood manner. [It does] an excellent job of covering a large and often confusing topic."
— American Reference Books Annual, 2000

Forensic Medicine Sourcebook

Basic Consumer Information for the Layperson about Forensic Medicine, Including Crime Scene Investigation, Evidence Collection and Analysis, Expert Testimony, Computer-Aided Criminal Identification, Digital Imaging in the Courtroom, DNA Profiling, Accident Reconstruction, Autopsies, Ballistics, Drugs and Explosives Detection, Latent Fingerprints, Product Tampering, and Questioned Document Examination

Along with Statistical Data, a Glossary of Forensics Terminology, and Listings of Sources for Further Help and Information

Edited by Annemarie S. Muth. 574 pages. 1999. 978-0-7808-0232-2.

"Given the expected widespread interest in its content and its easy to read style, this book is recommended for most public and all college and university libraries."
—E-Streams, Feb '01

"A wealth of information, useful statistics, references are up-to-date and extremely complete. This wonderful collection of data will help students who are interested in a career in any type of forensic field. It is a great resource for attorneys who need information about types of expert witnesses needed in a particular case. It also offers useful information for fiction and nonfiction writers whose work involves a crime. A fascinating compilation. All levels."
—CHOICE, Jan '00

"There are several items that make this book attractive to consumers who are seeking certain forensic data... This is a useful current source for those seeking general forensic medical answers."
—American Reference Books Annual, 2000

Gastrointestinal Diseases and Disorders Sourcebook, 2nd Edition

Basic Consumer Health Information about the Upper and Lower Gastrointestinal (GI) Tract, Including the Esophagus, Stomach, Intestines, Rectum, Liver, and Pancreas, with Facts about Gastroesophageal Reflux Disease, Gastritis, Hernias, Ulcers, Celiac Disease, Diverticulitis, Irritable Bowel Syndrome, Hemorrhoids, Gastrointestinal Cancers, and Other Diseases and Disorders Related to the Digestive Process

Along with Information about Commonly Used Diagnostic and Surgical Procedures, Statistics, Reports on Current Research Initiatives and Clinical Trials, a Glossary, and Resources for Additional Help and Information

Edited by Sandra J. Judd. 654 pages. 2006. 978-0-7808-0798-3.

575

"The text is designed for the general reader seeking information on prevention, disease warning signs, diagnostic and therapeutic questions... It is an excellent resource for the general reader to conveniently locate credible, coordinated and indexed information... The sourcebook will prove very helpful for patients, caregivers and should be available in every physician waiting room."
—*Doody's Review Service, 2006*

SEE ALSO *Diet and Nutrition Sourcebook, 3rd Edition, Digestive Diseases and Disorders Sourcebook*

Genetic Disorders Sourcebook, 4th Edition

Basic Consumer Health Information about Hereditary Diseases and Disorders, Including Facts about the Human Genome, Genetic Inheritance Patterns, Disorders Associated with Specific Genes, Such as Sickle Cell Disease, Hemophilia, and Cystic Fibrosis, Chromosome Disorders, Such as Down Syndrome, Fragile X Syndrome, and Turner Syndrome, and Complex Diseases and Disorders Resulting from the Interaction of Environmental and Genetic Factors, Such as Allergies, Cancer, and Obesity

Along with Facts about Genetic Testing, Suggestions for Parents of Children with Special Needs, Reports on Current Research Initiatives, a Glossary of Genetic Terminology, and Resources for Additional Help and Information

Edited by Sandra J. Judd. 600 pages. 2010. 978-0-7808-1076-1.

Head Trauma Sourcebook

Basic Information for the Layperson about Open-Head and Closed-Head Injuries, Treatment Advances, Recovery, and Rehabilitation

Along with Reports on Current Research Initiatives

Edited by Karen Bellenir. 414 pages. 1997. 978-0-7808-0208-7.

Headache Sourcebook

Basic Consumer Health Information about Migraine, Tension, Cluster, Rebound and Other Types of Headaches, with Facts about the Cause and Prevention of Headaches, the Effects of Stress and the Environment, Headaches during Pregnancy and Menopause, and Childhood Headaches

Along with a Glossary and Other Resources for Additional Help and Information

Edited by Dawn D. Matthews. 342 pages. 2002. 978-0-7808-0337-4.

"Highly recommended for academic and medical reference collections."
—*Library Bookwatch, Sep '02*

SEE ALSO *Pain Sourcebook, 3rd Edition*

Healthy Aging Sourcebook

Basic Consumer Health Information about Maintaining Health through the Aging Process, Including Advice on Nutrition, Exercise, and Sleep, Help in Making Decisions about Midlife Issues and Retirement, and Guidance Concerning Practical and Informed Choices in Health Consumerism

Along with Data Concerning the Theories of Aging, Different Experiences in Aging by Minority Groups, and Facts about Aging Now and Aging in the Future; and Featuring a Glossary, a Guide to Consumer Help, Additional Suggested Reading, and Practical Resource Directory

Edited by Jenifer Swanson. 537 pages. 1999. 978-0-7808-0390-9.

"Recommended reference source."
—*Booklist, Feb '00*

SEE ALSO *Adult Health Sourcebook, Physical and Mental Issues in Aging Sourcebook*

Healthy Children Sourcebook

Basic Consumer Health Information about the Physical and Mental Development of Children between the Ages of 3 and 12, Including Routine Health Care, Preventative Health Services, Safety and First Aid, Healthy Sleep, Dental Care, Nutrition, and Fitness, and Featuring Parenting Tips on Such Topics as Bedwetting, Choosing Day Care, Monitoring TV and Other Media, and Establishing a Foundation for Substance Abuse Prevention

Along with a Glossary of Commonly Used Pediatric Terms and Resources for Additional Help and Information.

Edited by Chad T. Kimball. 624 pages. 2003. 978-0-7808-0247-6.

"Should be required reading for parents and teachers."
—*E-Streams, Jun '04*

"It is hard to imagine that any other single resource exists that would provide such a comprehensive guide of timely information on health promotion and disease prevention for children aged 3 to 12."
—*American Reference Books Annual, 2004*

"This easy-to-read volume is a tremendous resource."
—*AORN Journal, May '05*

SEE ALSO *Childhood Diseases and Disorders Sourcebook, 2nd Edition*

Healthy Heart Sourcebook for Women

Basic Consumer Health Information about Cardiac Issues Specific to Women, Including Facts about Major Risk Factors and Prevention, Treatment and Control Strategies, and Important Dietary Issues

Along with a Special Section Regarding the Pros and Cons of Hormone Replacement Therapy and Its Impact on Heart Health, and Additional Help, Including Recipes, a Glossary, and a Directory of Resources

Edited by Dawn D. Matthews. 321 pages. 2000. 978-0-7808-0329-9.

"A good reference source and recommended for all public, academic, medical, and hospital libraries."
—*Medical Reference Services Quarterly, Summer '01*

"Contains very important information about coronary artery disease that all women should know. The information is current and presented in an easy-to-read format. The book will make a good addition to any library."
—*American Medical Writers Association Journal, Summer '00*

SEE ALSO *Cardiovascular Diseases and Disorders Sourcebook, 4th Edition, Women's Health Concerns Sourcebook, 3rd Edition*

Hepatitis Sourcebook

Basic Consumer Health Information about Hepatitis A, Hepatitis B, Hepatitis C, and Other Forms of Hepatitis, Including Autoimmune Hepatitis, Alcoholic Hepatitis, Nonalcoholic Steatohepatitis, and Toxic Hepatitis, with Facts about Risk Factors, Screening Methods, Diagnostic Tests, and Treatment Options

Along with Information on Liver Health, Tips for People Living with Chronic Hepatitis, Reports on Current Research Initiatives, a Glossary of Terms Related to Hepatitis, and a Directory of Sources for Further Help and Information

Edited by Sandra J. Judd. 570 pages. 2006. 978-0-7808-0749-5.

"The breadth of information found in this one book would not be readily found in another source. Highly recommended."
—*American Reference Books Annual, 2006*

SEE ALSO *Contagious Diseases Sourcebook, 2nd Edition*

Household Safety Sourcebook

Basic Consumer Health Information about Household Safety, Including Information about Poisons, Chemicals, Fire, and Water Hazards in the Home

Along with Advice about the Safe Use of Home Maintenance Equipment, Choosing Toys and Nursery Furniture, Holiday and Recreation Safety, a Glossary, and Resources for Further Help and Information

Edited by Dawn D. Matthews. 587 pages. 2002. 978-0-7808-0338-1.

"As a sourcebook on household safety this book meets its mark. It is encyclopedic in scope and covers a wide range of safety issues that are commonly seen in the home."
—*E-Streams, Jul '02*

Hypertension Sourcebook

Basic Consumer Health Information about the Causes, Diagnosis, and Treatment of High Blood Pressure, with Facts about Consequences, Complications, and Co-Occurring Disorders, Such as Coronary Heart Disease, Diabetes, Stroke, Kidney Disease, and Hypertensive Retinopathy, and Issues in Blood Pressure

Control, Including Dietary Choices, Stress Management, and Medications

Along with Reports on Current Research Initiatives and Clinical Trials, a Glossary, and Resources for Additional Help and Information

Edited by Dawn D. Matthews and Karen Bellenir. 588 pages. 2004. 978-0-7808-0674-0.

"Academic, public, and medical libraries will want to add the Hypertension Sourcebook to their collections."
—E-Streams, Aug '05

"The strength of this source is the wide range of information given about hypertension."
—American Reference Books Annual, 2005

SEE ALSO Stroke Sourcebook, 2nd Edition

Immune System Disorders Sourcebook, 2nd Edition

Basic Consumer Health Information about Disorders of the Immune System, Including Immune System Function and Response, Diagnosis of Immune Disorders, Information about Inherited Immune Disease, Acquired Immune Disease, and Autoimmune Diseases, Including Primary Immune Deficiency, Acquired Immunodeficiency Syndrome (AIDS), Lupus, Multiple Sclerosis, Type 1 Diabetes, Rheumatoid Arthritis, and Graves' Disease

Along with Treatments, Tips for Coping with Immune Disorders, a Glossary, and a Directory of Additional Resources

Edited by Joyce Brennfleck Shannon. 643 pages. 2005. 978-0-7808-0748-8.

"Highly recommended for academic and public libraries."
—American Reference Books Annual, 2006

"The updated second edition is a 'must' for any consumer health library seeking a solid resource covering the treatments, symptoms, and options for immune disorder sufferers... An excellent guide."
—MBR Bookwatch, Jan '06

SEE ALSO AIDS Sourcebook, 4th Edition, Arthritis Sourcebook, 3rd Edition

Infant and Toddler Health Sourcebook

Basic Consumer Health Information about the Physical and Mental Development of Newborns, Infants, and Toddlers, Including Neonatal Concerns, Nutrition Recommendations, Immunization Schedules, Common Pediatric Disorders, Assessments and Milestones, Safety Tips, and Advice for Parents and Other Caregivers

Along with a Glossary of Terms and Resource Listings for Additional Help

Edited by Jenifer Swanson. 570 pages. 2000. 978-0-7808-0246-9.

"As a reference for the general public, this would be useful in any library."
—E-Streams, May '01

"Recommended reference source."
—Booklist, Feb '01

Infectious Diseases Sourcebook

Basic Consumer Health Information about Non-Contagious Bacterial, Viral, Prion, Fungal, and Parasitic Diseases Spread by Food and Water, Insects and Animals, or Environmental Contact, Including Botulism, E. Coli, Encephalitis, Legionnaires' Disease, Lyme Disease, Malaria, Plague, Rabies, Salmonella, Tetanus, and Others, and Facts about Newly Emerging Diseases, Such as Hantavirus, Mad Cow Disease, Monkeypox, and West Nile Virus

Along with Information about Preventing Disease Transmission, the Threat of Bioterrorism, and Current Research Initiatives, with a Glossary and Directory of Resources for More Information

Edited by Karen Bellenir. 610 pages. 2004. 978-0-7808-0675-7.

"This reference continues the excellent tradition of the Health Reference Series in consolidating a wealth of information on a selected topic into a format that is easy to use and accessible to the general public."
—American Reference Books Annual, 2005

"Recommended for public and academic libraries."
—E-Streams, Jan '05

SEE ALSO Environmental Health Sourcebook, 3rd Edition

Injury and Trauma Sourcebook

Basic Consumer Health Information about the Impact of Injury, the Diagnosis and Treatment of Common and Traumatic Injuries, Emergency Care, and Specific Injuries Related to Home, Community, Workplace, Transportation, and Recreation

Along with Guidelines for Injury Prevention, a Glossary, and a Directory of Additional Resources

Edited by Joyce Brennfleck Shannon. 675 pages. 2002. 978-0-7808-0421-0.

"Practitioners should be aware of guides such as this in order to facilitate their use by patients and their families."
—Doody's Health Sciences Book Review Journal, Sep-Oct '02

"Recommended reference source."
—Booklist, Sep '02

"Highly recommended for academic and medical reference collections."
—Library Bookwatch, Sep '02

SEE ALSO Emergency Medical Services Sourcebook, Sports Injuries Sourcebook, 3rd Edition

Learning Disabilities Sourcebook, 3rd Edition

Basic Consumer Health Information about Dyslexia, Auditory and Visual Processing Disorders, Communication Disorders, Dyscalculia, Dysgraphia, and Other Conditions That Impede Learning, Including Attention Deficit/ Hyperactivity Disorder, Autism Spectrum Disorders, Hearing and Visual Impairments, Chromosome-Based Disorders, and Brain Injury

Along with Facts about Brain Function, Assessment, Therapy and Remediation, Accommodations, Assistive Technology, Legal Protections, and Tips about Family Life, School Transitions, and Employment Strategies, a Glossary of Related Terms, and Directories of Additional Resources

Edited by Joyce Brennfleck Shannon. 613 pages. 2009. 978-0-7808-1039-6.

"Intended to be a starting point for people who need to know about learning disabilities. Each chapter on a specific disability includes readable,

well-organized descriptions... The book is well indexed and a glossary is included. Chapters on organizations and helpful websites will aid the reader who needs more information."
—American Reference Books Annual, 2009

"This book provides the necessary information to better understand learning disabilities and work with children who have them... It would be difficult to find another book that so comprehensively explains learning disabilities without becoming incomprehensible to the average parent who needs this information."
—Doody's Review Service, 2009

SEE ALSO Attention Deficit Disorder Sourcebook, Autism and Pervasive Developmental Disorders Sourcebook

Leukemia Sourcebook

Basic Consumer Health Information about Adult and Childhood Leukemias, Including Acute Lymphocytic Leukemia (ALL), Chronic Lymphocytic Leukemia (CLL), Acute Myelogenous Leukemia (AML), Chronic Myelogenous Leukemia (CML), and Hairy Cell Leukemia, and Treatments Such as Chemotherapy, Radiation Therapy, Peripheral Blood Stem Cell and Marrow Transplantation, and Immunotherapy

Along with Tips for Life During and After Treatment, a Glossary, and Directories of Additional Resources

Edited by Joyce Brennfleck Shannon. 564 pages. 2003. 978-0-7808-0627-6.

"Unlike other medical books for the layperson... the language does not talk down to the reader... This volume is highly recommended for all libraries."
—American Reference Books Annual, 2004

"A fine title which ranges from diagnosis to alternative treatments, staging, and tips for life during and after diagnosis."
—The Bookwatch, Dec '03

SEE ALSO Blood & Circulatory Disorders Sourcebook, 3rd Edition, Cancer Sourcebook, 5th Edition

Liver Disorders Sourcebook

Basic Consumer Health Information about the Liver and How It Works; Liver Diseases, Including Cancer, Cirrhosis, Hepatitis, and

Toxic and Drug Related Diseases; Tips for Maintaining a Healthy Liver; Laboratory Tests, Radiology Tests, and Facts about Liver Transplantation

Along with a Section on Support Groups, a Glossary, and Resource Listings

Edited by Joyce Brennfleck Shannon. 580 pages. 2000. 978-0-7808-0383-1.

"This title is recommended for health sciences and public libraries with consumer health collections."
—E-Streams, Oct '00

"Recommended reference source."
—Booklist, Jun '00

SEE ALSO Gastrointestinal Diseases and Disorders Sourcebook, 2nd Edition, Hepatitis Sourcebook

■

Lung Disorders Sourcebook

Basic Consumer Health Information about Emphysema, Pneumonia, Tuberculosis, Asthma, Cystic Fibrosis, and Other Lung Disorders, Including Facts about Diagnostic Procedures, Treatment Strategies, Disease Prevention Efforts, and Such Risk Factors as Smoking, Air Pollution, and Exposure to Asbestos, Radon, and Other Agents

Along with a Glossary and Resources for Additional Help and Information

Edited by Dawn D. Matthews. 657 pages. 2002. 978-0-7808-0339-8.

"Highly recommended for academic and medical reference collections."
—Library Bookwatch, Sep '02

SEE ALSO Asthma Sourcebook, 2nd Edition, Respiratory Disorders Sourcebook, 2nd Edition

■

Medical Tests Sourcebook, 3rd Edition

Basic Consumer Health Information about X-Rays, Blood Tests, Stool and Urine Tests, Biopsies, Mammography, Endoscopic Procedures, Ultrasound Exams, Computed Tomography, Magnetic Resonance Imaging (MRI), Nuclear Medicine, Genetic Testing, Home-Use Tests, and More

Along with Facts about Preventive Care and Screening Test Guidelines, Screening and

Assessment Tests Associated with Such Specific Concerns as Cancer, Heart Disease, Allergies, Diabetes, Thyroid Disfunction, and Infertility, a Glossary of Related Terms, and a Directory of Resources for Additional Help and Information

Edited by Karen Bellenir. 627 pages. 2008. 978-0-7808-1040-2

"This volume has a wide scope that makes it useful... Can be a valuable reference guide."
—American Reference Books Annual, 2009

"Would be a valuable contribution to any consumer health or public library."
—Doody's Book Review Service, 2009

■

Men's Health Concerns Sourcebook, 3rd Edition

Basic Consumer Health Information about Wellness in Men and Gender-Related Differences in Health, With Facts about Heart Disease, Cancer, Traumatic Injury, and Other Leading Causes of Death in Men, Reproductive Concerns, Sexual Dysfunction, Disorders of the Prostate, Penis, and Testes, Sex-Linked Genetic Disorders, and Other Medical and Mental Concerns of Men

Along with Statistical Data, a Glossary of Related Terms, and a Directory of Resources for Additional Information

Edited by Sandra J. Judd. 632 pages. 2009. 978-0-7808-1033-4.

"A good addition to any reference shelf in academic, consumer health, or hospital libraries."
—ARBAOnline, Oct '09

SEE ALSO Prostate and Urological Disorders Sourcebook

■

Mental Health Disorders Sourcebook, 4th Edition

Basic Consumer Health Information about the Causes and Symptoms of Mental Health Problems, Including Depression, Bipolar Disorder, Anxiety Disorders, Posttraumatic Stress Disorder, Obsessive-Compulsive Disorder, Eating Disorders, Addictions, and Personality and Psychotic Disorders

Along with Information about Medications and Treatments, Mental Health Concerns in

Children, Adolescents, and Adults, Tips on Living with Mental Health Disorders, a Glossary of Related Terms, and a Directory of Resources for Additional Help and Information

Edited by Amy L. Sutton. 680 pages. 2009. 978-0-7808-1041-9.

"Mental health concerns are presented in everyday language and intended for patients and their families as well as the general public... This resource is comprehensive and up to date... The easy-to-understand writing style helps to facilitate assimilation of needed facts and specifics on often challenging topics."
—*ARBAOnline, Oct '09*

"No health collection should be without this resource, which will reach into many a general lending library as well."
—*Internet Bookwatch, Oct '09*

SEE ALSO *Depression Sourcebook, 2nd Edition, Stress-Related Disorders Sourcebook, 2nd Edition*

Mental Retardation Sourcebook

Basic Consumer Health Information about Mental Retardation and Its Causes, Including Down Syndrome, Fetal Alcohol Syndrome, Fragile X Syndrome, Genetic Conditions, Injury, and Environmental Sources

Along with Preventive Strategies, Parenting Issues, Educational Implications, Health Care Needs, Employment and Economic Matters, Legal Issues, a Glossary, and a Resource Listing for Additional Help and Information

Edited by Joyce Brennfleck Shannon. 627 pages. 2000. 978-0-7808-0377-0.

"Public libraries will find the book useful for reference and as a beginning research point for students, parents, and caregivers."
—*American Reference Books Annual, 2001*

"The strength of this work is that it compiles many basic fact sheets and addresses for further information in one volume. It is intended and suitable for the general public."
—*E-Streams, Nov '00*

"An invaluable overview."
—*Reviewer's Bookwatch, Jul '00*

Movement Disorders Sourcebook, 2nd Edition

Basic Consumer Health Information about the Symptoms and Causes of Movement Disorders, Including Parkinson Disease, Amyotrophic Lateral Sclerosis, Cerebral Palsy, Muscular Dystrophy, Multiple Sclerosis, Myasthenia, Myoclonus, Spina Bifida, Dystonia, Essential Tremor, Choreatic Disorders, Huntington Disease, Tourette Syndrome, and Other Disorders That Cause Slowed, Absent, or Excessive Movements

Along with Information about Surgical and Nonsurgical Interventions, Physical Therapies, Strategies for Independent Living, a Glossary of Related Terms, and a Directory of Resources for Additional Help and Information

Edited by Amy L. Sutton. 618 pages. 2009. 978-0-7808-1034-1.

"The second updated edition of Movement Disorders Sourcebook is a winner, providing the latest research and health findings on all kinds of movement disorders in children and adults... a top pick for any health or general lending library's health reference collection."
—*California Bookwatch, Aug '09*

SEE ALSO *Muscular Dystrophy Sourcebook*

Multiple Sclerosis Sourcebook

Basic Consumer Health Information about Multiple Sclerosis (MS) and Its Effects on Mobility, Vision, Bladder Function, Speech, Swallowing, and Cognition, Including Facts about Risk Factors, Causes, Diagnostic Procedures, Pain Management, Drug Treatments, and Physical and Occupational Therapies

Along with Guidelines for Nutrition and Exercise, Tips on Choosing Assistive Equipment, Information about Disability, Work, Financial, and Legal Issues, a Glossary of Related Terms, and a Directory of Additional Resources

Edited by Joyce Brennfleck Shannon. 553 pages. 2007. 978-0-7808-0998-7.

Muscular Dystrophy Sourcebook

Basic Consumer Health Information about Congenital, Childhood-Onset, and Adult-Onset

Forms of Muscular Dystrophy, Such as Duchenne, Becker, Emery-Dreifuss, Distal, Limb-Girdle, Facioscapulohumeral (FSHD), Myotonic, and Ophthalmoplegic Muscular Dystrophies, Including Facts about Diagnostic Tests, Medical and Physical Therapies, Management of Co-Occurring Conditions, and Parenting Guidelines

Along with Practical Tips for Home Care, a Glossary, and Directories of Additional Resources

Edited by Joyce Brennfleck Shannon. 552 pages. 2004. 978-0-7808-0676-4.

"This book is highly recommended for public and academic libraries as well as health care offices that support the information needs of patients and their families."
—E-Streams, Apr '05

"Excellent reference."
—The Bookwatch, Jan '05

SEE ALSO *Movement Disorders Sourcebook, 2nd Edition*

Obesity Sourcebook

Basic Consumer Health Information about Diseases and Other Problems Associated with Obesity, and Including Facts about Risk Factors, Prevention Issues, and Management Approaches

Along with Statistical and Demographic Data, Information about Special Populations, Research Updates, a Glossary, and Source Listings for Further Help and Information

Edited by Wilma Caldwell and Chad T. Kimball. 360 pages. 2001. 978-0-7808-0333-6.

"The book synthesizes the reliable medical literature on obesity into one easy-to-read and useful resource for the general public."
—American Reference Books Annual, 2002

"Well suited for the health reference collection of a public library or an academic health science library that serves the general population."
—E-Streams, Sep '01

Osteoporosis Sourcebook

Basic Consumer Health Information about Primary and Secondary Osteoporosis and Juvenile Osteoporosis and Related Conditions, Including Fibrous Dysplasia, Gaucher Disease, Hyperthyroidism, Hypophosphatasia,

Myeloma, Osteopetrosis, Osteogenesis Imperfecta, and Paget's Disease

Along with Information about Risk Factors, Treatments, Traditional and Non-Traditional Pain Management, a Glossary of Related Terms, and a Directory of Resources

Edited by Allan R. Cook. 568 pages. 2001. 978-0-7808-0239-1.

"This resource is recommended as a great reference source for public, health, and academic libraries, and is another triumph for the editors of Omnigraphics."
—American Reference Books Annual, 2002

"Will prove valuable to any library seeking to maintain a current, comprehensive reference collection of health resources... From prevention to treatment and associated conditions, this provides an excellent survey."
—The Bookwatch, Aug '01

SEE ALSO *Healthy Aging Sourcebook, Women's Health Concerns Sourcebook, 3rd Edition*

Pain Sourcebook, 3rd Edition

Basic Consumer Health Information about Acute and Chronic Pain, Including Nerve Pain, Bone Pain, Muscle Pain, Cancer Pain, and Disorders Characterized by Pain, Such as Arthritis, Temporomandibular Muscle and Joint (TMJ) Disorder, Carpal Tunnel Syndrome, Headaches, Heartburn, Sciatica, and Shingles, and Facts about Diagnostic Tests and Treatment Options for Pain, Including Over-the-Counter and Prescription Drugs, Physical Rehabilitation, Injection and Infusion Therapies, Implantable Technologies, and Complementary Medicine

Along with Tips for Living with Pain, a Glossary of Related Terms, and a Directory of Additional Resources

Edited by Joyce Brennfleck Shannon. 644 pages. 2008. 978-0-7808-1006-8.

"Excellent for ready-reference users and can be used for beginning students in health fields... appropriate for the consumer health collection in both public and academic libraries."
—American Reference Books Annual, 2009

SEE ALSO *Arthritis Sourcebook, 3rd Edition; Back and Neck Sourcebook, 2nd Edition;*

Headache Sourcebook; Sports Injuries Sourcebook, 3rd Edition

"Recommended for public libraries."
—American Reference Books Annual, 2000

SEE ALSO *Healthy Aging Sourcebook*

Pediatric Cancer Sourcebook

Basic Consumer Health Information about Leukemias, Brain Tumors, Sarcomas, Lymphomas, and Other Cancers in Infants, Children, and Adolescents, Including Descriptions of Cancers, Treatments, and Coping Strategies

Along with Suggestions for Parents, Caregivers, and Concerned Relatives, a Glossary of Cancer Terms, and Resource Listings

Edited by Edward J. Prucha. 575 pages. 1999. 978-0-7808-0245-2.

"An excellent source of information. Recommended for public, hospital, and health science libraries with consumer health collections."
—E-Streams, Jun '00

"A valuable addition to all libraries specializing in health services and many public libraries."
—American Reference Books Annual, 2000

SEE ALSO *Childhood Diseases and Disorders Sourcebook, 2nd Edition, Healthy Children Sourcebook*

Physical and Mental Issues in Aging Sourcebook

Basic Consumer Health Information on Physical and Mental Disorders Associated with the Aging Process, Including Concerns about Cardiovascular Disease, Pulmonary Disease, Oral Health, Digestive Disorders, Musculoskeletal and Skin Disorders, Metabolic Changes, Sexual and Reproductive Issues, and Changes in Vision, Hearing, and Other Senses

Along with Data about Longevity and Causes of Death, Information on Acute and Chronic Pain, Descriptions of Mental Concerns, a Glossary of Terms, and Resource Listings for Additional Help

Edited by Jenifer Swanson. 660 pages. 1999. 978-0-7808-0233-9.

"This is a treasure of health information for the layperson."
—CHOICE Health Sciences Supplement, May '00

Podiatry Sourcebook, 2nd Edition

Basic Consumer Health Information about Disorders, Diseases, and Deformities that Affect the Foot and Ankle, Including Sprains, Corns, Calluses, Bunions, Plantar Warts, Plantar Fasciitis, Neuromas, Clubfoot, Flat Feet, Achilles Tendonitis, and Much More

Along with Information about Selecting a Foot Care Specialist, Foot Fitness, Shoes and Socks, Diagnostic Tests and Corrective Procedures, Financial Assistance for Corrective Devices, a Glossary of Related Terms, and a Directory of Resources for Additional Help and Information

Edited by Ivy L. Alexander. 516 pages. 2007. 978-0-7808-0944-4.

"An excellent resource... Although there have been various types of 'foot books' published in the past, none are as comprehensive as this one. 5 Stars (out of 5)!"
—Doody's Review Service, 2007

"Perfect for both health libraries and general-interest lending collections."
—Internet Bookwatch, Jul '07

Pregnancy and Birth Sourcebook, 3rd Edition

Basic Consumer Health Information about Pregnancy and Fetal Development, Including Facts about Fertility and Conception, Physical and Emotional Changes during Pregnancy, Prenatal Care and Diagnostic Tests, High-Risk Pregnancies and Complications, Labor, Delivery, and the Postpartum Period

Along with Tips on Maintaining Health and Wellness during Pregnancy and Caring for Newborn Infants, a Glossary of Related Terms, and Directories of Resources for Additional Help and Information

Edited by Amy L. Sutton. 645 pages. 2009. 978-0-7808-1074-7.

SEE ALSO *Breastfeeding Sourcebook, Congenital Disorders Sourcebook, 2nd Edition, Family Planning Sourcebook, Women's Health Concerns Sourcebook, 3rd Edition*

Prostate and Urological Disorders Sourcebook

Basic Consumer Health Information about Urogenital and Sexual Disorders in Men, Including Prostate and Other Andrological Cancers, Prostatitis, Benign Prostatic Hyperplasia, Testicular and Penile Trauma, Cryptorchidism, Peyronie Disease, Erectile Dysfunction, and Male Factor Infertility, and Facts about Commonly Used Tests and Procedures, Such as Prostatectomy, Vasectomy, Vasectomy Reversal, Penile Implants, and Semen Analysis

Along with a Glossary of Andrological Terms and a Directory of Resources for Additional Information

Edited by Karen Bellenir. 604 pages. 2006. 978-0-7808-0797-6.

"Certain to be a popular pick among library reference holdings... No prior knowledge is assumed for any of the conditions or terms herein, making it a most accessible general-interest reference."
—*California Bookwatch, Apr '06*

SEE ALSO *Men's Health Concerns Sourcebook, 3rd Edition, Urinary Tract and Kidney Diseases and Disorders Sourcebook, 2nd Edition*

Prostate Cancer Sourcebook

Basic Consumer Health Information about Prostate Cancer, Including Information about the Associated Risk Factors, Detection, Diagnosis, and Treatment of Prostate Cancer

Along with Information on Non-Malignant Prostate Conditions, and Featuring a Section Listing Support and Treatment Centers and a Glossary of Related Terms

Edited by Dawn D. Matthews. 340 pages. 2001. 978-0-7808-0324-4.

"Recommended reference source."
—*Booklist, Jan '02*

"A valuable resource for health care consumers seeking information on the subject... All text is written in a clear, easy-to-understand language that avoids technical jargon. Any library that collects consumer health resources would strengthen their collection with the addition of the Prostate Cancer Sourcebook."
—*American Reference Books Annual, 2002*

SEE ALSO *Cancer Sourcebook, 5th Edition, Men's Health Concerns Sourcebook, 3rd Edition*

Rehabilitation Sourcebook

Basic Consumer Health Information about Rehabilitation for People Recovering from Heart Surgery, Spinal Cord Injury, Stroke, Orthopedic Impairments, Amputation, Pulmonary Impairments, Traumatic Injury, and More, Including Physical Therapy, Occupational Therapy, Speech/Language Therapy, Massage Therapy, Dance Therapy, Art Therapy, and Recreational Therapy

Along with Information on Assistive and Adaptive Devices, a Glossary, and Resources for Additional Help and Information

Edited by Dawn D. Matthews. 519 pages. 2000. 978-0-7808-0236-0.

"This is an excellent resource for public library reference and health collections."
—*American Reference Books Annual, 2001*

"Recommended reference source."
—*Booklist, May '00*

Respiratory Disorders Sourcebook, 2nd Edition

Basic Consumer Health Information about Infectious, Inflammatory, and Chronic Conditions Affecting the Lungs and Respiratory System, Including Pneumonia, Bronchitis, Influenza, Tuberculosis, Sarcoidosis, Asthma, Cystic Fibrosis, Chronic Obstructive Pulmonary Disease, Lung Abscesses, Pulmonary Embolism, Occupational Lung Diseases, and Other Bacterial, Viral, and Fungal Infections

Along with Facts about the Structure and Function of the Lungs and Airways, Methods of Diagnosing Respiratory Disorders, and Treatment and Rehabilitation Options, a Glossary of Related Terms, and a Directory of Resources for Additional Help and Information

Edited by Sandra L. Judd. 638 pages. 2008. 978-0-7808-1007-5.

"An excellent book for patients, their families, or for those who are just curious about respiratory disease. Public libraries and physician offices would find this a valuable resource as well. 4 Stars! (out of 5)"
—*Doody's Review Service, 2009*

"A great addition for public and school libraries because it provides concise health information... readers can start with this reference source and get satisfactory answers before proceeding to other medical reference tools for

more in depth information... A good guide for health education on lung disorders."
—*American Reference Books Annual, 2009*

SEE ALSO Asthma Sourcebook, 2nd Edition, Lung Disorders Sourcebook

Sexually Transmitted Diseases Sourcebook, 4th Edition

Basic Consumer Health Information about Chlamydial Infections, Gonorrhea, Hepatitis, Herpes, HIV/AIDS, Human Papillomavirus, Pubic Lice, Scabies, Syphilis, Trichomoniasis, Vaginal Infections, and Other Sexually Transmitted Diseases, Including Facts about Risk Factors, Symptoms, Diagnosis, Treatment, and the Prevention of Sexually Transmitted Infections

Along with Updates on Current Research Initiatives, a Glossary of Related Terms, and Resources for Additional Help and Information

Edited by Laura Larsen. 623 pages. 2009. 978-0-7808-1073-0.

"**Extremely beneficial... The question-and-answer format along with the index and table of contents make this well-organized resource extremely easy to reference, read, and comprehend... an invaluable medical reference source for lay readers, and a highly appropriate addition for public library collections, health clinics, and any library with a consumer health collection**"
—*ARBAOnline, Oct '09*

SEE ALSO AIDS Sourcebook, 4th Edition, Contagious Diseases Sourcebook, 2nd Edition, Men's Health Concerns Sourcebook, 3rd Edition, Women's Health Concerns Sourcebook, 3rd Edition

Sleep Disorders Sourcebook, 3rd Edition

Basic Consumer Health Information about Sleep Disorders, Including Insomnia, Sleep Apnea and Snoring, Jet Lag and Other Circadian Rhythm Disorders, Narcolepsy, and Parasomnias, Such as Sleep Walking and Sleep Talking, and Featuring Facts about Other Health Problems that Affect Sleep, Why Sleep Is Necessary, How Much Sleep Is Needed, the Physical and Mental Effects of Sleep Deprivation, and Pediatric Sleep Issues

Along with Tips for Diagnosing and Treating Sleep Disorders, a Glossary of Related Terms, and a List of Resources for Additional Help and Information

Edited by Sandra J. Judd. 600 pages. 2010. 978-0-7808-1084-6.

Smoking Concerns Sourcebook

Basic Consumer Health Information about Nicotine Addiction and Smoking Cessation, Featuring Facts about the Health Effects of Tobacco Use, Including Lung and Other Cancers, Heart Disease, Stroke, and Respiratory Disorders, Such as Emphysema and Chronic Bronchitis

Along with Information about Smoking Prevention Programs, Suggestions for Achieving and Maintaining a Smoke-Free Lifestyle, Statistics about Tobacco Use, Reports on Current Research Initiatives, a Glossary of Related Terms, and Directories of Resources for Additional Help and Information

Edited by Karen Bellenir. 595 pages. 2004. 978-0-7808-0323-7.

"**Provides everything needed for the student or general reader seeking practical details on the effects of tobacco use.**"
—*The Bookwatch, Mar '05*

"**Public libraries and consumer health care libraries will find this work useful.**"
—*American Reference Books Annual, 2005*

SEE ALSO Respiratory Disorders Sourcebook, 2nd Edition

Sports Injuries Sourcebook, 3rd Edition

Basic Consumer Health Information about Sprains and Strains, Fractures, Growth Plate Injuries, Overtraining Injuries, and Injuries to the Head, Face, Shoulders, Elbows, Hands, Spinal Column, Knees, Ankles, and Feet, and with Facts about Heat-Related Illness, Steroids and Sport Supplements, Protective Equipment, Diagnostic Procedures, Treatment Options, and Rehabilitation

Along with a Glossary of Related Terms and a Directory of Resources for Additional Help and Information

Edited by Sandra J. Judd. 623 pages. 2007. 978-0-7808-0949-9.

SEE ALSO Fitness and Exercise Sourcebook, 3rd Edition, Podiatry Sourcebook, 2nd Edition

Stress-Related Disorders Sourcebook, 2nd Edition

Basic Consumer Health Information about Stress and Stress-Related Disorders, Including Types of Stress, Sources of Acute and Chronic Stress, the Impact of Stress on the Body's Systems, and Mental and Emotional Health Problems Associated with Stress, Such as Depression, Anxiety Disorders, Substance Abuse, Posttraumatic Stress Disorder, and Suicide

Along with Advice about Getting Help for Stress-Related Disorders, Information about Stress Management Techniques, a Glossary of Stress-Related Terms, and a Directory of Resources for Additional Help and Information

Edited by Amy L. Sutton. 608 pages. 2007. 978-0-7808-0996-3.

"Accessible to the lay reader. Highly recommended for medical and psychiatric collections."
—Library Journal, Mar '08

"Well-written for a general readership, the 2ⁿᵈ Edition of Stress-Related Disorders Sourcebook is a useful addition to the health reference literature."
—American Reference Books Annual, 2008

SEE ALSO Mental Health Disorders Sourcebook, 4th Edition

Stroke Sourcebook, 2nd Edition

Basic Consumer Health Information about Stroke, Including Ischemic, Hemorrhagic, and Mini Strokes, as Well as Risk Factors, Prevention Guidelines, Diagnostic Tests, Medications and Surgical Treatments, and Complications of Stroke

Along with Rehabilitation Techniques and Innovations, Tips on Staying Healthy and Maintaining Independence after Stroke, a Glossary of Related Terms, and a Directory of Resources for Stroke Survivors and Their Families

Edited by Amy L. Sutton. 626 pages. 2008. 978-0-7808-1035-8.

"An encyclopedic handbook on stroke that is written in a language the layperson can understand... This is one of the most helpful, readable books on stroke. This volume is highly recommended and should be in every medical, hospital and public library; in addition, every family practitioner should have a copy in his or her office."
—American Reference Books Annual, 2009

SEE ALSO Brain Disorders Sourcebook, 3rd Edition, Hypertension Sourcebook

Surgery Sourcebook, 2nd Edition

Basic Consumer Health Information about Common Inpatient and Outpatient Surgeries, Including Critical Care and Trauma, Gastrointestinal, Gynecologic and Obstetric, Cardiac and Vascular, Neurologic, Ophthalmologic, Orthopedic, Reconstructive and Cosmetic, and Other Major and Minor Surgeries

Along with Information about Anesthesia and Pain Relief Options, Risks and Complications, Postoperative Recovery Concerns, and Innovative Surgical Techniques and Tools, a Glossary of Related Terms, and a Directory of Additional Resources

Edited by Amy L. Sutton. 645 pages. 2008. 978-0-7808-1004-4.

"Large public libraries and medical libraries would benefit from this material in their reference collections."
—American Reference Books Annual, 2009

SEE ALSO Cosmetic and Reconstructive Surgery Sourcebook, 2nd Edition

Thyroid Disorders Sourcebook

Basic Consumer Health Information about Disorders of the Thyroid and Parathyroid Glands, Including Hypothyroidism, Hyperthyroidism, Graves Disease, Hashimoto Thyroiditis, Thyroid Cancer, and Parathyroid Disorders, Featuring Facts about Symptoms, Risk Factors, Tests, and Treatments

Along with Information about the Effects of Thyroid Imbalance on Other Body Systems, Environmental Factors That Affect the Thyroid Gland, a Glossary, and a Directory of Additional Resources

Edited by Joyce Brennfleck Shannon. 573 pages. 2005. 978-0-7808-0745-7.

"Recommended for consumer health collections."
—*American Reference Books Annual, 2006*

"Highly recommended pick for Basic Consumer health reference holdings at all levels."
—*The Bookwatch, Aug '05*

SEE ALSO *Endocrine and Metabolic Disorders Sourcebook, 2nd Edition*

Transplantation Sourcebook
Basic Consumer Health Information about Organ and Tissue Transplantation, Including Physical and Financial Preparations, Procedures and Issues Relating to Specific Solid Organ and Tissue Transplants, Rehabilitation, Pediatric Transplant Information, the Future of Transplantation, and Organ and Tissue Donation

Along with a Glossary and Listings of Additional Resources

Edited by Joyce Brennfleck Shannon. 610 pages. 2002. 978-0-7808-0322-0.

"Recommended for libraries with an interest in offering consumer health information."
—*E-Streams, Jul '02*

"This is a unique and valuable resource for patients facing transplantation and their families."
—*Doody's Review Service, Jun '02*

Traveler's Health Sourcebook
Basic Consumer Health Information for Travelers, Including Physical and Medical Preparations, Transportation Health and Safety, Essential Information about Food and Water, Sun Exposure, Insect and Snake Bites, Camping and Wilderness Medicine, and Travel with Physical or Medical Disabilities

Along with International Travel Tips, Vaccination Recommendations, Geographical Health Issues, Disease Risks, a Glossary, and a Listing of Additional Resources

Edited by Joyce Brennfleck Shannon. 619 pages. 2000. 978-0-7808-0384-8.

"Recommended reference source."
—*Booklist, Feb '01*

"This book is recommended for any public library, any travel collection, and especially any collection for the physically disabled."
—*American Reference Books Annual, 2001*

SEE ALSO *Worldwide Health Sourcebook*

Urinary Tract and Kidney Diseases and Disorders Sourcebook, 2nd Edition
Basic Consumer Health Information about the Urinary System, Including the Bladder, Urethra, Ureters, and Kidneys, with Facts about Urinary Tract Infections, Incontinence, Congenital Disorders, Kidney Stones, Cancers of the Urinary Tract and Kidneys, Kidney Failure, Dialysis, and Kidney Transplantation

Along with Statistical and Demographic Information, Reports on Current Research in Kidney and Urologic Health, a Summary of Commonly Used Diagnostic Tests, a Glossary of Related Terms, and a Directory of Resources for Additional Help and Information

Edited by Ivy L. Alexander. 621 pages. 2005. 978-0-7808-0750-1.

"A good choice for a consumer health information library or for a medical library needing information to refer to their patients."
—*American Reference Books Annual, 2006*

SEE ALSO *Prostate and Urological Disorders Sourcebook*

Vegetarian Sourcebook
Basic Consumer Health Information about Vegetarian Diets, Lifestyle, and Philosophy, Including Definitions of Vegetarianism and Veganism, Tips about Adopting Vegetarianism, Creating a Vegetarian Pantry, and Meeting Nutritional Needs of Vegetarians, with Facts Regarding Vegetarianism's Effect on Pregnant and Lactating Women, Children, Athletes, and Senior Citizens

Along with a Glossary of Commonly Used Vegetarian Terms and Resources for Additional Help and Information

Edited by Chad T. Kimball. 337 pages. 2002. 978-0-7808-0439-5.

"Organizes into one concise volume the answers to the most common questions concerning vegetarian diets and lifestyles. This title is recommended for public and secondary school libraries."

—E-Streams, Apr '03

"Invaluable reference for public and school library collections alike."
—Library Bookwatch, Apr '03

"The articles in this volume are easy to read and come from authoritative sources. The book does not necessarily support the vegetarian diet but instead provides the pros and cons of this important decision... Recommended for public libraries and consumer health libraries."
—American Reference Books Annual, 2003

SEE ALSO *Diet and Nutrition Sourcebook, 3rd Edition*

■

Women's Health Concerns Sourcebook, 3rd Edition

Basic Consumer Health Information about Issues and Trends in Women's Health and Health Conditions of Special Concern to Women, Including Endometriosis, Uterine Fibroids, Menstrual Irregularities, Menopause, Sexual Dysfunction, Infertility, Cancer in Women, and Other Such Chronic Disorders as Lupus, Fibromyalgia, and Thyroid Disease

Along with Statistical Data, Tips for Maintaining Wellness, a Glossary, and a Directory of Resources for Further Help and Information

Edited by Sandra J. Judd. 679 pages. 2009. 978-0-7808-1036-5.

"This useful resource provides information about a wide range of topics that will help women understand their bodies, prevent or treat disease, and maintain health... A detailed index helps readers locate information. This is a useful addition to public and consumer health library collections"
—ARBAOnline, Jun '09

SEE ALSO *Breast Cancer Sourcebook, 3rd Edition, Cancer Sourcebook for Women, 4th Edition, Healthy Heart Sourcebook for Women*

■

Workplace Health and Safety Sourcebook

Basic Consumer Health Information about Workplace Health and Safety, Including the Effect of Workplace Hazards on the Lungs,

Skin, Heart, Ears, Eyes, Brain, Reproductive Organs, Musculoskeletal System, and Other Organs and Body Parts

Along with Information about Occupational Cancer, Personal Protective Equipment, Toxic and Hazardous Chemicals, Child Labor, Stress, and Workplace Violence

Edited by Chad T. Kimball. 610 pages. 2000. 978-0-7808-0231-5.

"As a reference for the general public, this would be useful in any library."
—E-Streams, Jun '01

"Provides helpful information for primary care physicians and other caregivers interested in occupational medicine... General readers; professionals."
—CHOICE, May '01

■

Worldwide Health Sourcebook

Basic Information about Global Health Issues, Including Malnutrition, Reproductive Health, Disease Dispersion and Prevention, Emerging Diseases, Risky Health Behaviors, and the Leading Causes of Death

Along with Global Health Concerns for Children, Women, and the Elderly, Mental Health Issues, Research and Technology Advancements, and Economic, Environmental, and Political Health Implications, a Glossary, and a Resource Listing for Additional Help and Information

Edited by Joyce Brennfleck Shannon. 597 pages. 2001. 978-0-7808-0330-5.

"Named an Outstanding Academic Title."
—CHOICE, Jan '02

"Yet another handy but also unique compilation in the extensive Health Reference Series, this is a useful work because many of the international publications reprinted or excerpted are not readily available. Highly recommended."
—CHOICE, Nov '01

SEE ALSO *Traveler's Health Sourcebook*

Teen Health Series
Complete Catalog
List price $69 per volume. School and library price $62 per volume.

Abuse and Violence Information for Teens
Health Tips about the Causes and Consequences of Abusive and Violent Behavior
Including Facts about the Types of Abuse and Violence, the Warning Signs of Abusive and Violent Behavior, Health Concerns of Victims, and Getting Help and Staying Safe

Edited by Sandra Augustyn Lawton. 411 pages. 2008. 978-0-7808-1008-2.

"A useful resource for schools and organizations providing services to teens and may also be a starting point in research projects."
—*Reference and Research Book News, Aug '08*

"Violence is a serious problem for teens... This resource gives teens the information they need to face potential threats and get help—either for themselves or for their friends."
—*American Reference Books Annual, 2009*

Accident and Safety Information for Teens
Health Tips about Medical Emergencies, Traumatic Injuries, and Disaster Preparedness
Including Facts about Motor Vehicle Accidents, Burns, Poisoning, Firearms, Natural Disasters, National Security Threats, and More

Edited by Karen Bellenir. 420 pages. 2008. 978-0-7808-1046-4.

"Aimed at teenage audiences, this guide provides practical information for handling a comprehensive list of emergencies, from sport injuries and auto accidents to alcohol poisoning and natural disasters."
—*Library Journal, Apr 1, '09*

"Useful in the young adult collections of public libraries as well as high school libraries."
—*American Reference Books Annual, 2009*

SEE ALSO Sports Injuries Information for Teens, 2nd Edition

Alcohol Information for Teens, 2nd Edition
Health Tips about Alcohol and Alcoholism
Including Facts about Alcohol's Effects on the Body, Brain, and Behavior, the Consequences of Underage Drinking, Alcohol Abuse Prevention and Treatment, and Coping with Alcoholic Parents

Edited by Lisa Bakewell. 410 pages. 2009. 978-0-7808-1043-3.

"This handbook, written for a teenage audience, provides information on the causes, effects, and preventive measures related to alcohol abuse among teens... The chapters are quick to make a connection to their teenage reading audience. The prose is straightforward and the book lends itself to spot reading. It should be useful both for practical information and for research, and it is suitable for public and school libraries."
—*ARBAOnline, Jun '09*

SEE ALSO Drug Information for Teens, 2nd Edition

Allergy Information for Teens
Health Tips about Allergic Reactions Such as Anaphylaxis, Respiratory Problems, and Rashes
Including Facts about Identifying and Managing Allergies to Food, Pollen, Mold, Animals, Chemicals, Drugs, and Other Substances

Edited by Karen Bellenir. 410 pages. 2006. 978-0-7808-0799-0.

"This is a comprehensive, readable text on the subject of allergic diseases in teenagers. 5 Stars (out of 5)!"
—*Doody's Review Service, Jun '06*

"This authoritative and useful self-help title is a solid addition to YA collections, whether for personal interest or reports."
—*School Library Journal, Jul '06*

Asthma Information for Teens, 2nd Ed.
Health Tips about Managing Asthma and Related Concerns

Including Facts about Asthma Causes, Triggers and Symptoms, Diagnosis, and Treatment

Edited by Kim Wohlenhaus. 400 pages. 2010. 978-0-7808-1086-0.

▓

Body Information for Teens
Health Tips about Maintaining Well-Being for a Lifetime
Including Facts about the Development and Functioning of the Body's Systems, Organs, and Structures and the Health Impact of Lifestyle Choices

Edited by Sandra Augustyn Lawton. 458 pages. 2007. 978-0-7808-0443-2.

▓

Cancer Information for Teens, 2nd Edition
Health Tips about Cancer Awareness, Symptoms, Prevention, Diagnosis, and Treatment
Including Facts about Common Cancers Affecting Teens, Causes, Detection, Coping Strategies, Clinical Trials, Nutrition and Exercise, Cancer in Friends or Family, and More

Edited by Karen Bellenir and Lisa Bakewell. 445 pages. 2010. 978-0-7808-1085-3.

▓

Complementary and Alternative Medicine Information for Teens
Health Tips about Non-Traditional and Non-Western Medical Practices
Including Information about Acupuncture, Chiropractic Medicine, Dietary and Herbal Supplements, Hypnosis, Massage Therapy, Prayer and Spirituality, Reflexology, Yoga, and More

Edited by Sandra Augustyn Lawton. 407 pages. 2007. 978-0-7808-0966-6.

"This volume covers CAM specifically for teenagers but of general use also. It should be a welcome addition to both public and academic libraries."
—*American Reference Books Annual, 2008*

"This volume provides a solid foundation for further investigation of the subject, making it useful for both public and high school libraries."
—*VOYA: Voice of Youth Advocates, Jun '07*

Diabetes Information for Teens
Health Tips about Managing Diabetes and Preventing Related Complications
Including Information about Insulin, Glucose Control, Healthy Eating, Physical Activity, and Learning to Live with Diabetes

Edited by Sandra Augustyn Lawton. 410 pages. 2006. 978-0-7808-0811-9.

"A comprehensive instructional guide for teens... some of the material may also be directed towards parents or teachers. 5 stars (out of 5)!"
—*Doody's Review Service, 2006*

"Students dealing with their own diabetes or that of a friend or family member or those writing reports on the topic will find this a valuable resource."
—*School Library Journal, Aug '06*

"This text is directed to the teen population and would be an excellent library resource for a health class or for the teacher as a reference for class preparation. It can, however, serve a much wider audience. The clinical educator on diabetes may find it valuable to educate the newly diagnosed client regardless of age. It also would be an excellent reference and education tool for a preventive medicine seminar on diabetes."
—*Physical Therapy, Mar '07*

▓

Diet Information for Teens, 2nd Edition
Health Tips about Diet and Nutrition
Including Facts about Dietary Guidelines, Food Groups, Nutrients, Healthy Meals, Snacks, Weight Control, Medical Concerns Related to Diet, and More

Edited by Karen Bellenir. 432 pages. 2006. 978-0-7808-0820-1.

"A very quick and pleasant read in spite of the fact that it is very detailed in the information it gives... A book for anyone concerned about diet and nutrition."
—*American Reference Books Annual, 2007*

SEE ALSO *Eating Disorders Information for Teens, 2nd Edition*

▓

Drug Information for Teens, 2nd Edition

Health Tips about the Physical and Mental Effects of Substance Abuse

Including Information about Marijuana, Inhalants, Club Drugs, Stimulants, Hallucinogens, Opiates, Prescription and Over-the-Counter Drugs, Herbal Products, Tobacco, Alcohol, and More

Edited by Sandra Augustyn Lawton. 468 pages. 2006. 978-0-7808-0862-1.

"As with earlier installments in Omnigraphics' Teen Health Series, Drug Information for Teens is designed specifically to meet the needs and interests of middle and high school students... Strongly recommended for both academic and public libraries."

—*American Reference Books Annual, 2007*

"Solid thoughtful advice is given about how to handle peer pressure, drug-related health concerns, and treatment strategies."

—*School Library Journal, Dec '06*

SEE ALSO *Alcohol Information for Teens, 2nd Edition, Tobacco Information for Teens, 2nd Edition*

Eating Disorders Information for Teens, 2nd Edition

Health Tips about Anorexia, Bulimia, Binge Eating, And Other Eating Disorders

Including Information about Risk Factors, Diagnosis and Treatment, Prevention, Related Health Concerns, and Other Issues

Edited by Sandra Augustyn Lawton. 377 pages. 2009. 978-0-7808-1044-0.

"This handy reference offers basic information and addresses specific disorders, consequences, prevention, diagnosis and treatment, healthy eating, and more. It is written in a conversational style that is easy to understand... Will provide plenty of facts for reports as well as browsing potential for students with an interest in the topic."

—*School Library Journal, Jun '09*

"Written in a straightforward style that will appeal to its teenage audience. The author does not play down the danger of living with an eating disorder and urges those struggling with this problem to seek professional help.

This work, as well as others in this series, will be a welcome addition to high school and undergraduate libraries."

—*American Reference Books Annual, 2009*

SEE ALSO *Diet Information for Teens, 2nd Edition*

Fitness Information for Teens, 2nd Edition

Health Tips about Exercise, Physical Well-Being, and Health Maintenance

Including Facts about Conditioning, Stretching, Strength Training, Body Shape and Body Image, Sports Nutrition, and Specific Activities for Athletes and Non-Athletes

Edited by Lisa Bakewell. 432 pages. 2009. 978-0-7808-1045-7.

"This no-nonsense guide packs a great deal into its pages... This is a helpful reference for basic diet and exercise information for health reports or personal use."

—*School Library Journal, April 2009*

"An excellent source for general information on why teens should be active, making time to exercise, the equipment people might need, various types of activities to try, how to maintain health and wellness, and how to avoid barriers to becoming healthier... This would still be an excellent addition to a public library ready-reference collection or a high school health library collection."

—*American Reference Books Annual, 2009*

"This easy to read, well-written, up-to-date overview of fitness for teenagers provides excellent wellness and exercise tips, information, and directions... It is a useful tool for them to obtain a base knowledge in fitness topics and different sports."

—*Doody's Review Service, 2009*

SEE ALSO *Diet Information for Teens, 2nd Edition, Sports Injuries Information for Teens, 2nd Edition*

Learning Disabilities Information for Teens

Health Tips about Academic Skills Disorders and Other Disabilities That Affect Learning

Including Information about Common Signs of Learning Disabilities, School Issues, Learning to Live with a Learning Disability, and Other Related Issues

Edited by Sandra Augustyn Lawton. 400 pages. 2006. 978-0-7808-0796-9.

"This book provides a wealth of information for any reader interested in the signs, causes, and consequences of learning disabilities, as well as related legal rights and educational interventions... Public and academic libraries should want this title for both students and general readers."
—*American Reference Books Annual, 2006*

Mental Health Information for Teens, 3rd Edition
Health Tips about Mental Wellness and Mental Illness
Including Facts about Mental and Emotional Health, Depression and Other Mood Disorders, Anxiety Disorders, Behavior Disorders, Self-Injury, Psychosis, Schizophrenia, and More

Edited by Karen Bellenir. 400 pages. 2010. 978-0-7808-1087-7.

SEE ALSO *Stress Information for Teens, Suicide Information for Teens, 2nd Edition*

Pregnancy Information for Teens
Health Tips about Teen Pregnancy and Teen Parenting
Including Facts about Prenatal Care, Pregnancy Complications, Labor and Delivery, Postpartum Care, Pregnancy-Related Lifestyle Concerns, and More

Edited by Sandra Augustyn Lawton. 434 pages. 2007. 978-0-7808-0984-0.

Sexual Health Information for Teens, 2nd Edition
Health Tips about Sexual Development, Reproduction, Contraception, and Sexually Transmitted Infections
Including Facts about Puberty, Sexuality, Birth Control, Chlamydia, Gonorrhea, Herpes, Human Papillomavirus, Syphilis, and More

Edited by Sandra Augustyn Lawton. 430 pages. 2008. 978-0-7808-1010-5.

"This offering represents the most up-to-date information available on an array of topics including abstinence-only sexual education and pregnancy-prevention methods... The range of coverage—from puberty and anatomy to sexually transmitted diseases—is thorough and extensive. Each chapter includes a bibliographic citation, and the three back sections containing additional resources, further reading, and the index are all first-rate... This volume will be well used by students in need of the facts, whether for educational or personal reasons."
—*School Library Journal, Nov '08*

"Presents information related to the emotional, physical, and biological development of both males and females that occurs during puberty. It also strives to address some of the issues and questions that may arise... The text is easy to read and understand for young readers, with satisfactory definitions within the text to explain new terms."
—*American Reference Books Annual, 2009*

Skin Health Information for Teens, 2nd Edition
Health Tips about Dermatological Concerns and Skin Cancer Risks
Including Facts about Acne, Warts, Hives, and Other Conditions and Lifestyle Choices, Such as Tanning, Tattooing, and Piercing, That Affect the Skin, Nails, Scalp, and Hair

Edited by Edited by Kim Wohlenhaus. 418 pages. 2009. 978-0-7808-1042-6.

"The material in this work will be easily understood by teenagers and young adults. The publisher has liberally used bulleted lists and sidebars to keep the reader's attention... A useful addition to school and public library collections."
—*ARBAOnline, Oct '09*

Sleep Information for Teens
Health Tips about Adolescent Sleep Requirements, Sleep Disorders, and the Effects of Sleep Deprivation
Including Facts about Why People Need Sleep, Sleep Patterns, Circadian Rhythms, Dreaming, Insomnia, Sleep Apnea, Narcolepsy, and More

Edited by Karen Bellenir. 355 pages. 2008. 978-0-7808-1009-9.

"Clear, concise, and very readable and would be a good source of sleep information for anyone—not just teenagers. This work is highly recommended for medical libraries, public school libraries, and public libraries."
—*American Reference Books Annual, 2009*

SEE ALSO *Body Information for Teens*

Sports Injuries Information for Teens, 2nd Edition
Health Tips about Acute, Traumatic, and Chronic Injuries in Adolescent Athletes
Including Facts about Sprains, Fractures, and Overuse Injuries, Treatment, Rehabilitation, Sport-Specific Safety Guidelines, Fitness Suggestions, and More

Edited by Karen Bellenir. 429 pages. 2008. 978-0-7808-1011-2.

"An engaging selection of informative articles about the prevention and treatment of sports injuries... The value of this book is that the articles have been vetted and are often augmented with inserts of useful facts, definitions of technical terms, and quick tips. Sensitive topics like injuries to genitalia are discussed openly and responsibly. This revised edition contains updated articles and defines sport more broadly than the first edition."
—*School Library Journal, Nov '08*

"This work will be useful in the young adult collections of public libraries as well as high school libraries... A useful resource for student research."
—*American Reference Books Annual, 2009*

SEE ALSO *Accident and Safety Information for Teens*

Stress Information for Teens
Health Tips about the Mental and Physical Consequences of Stress
Including Information about the Different Kinds of Stress, Symptoms of Stress, Frequent Causes of Stress, Stress Management Techniques, and More

Edited by Sandra Augustyn Lawton. 392 pages. 2008. 978-0-7808-1012-9.

"Understanding what stress is, what causes it, how the body and the mind are impacted by it, and what teens can do are the general categories addressed here... The chapters are brief but informative, and the list of community-help organizations is exhaustive. Report writers will find information quickly and easily, as will those who have personal concerns. The print is clear and the format is readable, making this an accessible resource for struggling readers and researchers."
—*School Library Journal, Dec '08*

"The articles selected will specifically appeal to young adults and are designed to answer their most common questions."
— *American Reference Books Annual, 2009*

SEE ALSO *Mental Health Information for Teens, 3rd Edition*

Suicide Information for Teens, 2nd Edition
Health Tips about Suicide Causes and Prevention
Including Facts about Depression, Risk Factors, Getting Help, Survivor Support, and More

Edited by Kim Wohlenhaus. 400 pages. 2010. 978-0-7808-1088-4.

SEE ALSO *Mental Health Information for Teens, 3rd Edition*

Tobacco Information for Teens, 2nd Edition
Health Tips about the Hazards of Using Cigarettes, Smokeless Tobacco, and Other Nicotine Products
Including Facts about Nicotine Addiction, Nicotine Delivery Systems, Secondhand Smoke, Health Consequences of Tobacco Use, Related Cancers, Smoking Cessation, and Tobacco Use Statistics

Edited by Karen Bellenir. 400 pages. 2010. 978-0-7808-1153-9.

SEE ALSO *Drug Information for Teens, 2nd Edition*

Health Reference Series

Adolescent Health Sourcebook, 3rd Edition

Adult Health Concerns Sourcebook

AIDS Sourcebook, 4th Edition

Alcoholism Sourcebook, 3rd Edition

Allergies Sourcebook, 3rd Edition

Alzheimer Disease Sourcebook, 4th Edition

Arthritis Sourcebook, 3rd Edition

Asthma Sourcebook, 2nd Edition

Attention Deficit Disorder Sourcebook

Autism & Pervasive Developmental Disorders Sourcebook

Back & Neck Sourcebook, 2nd Edition

Blood & Circulatory Disorders Sourcebook, 3rd Edition

Brain Disorders Sourcebook, 3rd Edition

Breast Cancer Sourcebook, 3rd Edition

Breastfeeding Sourcebook

Burns Sourcebook

Cancer Sourcebook for Women, 4th Edition

Cancer Sourcebook, 5th Edition

Cancer Survivorship Sourcebook

Cardiovascular Disorders Sourcebook, 4th Edition

Caregiving Sourcebook

Child Abuse Sourcebook

Childhood Diseases & Disorders Sourcebook, 2nd Edition

Colds, Flu & Other Common Ailments Sourcebook

Communication Disorders Sourcebook

Complementary & Alternative Medicine Sourcebook, 4th Edition

Congenital Disorders Sourcebook, 2nd Edition

Contagious Diseases Sourcebook

Cosmetic & Reconstructive Surgery Sourcebook, 2nd Edition

Death & Dying Sourcebook, 2nd Edition

Dental Care & Oral Health Sourcebook, 3rd Edition

Depression Sourcebook, 2nd Edition

Dermatological Disorders Sourcebook, 2nd Edition

Diabetes Sourcebook, 4th Edition

Diet & Nutrition Sourcebook, 3rd Edition

Digestive Diseases & Disorder Sourcebook

Disabilities Sourcebook

Disease Management Sourcebook

Domestic Violence Sourcebook, 3rd Edition

Drug Abuse Sourcebook, 3rd Edition

Ear, Nose & Throat Disorders Sourcebook, 2nd Edition

Eating Disorders Sourcebook, 3rd Edition

Emergency Medical Services Sourcebook

Endocrine & Metabolic Disorders Sourcebook, 2nd Edition

Environmental Health Sourcebook, 3rd Edition

Ethnic Diseases Sourcebook

Eye Care Sourcebook, 3rd Edition

Family Planning Sourcebook

Fitness & Exercise Sourcebook, 4th Edition

Food Safety Sourcebook

Forensic Medicine Sourcebook

Gastrointestinal Diseases & Disorders Sourcebook, 2nd Edition

Genetic Disorders Sourcebook, 3rd Edition

Head Trauma Sourcebook

Headache Sourcebook

Health Insurance Sourcebook

Healthy Aging Sourcebook

Healthy Children Sourcebook

Healthy Heart Sourcebook for Women

Hepatitis Sourcebook

Household Safety Sourcebook

Hypertension Sourcebook

Immune System Disorders Sourcebook, 2nd Edition

Infant & Toddler Health Sourcebook

Infectious Diseases Sourcebook

Injury & Trauma Sourcebook